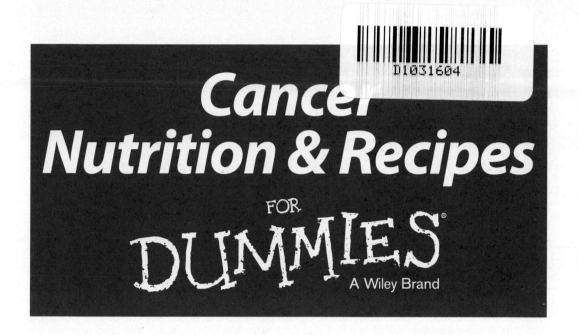

Cancer Nutrition & Recipes

FOR DUMMIES®

A Wiley Brand

by Maurie Markman, MD;
Carolyn Lammersfeld, RD;
and Christina Torster Loguidice

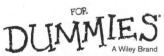

FOR DUMMIES®
A Wiley Brand

Cancer Nutrition & Recipes For Dummies®

Published by
John Wiley & Sons, Inc.
111 River Street
Hoboken, NJ 07030-5774
www.wiley.com

Contents at a Glance

Recipes at a Glance

To help with fatigue

To help with indigestion

To help with low appetite

To help with nausea

To help with sore mouth/throat

To help with taste/smell changes

To help with unintended weight loss

Table of Contents

Introduction

● ●

*A*lmost no words generate more fear than "You have cancer." Suddenly, the future feels uncertain, and you're flooded with all kinds of over-whelming emotions — from shock, to fear, to anger, to sadness. This is a normal part of coming to terms with your diagnosis. During this time, you may think about how other family members or friends went through their cancer diagnoses. Some may have been cured, providing you with a sense of hope; others may have ultimately succumbed to their illness, leaving you filled with dread.

But a cancer diagnosis today doesn't mean the same thing it meant even five years ago. The medical community's understanding of cancer is growing by leaps and bounds, enabling us to provide better treatments than ever before, and they'll only continue to improve. Today we also know that everyone's cancer is different, so even if you're told your prognosis is poor, remember that you're not marked with an expiration date.

After you come to terms with your diagnosis, you may wonder what you can do to improve your outcomes. Depending on what type of cancer you have, you may not have much choice when it comes to your treatments, leaving you feeling like a crash-test dummy strapped in for a wild ride. But you do have control over what you eat, which can give you a sense of empowerment and stability. Optimizing what you eat and your nutrient intake during and after your cancer journey can play an integral role in

- ✔ Combating the side effects of treatment
- ✔ Preventing infections when your immune system is compromised
- ✔ Giving your body the reserves it needs to fight the cancer and prevent a secondary cancer, a recurrence, or another chronic illness like heart disease or diabetes

Plus, it'll help you feel better and more energetic.

And that's what this book is meant to do: help empower you through nutrition. Depending on where you are on your cancer journey, your nutritional needs vary. You may also be struggling with side effects that make eating a challenge, such as loss of appetite. This can be overwhelming, leaving you wondering what you can and should eat to get you through these times. But this book is here to help. Think of it as a friend, guiding and supporting you through your changing needs, from diagnosis, through treatment, through recovery.

About This Book

To ensure that you eat properly during your cancer journey, you need to understand how cancer and its treatments affect nutritional demands. You also need a basic understanding of nutrients and how to monitor your nutrient intake. This book provides all this information in simple, easy-to-understand terms. And to help you put the information into practice, we provide more than 80 tasty and nutrient-packed recipes for meals, snacks, and desserts. Although these recipes appear in a cancer nutrition book, they can be enjoyed by anyone.

In this book, we also provide guidance on tools you can consider purchasing to simplify meal preparation, review cooking methods that help foods retain their nutrients, and examine ways to organize your kitchen to help you optimize nutrition and food safety, while being friendly for those times when you're dealing with side effects. If you want to adopt a healthy lifestyle beyond your eating, we offer some lifestyle recommendations to decrease cancer risk as well.

In the recipes, we use the following conventions, unless otherwise stated:

- All butter is unsalted.
- All eggs are large.
- All onions are yellow.
- All broths and stocks are low fat and low sodium.
- All milk and dairy products are low fat.
- All dry ingredient measurements are level.
- All temperatures are Fahrenheit.

All vegetarian recipes are preceded with a ↻ icon in the lists of recipes at the beginning of every chapter, as well as in the Recipes at a Glance, before the Table of Contents.

Within this book, you may note that some web addresses break across two lines of text. If you're reading this book in print and want to visit one of these web pages, simply key in the web address exactly as it's noted in the text, pretending as though the line break doesn't exist. If you're reading this as an e-book, you've got it easy — just click the web address to be taken directly to the web page.

Foolish Assumptions

As we wrote this book, we assumed the following about you:

- ✔ You or someone you love has received a cancer diagnosis or is at high risk of developing cancer.

- ✔ You're interested in understanding cancer and nutrition, including how cancer and its treatments can affect your nutritional needs.

- ✔ You want to understand how you can eat optimally during your cancer journey, whether you've just been diagnosed, are actively undergoing treatment, or are a survivor.

- ✔ You're interested in living healthier, but you aren't sure how to go about it.

- ✔ You want truthful information and not a bunch of hype.

Regardless of why you're reading this book, you can assume the following about us: We've made every effort to provide you with the latest and most widely supported cancer nutrition information in a way that's easy to understand and put into practice.

Icons Used in This Book

This book contains several icons that are intended to help you locate key ideas and information. The icons you'll see include the following:

The Tip icon appears next to information that can make your life easier or save you time.

The Remember icon points to important information that you won't want to forget. By flipping through this book and reading all the information next to this icon, you'll extract the most essential points we're trying to make.

The Warning icon alerts you to potential hazards, so be sure to look out for it and heed any information associated with it.

Paragraphs marked by the Technical Stuff icon are really interesting (at least to us), but you don't have to read them word for word to grasp the core concepts. In fact, you can skip right over them if you think the information contains more detail than you need.

Beyond the Book

In addition to the material in the print or e-book you're reading right now, this product comes with some access-anywhere goodies on the web. Check out the free Cheat Sheet at www.dummies.com/cheatsheet/cancer nutritionrecipes for tips on combatting treatment-related side effects (everything from nausea to a sore mouth or throat to taste changes) through the foods you eat, advice on staying active during treatment, and more.

Where to Go from Here

If you read the entire book cover to cover, you won't be disappointed, but we've organized the book so that you can dive in wherever you want and get the information you need. If you prefer to read only certain sections, you can use the Table of Contents to locate broad categories or subjects, or you can refer to the Index when you want to drill down to key terms or ideas. If you're looking for a recipe to ease a symptom you're experiencing (for example, nausea), the Recipes at a Glance points you in the right direction. Of course, you also can just flip through the book and read whatever catches your eye.

No matter how you decide to read this book, we recommend that you personalize it by highlighting text, writing questions in the margins, or putting sticky notes on pages that contain information that resonates with you or that you want to ask your oncologist or healthcare team about.

If you try a recipe in Part III, consider noting any substitutions you made, what you thought of the recipe, and how the recipe made you feel. If a recipe doesn't sit well with you, you may want to avoid making it again or wait a while before doing so. Finally, consider adding sticky notes to your favorite recipes so that you can easily find them again. Enjoy!

Part I
Getting Started with Cancer Nutrition

For Dummies can help you get started with lots of subjects. Visit www.dummies.com to learn more and do more with *For Dummies*.

In this part . . .

- Find out about cancer and the terminology that surrounds it.
- Meet the healthcare providers who may treat you and find out about the treatments you may receive.
- Get clear on the common physical and emotional effects of cancer, their treatments, and how to overcome them.
- Discover the importance of nutrition and why it's a powerful weapon in your cancer-fighting arsenal.
- See how you can overcome any treatment-related obstacles that impede your ability to nourish yourself.

Chapter 1

The 4-1-1 on Cancer

*E*veryone knows someone who's had cancer. In the United States, approximately one in two men and one in three women will develop some form of cancer during their lifetimes. But cancer isn't one disease — it's actually a wide spectrum of diseases, ranging from conditions that can be easily managed with surgery to illnesses that require extensive treatments, including surgery, radiation, and chemotherapy.

So, what exactly is cancer? How does it develop? Why are some cancers cured, but others progress despite the best available treatment? Why are some cancers found early, when they're confined to one specific region of the body, while others aren't found until they're widespread?

If you or your loved one received a cancer diagnosis, these questions were probably rolling around in your head at some point. In this chapter, we answer some of these important, yet often complex, questions so that you understand what a cancer diagnosis really means.

A Primer on the "Big C"

Ever have a symptom and go online to see what it may be? We've all done it, and no possibility of what that symptom might indicate instills more fear than the word *cancer*. After the diagnosis is made, you have an even greater thirst for information. Being educated about your disease is essential. Studies indicate that educated patients are more compliant with their treatments and have better outcomes, which is what you want! But to have real knowledge, you need to be able to distinguish fact from fiction — and with cancer, there's a lot of fiction out there. So, in this section, we give you a quick overview of cancer, answering the key questions, so that you're truly educated about your disease and the cancer landscape you'll be traversing.

What is cancer?

In the early development of our understanding of cancer, most researchers thought that it resulted from cells no longer being under the control of normal growth factors and immune regulation, causing them to suddenly grow wildly. If the cancer couldn't be removed completely with surgery, it would spread and cause the patient to die. Although this explanation does appear to describe the course of *some* malignancies, the scientific and medical communities now know that cancer is actually a far more complex and remarkably diverse group of medical conditions. In fact, even two seemingly similar cancers — like two breast cancers or two colorectal cancers — may actually be quite different, causing them to respond differently to the same treatments.

As a result, we can't describe every type of cancer in this book — that would be akin to trying to describe every snowflake that falls from the sky. So, for our purposes, it's fair to simplify things by saying that cancer is characterized by the growth of abnormal cells, their invasion into surrounding tissue, and, ultimately, their spread to other regions of the body if not caught early enough. This process occurs because these abnormal cells (also called *cancerous cells* or *malignant cells*) have somehow lost their ability to appropriately respond to the extensive network of highly complex regulatory mechanisms whose primary purpose is to ensure the normal functioning of the particular tissue. (For more on the definition of *malignant,* see the nearby sidebar, "Building your cancer vocabulary.")

How does cancer develop?

Cancer is caused by changes in a cell's DNA (its genetic blueprint), leading to cellular mutations. Some of these mutations may be genetic (inherited from our parents), while others may be caused by exposure to *carcinogens* (cancer-causing substances). But although all cancers are caused by mutations, not all mutations cause cancer. Mutations within genes of normal cells occur quite regularly, particularly when cells divide to increase their numbers, and most mutations are harmless. The increase in the number of cells in a given tissue may be due to any of the following:

- **The normal process of growth of the individual:** This kind of cell division occurs during childhood.

- **As part of the repair of damaged tissue:** When you have a cut on your hand or surgery for a broken leg, cells divide to repair the tissue that was damaged.

✔ **As a component of the body's strategy to successfully combat external threats:** For example, there is an increase in immune cells after infection by bacteria or a virus, or the body is exposed to carcinogens that cause mutations, affect hormone levels, or impair the immune response.

Building your cancer vocabulary

If you find that your oncologist or anyone else on your treatment team is using words that you don't understand, ask for clarification and be sure to write it down. When you get home, you can look up that word online and familiarize yourself with what it means.

It would be impossible for us to outline all the cancer terms you'll be encountering. We'd need volumes for that, and you don't need us to provide you with a dictionary anyway. But what we can provide you with is some of the terminology that you may encounter with regard to your tumor:

✔ *Benign* **versus** *malignant:* A *benign* tumor is a mass that grows locally, does not invade surrounding tissue, and, in most cases, doesn't spread to distant sites. Such tumors may also be referred to as *noncancerous* or *nonmalignant*. In contrast, *malignant* tumors can invade surrounding normal tissue and spread to distant sites.

Although most people are relieved when they hear that their tumor is benign, depending on its location, benign tumors can still cause considerable harm. For example, a benign tumor in the brain may destroy normal tissue as it grows. In contrast, some malignant tumors may be easily removed through surgical excision and require no further treatment, such as in many cases of basal cell carcinoma of the skin. So, as you can see, *benign* and *malignant* can be relative terms.

However, in most circumstances, benign tumors can be removed surgically and don't require subsequent external radiation, and there is no role for chemotherapy when it comes to these tumors.

✔ *Noninvasive* **and** *locally invasive* **versus** *metastatic: Noninvasive tumors* are generally considered superficial cancers because the tumor cells haven't spread into the surrounding tissue, whereas *locally invasive* cancer has spread beyond the confines of its own tissue space and directly into the surrounding tissues where it's not normally present. *Metastatic* cancer means the cancer has spread to sites beyond its tissue of origin. This may be to local lymph nodes or to distant organs. The method of spread may be by growth of the cancer into surrounding organs or spread to the lymph nodes or the blood.

✔ *Primary tumor* **versus** *secondary tumor: Primary tumor* refers to what is believed to be the initial site of the malignancy, while *secondary tumor* or *metastatic site(s)* refers to locations where the tumor may have spread.

It may not always be easy to distinguish between the primary and secondary tumor sites. This is particularly the case when the cancer is found in multiple sites at diagnosis and one of a number of locations might have been the "primary site." In general, in this situation, the most important reason to know the primary site is to determine the most effective treatment program.

The complex system of normal regulatory mechanisms present within all of us allows for necessary cellular growth. When the required task has been completed, that same system slows the growth rate. This process occurs in every tissue in the body and is constantly in operation. Unfortunately, in some people, this complex regulatory system fails to keep this growth and spread in complete check, and a cancerous growth develops.

All cancers have some degree of genetic abnormality compared with the corresponding normal tissue. In some situations, there may be a single well-defined event that led to the cancer, but most often there are large numbers of changes from the normal condition, frequently making it very difficult to know which specific mutation or alteration is actually responsible for the initial development of the malignancy or driving its progression. Most cancers require a number of specific events to occur before a given cell becomes malignant.

Therefore, the body may actually have a number of opportunities to control the cancer before it becomes widespread in the body, and this is also why cancer screenings are so important. When regular cancer screenings are undertaken, a cancer may be detected before it has acquired the ability to invade surrounding tissue or spread throughout the body.

Genetic abnormalities develop over a long period of time, usually years or even decades. So, although it may feel like your cancer started and progressed quite suddenly, depending on your tumor, this process may have been going on for many years.

Why aren't all cancers created equal?

You can better appreciate the tremendous variation in the rate of development, growth, and spread of cancer when you consider

- ✔ The remarkable complexity of the genetic background of individual cancers
- ✔ The differences in an individual patient's own biological mechanism that attempts to respond to the presence of the cancer (which may include various immune mechanisms or changes in growth factors that may still influence the rate of tumor growth and spread even after the malignancy has been established)

Certain cancers, by their very nature, are widespread at diagnosis (such as blood cancers), while others are more easily detected because they can be directly observed by the individual (such as skin cancers), by a physical examination (such as breast cancer), by imaging procedures (such as breast and lung cancers), or by blood tests (such as prostate cancer).

In addition, some cancers appear to maintain some degree of the normal mechanisms of control and are, in general, more likely to progress slowly, whereas other cancers appear to have lost all ability to respond to any normal control mechanisms. Examination of the actual cancer tissue under the microscope can often provide a clue to the anticipated prognosis of a given cancer. Tumors that are described as being *well-differentiated* or *low-grade* appear (under the microscope) to have characteristics of a malignancy, but they also continue to have features that are similar to the normal cells in that particular tissue. Conversely, cancers that are described as being *poorly differentiated, undifferentiated,* or *high-grade* are likely to have a more aggressive clinical course. Again, the thought here is that the body's normal regulatory mechanisms are less able to impact the progress of the cancer in the poorly differentiated state.

Other factors that are likely to influence the behavior of your cancer include

- ✔ **Your age:** As you age, you have more of the other risk factors for cancer, you've been exposed to possible carcinogens for longer, and your cellular repair mechanisms are likely to be less effective.

- ✔ **Any underlying immune deficiency problems:** Immune problems can compromise your body's ability to control the cancer's spread.

- ✔ **Your underlying nutritional state:** Nutritional deficiencies can impair immunological and other essential internal regulatory strategies.

Which factors increase the risk of cancer?

When it comes to cancer, a *risk factor* is a feature present within an individual that is associated with a statistically greater risk for the development of the disease, but is itself not necessarily the cause of the disease. For example, it has been shown that women who are obese have an increased risk of breast cancer. The weight itself likely isn't the *cause* of the cancer; instead, it's the fact that these women have higher levels of estrogen bathing the normal breast tissue, which, over a period of many years, may increase the potential for the development of breast cancer.

In the following sections, we cover the major risk factors for cancer.

Smoking

Without any possible question, the single most important risk factor for the development of cancer is tobacco exposure. Research has shown that tobacco contains thousands of different chemicals, and more than 40 of these chemicals have been documented to be possible carcinogens.

Although cigarette smoking is the major cause of lung cancer (the single most deadly cancer in both men and women) and cancers in the head and neck regions, it's also a major risk factor for the development of cancers of the esophagus, stomach, pancreas, colon, liver, kidney, bladder, and cervix. In addition, exposure to secondhand smoke, resulting from regular close contact with a smoker, has been estimated to result in more than 3,000 cancer deaths in the United States each year.

Nutrition

Another major risk factor is nutrition. As many as one-third of all cancers in the United States are thought to be related to a nutritional factor, which may include obesity, poor diet, and lack of adequate physical activity. Cancers that have been most strongly correlated with obesity include malignancies of the uterus, breast (in postmenopausal women), colon, esophagus, kidney, and gallbladder. Other sites where existing data are not quite as compelling regarding obesity as a risk factor include blood cancers and malignancies of the liver, pancreas, and stomach.

Alcohol

Excessive alcohol consumption has been identified to be a major risk factor for the development of cancers in the head and neck region, liver, esophagus, and breast.

Infectious diseases

Exposure to particular infectious diseases has also been shown to be a highly relevant risk factor for certain malignant conditions.

Studies have unequivocally shown that essentially all cervical cancers develop following exposure to, and persistence of, human papillomavirus (HPV). HPV has also been linked to *oropharyngeal cancer* (cancer of the head and neck), whereas the hepatitis virus is a major cause of liver cancer. Additional viruses known to be associated with the development of cancer include the human immunodeficiency virus (HIV) and *Helicobacter pylori,* an important cause of stomach cancer and a particular type of lymphoma.

Other risk factors

Other recognized cancer risk factors include

- Exposure to ionizing radiation — either intentional (for therapeutic or diagnostic purposes) or accidental exposure (such as from radon gas; see Chapter 17)
- Certain medications, including chemotherapy drugs
- Exposure to chemicals

What does cancer feel like?

Providing a simple characterization of what your cancer may feel like when it develops and progresses is difficult.

Some cancers can present quite dramatically due to their location in the body or can impact normal body function. For example, if you have a large colon cancer, it may cause an obstruction of the bowel, resulting in pain or an inability to have a normal bowel movement. If you have acute leukemia, you may have a high fever (due to infection and a very low concentration of normal white blood cells capable of fighting the infection) or spontaneous bleeding or bruising (due to a very low level of *platelets,* which are the cells responsible for preventing this process).

Conversely, your cancer may initially cause no symptoms and you may discover it by chance, such as by feeling an abnormal lump or mass under the skin while bathing. Or it may be found on a routine screening test, such as through a Pap smear, mammogram, or prostate-specific antigen (PSA) test.

Some cancers that result in absolutely no symptoms in their early stages may cause modest or even severe symptoms if detected later during their course. For example, if prostate cancer is found early through screening, you may have no or only minor urinary symptoms, but if it's found at a late stage, you may have considerable bone pain if the cancer has spread to your bones.

Most symptoms are not specific to cancer (as anyone who's spent any time looking up symptoms on WebMD can tell you). For example, if you have severe abdominal pain, it may be colon cancer or another cancer, but it may also be due to another serious medical condition (such as appendicitis or diverticulitis) or possibly something less serious (like severe constipation). And even if a cancer is ultimately discovered, the particular symptoms may not be helpful in defining the specific type of cancer. For example, abdominal pain may be caused by cancers of the colon, stomach, liver, ovary, uterus, pancreas, and other malignancies that may have spread to this location (such as breast cancer). Finally, no matter what your symptoms, they aren't necessarily indicative of your prognosis.

Coming to Terms with Your Diagnosis

When you received your cancer diagnosis, it may have felt like the end of the world, or maybe you found yourself living in a haze for a while. Perhaps you had nightmares about it, only to find that when you woke up, the nightmare wasn't over. Coming to terms with a cancer diagnosis takes time. Your mind has a lot to process, so you'll feel many things: fear, anxiety, hopelessness, sadness. If your prognosis is good and there's a good chance for a cure, then these emotions may not be as severe, but if your prognosis is uncertain or appears poor, these feelings may be magnified.

In this section, we examine the emotional side of a cancer diagnosis and how to deal with your emotions and telling your loved ones. We also look at where you can find additional emotional support and how to get yourself prepared for what lies ahead.

Processing your emotions

We can't overstate the profound impact the word *cancer* has, particularly when you're on the receiving end of the diagnosis. But despite the natural fear generated by this diagnosis, most people with cancer today will, in fact, be *cured* of their illness. Cancer is no longer the death sentence it once was, and, for some, the diagnosis brings a whole new meaning to life.

The process of cancer management is a journey, with the diagnosis only being the first stop. You'll experience a whole range of emotions as you work toward recovery. That's completely natural. But regardless of where you are and any frustrations and setbacks you may encounter along the way, trying to remain optimistic is important, even if your prognosis doesn't seem favorable. Remember that no one comes with an expiration date! And some evidence suggests that optimism can be an important key to good outcomes.

And there's good reason to be optimistic. These days, treatment can be highly successful in relieving and preventing symptoms, improving overall quality of life, substantially extending survival, and, in many settings, actually eliminating the disease. In fact, the very term *survivorship* has been developed to describe the process of recuperation. The idea is that you begin this journey the day the diagnosis is made and continue to concentrate your personal efforts on the goal of survival, whether you're ultimately cured or you end up living with your cancer.

With all the treatments these days, even if you can't be cured, chances are good that there's a treatment that can extend your life for many years to come. Plus, new treatments are constantly under investigation and being approved. So, there's considerable hope when you find yourself duking it out in the cancer arena.

Now, we're not saying you should be happy about having cancer or feel good about it. We're also not saying the road will be easy. Under some conditions, it may be very difficult — perhaps the greatest challenge you've ever faced. It's okay for you to cry and be angry. Letting out those emotions is better than keeping them bottled up inside. But it's also critical not to let your emotions impede your ability to progress down the cancer treatment road.

Telling family and friends

Informing your family and friends that you have cancer isn't easy, particularly if your suggested prognosis is less than optimal.

Saying the words may be difficult, but remember that these are the people who love and understand you most, and they want nothing more than to provide you with support. They'll understand if you need to say the words through tears, by cracking a joke, or by sounding very matter of fact. But no matter how you tell them, the best thing you can do is be honest with them, while also letting them know what you need. Just like you, they may feel afraid, angry, and helpless. They may also be concerned about saying the wrong things. By involving them in your cancer journey and letting them know what you need, you may just strengthen the bonds with the people you're closest to.

Finding the support you need

Your family and close friends may provide you with all the support you need to get through your cancer journey. After all, they can serve as a sounding board for your diagnosis, prognosis, and experiences; help you with chores if you're too tired to do them yourself; and just provide you with love and support (for example, by holding your hand if you need it). But if this support isn't enough for you, or if you want to connect with others who already have or are currently walking the cancer road, you may want to look into support groups. Numerous options are available, from faith-based groups to cancer-specific support groups. Some support groups regularly meet in person, whereas others are web based, allowing you to connect with people through message boards, video chats, text chats, and other means. The American Cancer Society maintains a list of organizations that provide support groups at www.cancer.org/treatment/supportprogramsservices.

In some circumstances, you may consider seeking assistance from a medical professional, such as a psychologist, social worker, or counselor. Cancer can lead to a range of emotions, and a therapist may be able to help guide you through these emotions and provide you with new insights. If your emotions are preventing you from moving forward with treatment (for example, because you're afraid of the side effects), seeking support is especially important, because delaying treatment can lead to poor outcomes.

Your cancer center may have a therapist on staff who you could speak with. If not, your oncologist or healthcare team can point you in the right direction.

Getting prepared

There's no simple formula for preparing for the future, but obtaining as much helpful information regarding your particular cancer type and available therapeutic options is an essential first step. By being well informed, you're in the best position to work with your healthcare team to optimize your treatments.

So, where to get such information? Getting it from reputable sources is critical. Fortunately, there are many of them. First and foremost, your healthcare providers — both your primary-care doctor and specialty medical team — should be able to provide you with important information or point you in the right direction. The Internet is also increasingly serving as a vital source of information for people with serious medical conditions, including cancer. When seeking information online, look to government sites (like the National Cancer Institute; `www.cancer.gov`), cancer organizations (like the American Cancer Society; `www.cancer.org`), professional medical organizations (like the American Society of Clinical Oncology; `www.asco.org`), and treatment center websites (like the Cancer Treatment Centers of America; `www.cancercenter.com`).

When your treatment plan is developed, take the time to understand it. Don't hesitate to ask questions. When it comes to cancer and its management, there are simply no silly or stupid questions, and don't let anyone tell you otherwise!

Understanding the Types of Cancer

As we mention at the beginning of this chapter, cancer isn't just one disease — it's actually a host of different diseases, all involving some form of abnormal cellular development. But to better classify cancer, its *primary site* (where in the body the cancer first developed) and *histological type* (type of tissue from which it originated) are considered. In this section, we look at the common types of cancer. (For more on primary tumors, see the "Building your cancer vocabulary" sidebar, earlier in this chapter.)

Carcinoma

Carcinoma refers to a group of malignant conditions whose normal tissue of origin serves as the lining cells (inner or outer surfaces) of a particular organ. These cells are known as *epithelial cells*. Carcinomas are by far the most frequent cancers seen in both men and women, and they affect common primary sites, such as the breasts, lungs, colon, prostate, and pancreas.

Surgical removal, if possible, is the primary treatment of a localized carcinoma. If your oncologist is concerned that residual local cancer may remain, you may be given radiation treatment to the region where the tumor was located. If there is no definite evidence that the cancer has spread beyond the local or regional area, but there's a risk of malignant cells having spread to other areas of the body before treatment was undertaken, chemotherapy (called *adjuvant chemotherapy*) may be given.

If surgically removing a carcinoma isn't possible because of its size or a medical condition that makes surgery dangerous (such as pre-existing severe heart disease), the cancer may be managed with external radiation. And if there is concern that the cancer may have spread beyond the local area, adjuvant chemotherapy may also be administered.

A relatively recent approach for treating several types of carcinomas (like those of the breast, head and neck, and ovaries) has been to administer chemotherapy *before* surgical treatment (called *neoadjuvant chemotherapy*). The goal here is to decrease the size of the cancer before surgery, with the specific purpose of reducing the amount of normal tissue that must be removed and potentially increasing the size of the patient population that may benefit from definitive local therapy.

Sarcoma

Compared with carcinomas, sarcomas are uncommon malignancies. In addition, they comprise a rather heterogeneous group of cancers, which are characterized by the fact that they've arisen from the middle of tissues, or the supporting cells in those tissues. Sarcomas can develop from fat, muscle, cartilage, bone, and vascular tissue.

The names of sarcomas include information regarding the cell of origin. For example, sarcomas arising from bone are called *osteosarcomas,* while sarcomas developing from fat cells are called *liposarcomas.*

The principal treatment approach is surgery, if possible. Local radiation is used if residual cancer is a concern. With the important exception of osteosarcomas, the role of chemotherapy as an adjuvant treatment or to manage metastatic sarcomas in adults is limited. (For more on the definition of *metastatic,* see the "Building your cancer vocabulary" sidebar, earlier in this chapter.) In contrast, children or young adults with sarcomas are likely to receive chemotherapy because they tend to respond very well to it.

Myeloma

Multiple myeloma is a cancer that develops in the bone marrow from a normal cell population known as *plasma cells.* Plasma cells have a critical role to play in normal antibody formation. Multiple myeloma often causes the blood and urine to contain a high concentration of an abnormal protein, which can be measured to evaluate the response of the illness to treatment.

Although multiple myeloma is uncommon (accounting for only 1 percent of all cancers), it's the second most frequently observed malignant condition developing from bone marrow cells. Multiple myeloma is frequently associated with anemia, problems with kidney function, and elevated blood calcium levels.

Over the past decade, outcomes following multiple myeloma treatment have substantially improved. Routine treatment for the malignancy includes the use of steroids, standard chemotherapy drugs, and two new drug classes known as *immunomodulatory drugs* and *proteasome inhibitors.* External radiation may be given, particularly in the management of painful bone lesions, and bone marrow or stem cell transplantation may be used in select cases.

Leukemia

Leukemia refers to a group of cancers arising from two normal cellular populations in the bone marrow: granulocytes and lymphocytes. The major role of *granulocytes* is to prevent illness from exposure to *pathogens* (disease-causing agents) in the environment, while *lymphocytes* play a major role in *immunoregulation* (control of specific mechanisms that affect immune responses) and also help with controlling certain types of infections.

The terms *acute* and *chronic* are added to the particular cellular type of leukemia to identify how involved the most immature cell population is:

- ✔ **Acute:** Acute leukemia has a substantial percentage of such immature cells and tends to progress very rapidly if chemotherapy isn't given. In fact, acute leukemia is frequently considered a medical emergency, often requiring hospitalization and initiation of therapy within hours of the time the diagnosis is made.

- ✔ **Chronic:** Chronic leukemia has much lower percentage of immature cells and a far higher proportion of more mature cells. It tends to progress more slowly and may not cause symptoms for years.

The distinction between acute and chronic leukemias is principally based on the percentage of immature cells versus mature cells, rather than the actual number of abnormal cells found in the blood or bone marrow.

In addition to being classified as acute or chronic, leukemia may be lymphocytic/lymphoblastic or myelogenous:

- ✔ Lymphocytic/lymphoblastic leukemia affects white blood cells called *lymphocytes.*
- ✔ Myelogenous leukemia affects white blood cells called *myelocytes.*

The four main types of leukemia are acute lymphoblastic leukemia (ALL), acute myelogenous leukemia (AML), chronic lymphocytic leukemia (CLL), and chronic myelogenous leukemia (CML).

Many patients with leukemia have a low concentration of normal bone marrow cells, leading to anemia (because of reduced red blood cell counts), infection (because of a reduced number of granulocytes), and bleeding (because of reduced platelet counts). The severity of the leukemia is greatly influenced by the disease's impact on the ability of the bone marrow to make normal cells.

In the past, all leukemias were managed in a similar manner, with all patients receiving chemotherapy. There was no difference in the class of drugs used, but the intensity of treatment may have varied. However, the discovery of a specific molecular abnormality in most patients with CML and the development of new "targeted" agents, such as imatinib, directed at this abnormality have significantly improved the prognosis of this cancer. Today, most patients survive more than eight to ten years following their initial diagnosis.

In addition, most children with ALL, which is the most frequent type of leukemia in this age group, are able to be cured of their illness. Although this outcome is less common for adults with either AML or ALL, it is possible.

Lymphoma

Lymphomas are malignancies of *lymphocytes* (the cells responsible for immunoregulation and control of certain infectious organisms). Lymphomas are divided into two major categories: Hodgkin's disease and non-Hodgkin's disease.

Although lymphomas appear to originate from lymph tissue, the same cellular population can be present in the bone marrow and blood.

In some situations, the decision to classify a particular cancer as being a lymphoma versus a CLL (with excessive concentrations of mature-appearing lymphocytes present in the blood) may be based on the relative importance of blood versus tissue involvement by the process.

Making matters even more complex, lymph tissue can normally be found outside the lymph nodes. As a result, it's possible to have lymphomas arise in organs such as the stomach, bone, brain, and colon. Lymphomas that develop in one body region may also commonly spread to the bone, bone marrow, lungs, liver, and brain.

Treatment of lymphomas includes chemotherapy, radiation, immunotherapy, and bone marrow or stem cell transplantation. The prognosis depends on how widespread the disease is and how well it responds to treatment. The goal of therapy is also influenced by the specific type of lymphoma. Some forms can be cured by current therapy, whereas other subgroups may not be curable (but it may still be possible to control symptoms for an extended period of time in such cases).

Mixed types

Microscopic examination (also called *pathological review*) may reveal that a particular cancer is composed of several cellular elements. For example, a lung cancer may be found to have both a squamous cell carcinoma and an adenocarcinoma. This may be due to the fact that a particular cancer actually develops from a very early (immature) cell population and subsequently attempts to differentiate into more mature cells involving more than one "normal" pathway. So, what's seen under the microscope is not the actual malignant cell, but the end result of this unsuccessful differentiation process. So-called *mixed tumors* are also seen in sarcomas and germ cell tumors, likely for similar reasons.

In other cases, two separate cancers are found, with one cancer being a primary lesion in the organ and the second being metastatic disease from another site. Or two apparently independent primary cancers may be found at the same time in neighboring tissues. This unusual pattern has been observed in some women, who appear to develop simultaneous cancers in both the ovaries and the uterus. This outcome is thought to result from what has been dubbed a *field defect,* with the same environmental factors interacting upon a susceptible genetic background, leading to the two organs developing malignancies in roughly the same time period.

Other types

A number of additional less common malignancies can involve multiple sites in the body. When a diagnosis of cancer is made, one of the first problems that needs to be solved is determining what part of the body the process began in. Because cancer may spread to distant locations, the discovery of a mass in a lung doesn't necessarily mean the patient has "lung cancer"; if this occurs in the liver, it doesn't necessarily mean that the patient has "liver cancer."

To determine the best therapy, doctors need to know the location(s) of the tumor(s) and where the cancer started. For example, the chemotherapy used in the treatment of breast cancer (that may have spread to the liver or lungs) is very different from what would be used if the cancer in the breast is actually a liver or lung cancer.

Certain relatively uncommon conditions clearly behave like a malignancy, but under the microscope the *pathologist* (doctor who interprets changes caused by disease in tissues and body fluids to make a diagnosis) is unable to classify the condition as falling into this group of illnesses. So, in rare situations, tumors that appear to be "benign" have been documented to have spread to other parts of the body, and tumors that are "noninvasive" may be found in multiple locations (see the "Building your cancer vocabulary" sidebar, earlier in this chapter). This experience emphasizes the complexity of cancer and the need for scientists to continue to learn more about this group of diseases to ultimately improve treatments and outcomes.

Grasping the Diagnostic Tests

On your way to getting your cancer diagnosis, you probably felt like a pin cushion, constantly being poked and prodded. You may have also been stuffed into or squeezed by various machines to get a closer look at your body tissues. During your cancer treatment, you'll experience more of this. These events are never fun and may leave you feeling anxious, but they're important for getting a more accurate clinical picture of your cancer so that it can be treated optimally while minimizing the risk of side effects.

In this section, we take a closer look at some of the types of tests you'll undergo on your cancer journey. If you understand them a bit better, maybe they won't be quite so scary.

Blood tests

A variety of blood tests are often used to help make an initial diagnosis of cancer. But although certain blood tests may be very helpful in suggesting the presence of cancer, the "gold standard" for diagnosing a malignancy is a formal analysis of a tissue sample (or blood) under the microscope by a pathologist (see "Biopsies," later in this chapter).

Specific examples of useful blood tests in the diagnosis of cancer include the PSA test for prostate cancer (although some recent debate has been raised after an expert panel recommended against performing the test in men of any age group) and the CA-125 test for ovarian cancer. Again, finding abnormal blood levels in these particular tests would lead to further evaluation and, most likely, a tissue biopsy (for example, of the prostate or a mass in the abdomen) to make a definitive diagnosis.

Blood tests are also useful in determining whether a particular cancer may have spread to other locations in your body. For example, certain abnormalities in what are often called "liver function tests" may suggest that your malignancy has spread to your liver. They can also be very helpful in evaluating your ability to undergo specific treatments. For example, abnormal "kidney function tests" may indicate a preexisting kidney problem that may make it difficult to administer certain chemotherapy agents due to the risk of serious side effects.

In addition, after the diagnosis is made, the actual level of a particular blood test may be used to monitor the course of the illness. These are called *tumor markers*. For example, if you have ovarian cancer, monitoring your blood level of CA-125 is a useful approach to determine the effectiveness of your chemotherapy regimen.

Imaging studies

As with blood tests, imaging studies can be very helpful, but they aren't considered (except in very rare situations) diagnostic of cancer. However, they can clearly show the site of a primary tumor and of possible locations of secondary tumors (see the "Building your cancer vocabulary" sidebar, earlier in this chapter, for more on primary and secondary tumors). Examples of imaging tests used to assess for cancer include mammograms for breast cancer, chest X-rays and computed tomography (CT) scans for lung cancer, abdominal CT scans for ovarian and pancreatic cancer, and magnetic resonance imaging (MRI) for brain cancers.

As with blood tests, imaging studies can monitor your response to treatment and identify any disease progression. One of the most exciting developments in the area of cancer diagnosis over the past decade has been advancement in the imaging technologies designed to find and monitor malignant disease — for example, the advent of positron emission tomography (PET) scanning, which, unlike CT scans and MRIs that look at the body's anatomy, produces a three-dimensional picture of functional processes in the body.

Biopsies

The "gold standard" for the diagnosis of cancer is the careful analysis of actual tumor tissue under the microscope by a pathologist. This requires a piece of tissue (or blood, in the case of leukemias and other bone marrow diseases) to be obtained for this specific purpose.

Although the biopsy material may come from your tumor following a surgery that was planned to remove the malignancy, in most circumstances, you'll undergo a biopsy before such surgery. This is because confirming the diagnosis in advance permits you and your doctor to discuss and decide upon the best strategy based on the biopsy results. For example, if you undergo a needle biopsy of a breast lump you discovered in the shower one day, certain important features of your cancer, such as the presence or absence of certain receptors, will influence the treatment options that are available to you.

An initial attempt to get enough material for a definitive diagnosis sometimes isn't successful. This situation may occur for several reasons. For example, an insufficient amount of tissue may have been obtained; the sample may have appeared "normal," but it's suspected that the actual cancer site was missed in the biopsy attempt; or the cells may have been *necrotic* (dead or dying cells with insufficient features to permit a diagnosis). In such cases, you may need to undergo a second biopsy.

Getting a Handle on Cancer Staging

Staging is a way to describe the severity of your cancer based on the extent of your original (primary) tumor and whether your cancer has spread to other areas of your body. Staging is important because it can enable your oncologist to work with you to develop an appropriate treatment plan. It can also help give some indication of your prognosis. But remember, no one can tell you for sure what your prognosis will be.

Staging is important language when it comes to cancer, so this section fills you in on everything you need to know about it, including how cancer is staged and what these stages mean.

How cancer is staged

There is a well-established cancer "staging system" that is widely used by oncologists, which is both a good thing and a bad thing. It's a good thing because oncologists and pathologists around the world generally agree with the system. As a result, you can be confident that if you're given a "stage" for your cancer after a definitive evaluation by your oncologist, you would have received that same stage had that evaluation been conducted by another oncologist. This is because doctors follow agreed-upon criteria for staging, which is as follows:

- ✔ **Stage 0:** The cancer is noninvasive.
- ✔ **Stages I, II, and III:** The higher the number, the more extensive the disease. The tumor may be larger or may have spread beyond the organ in which it first developed to nearby lymph nodes and/or organs adjacent to the location of the primary tumor.
- ✔ **Stage IV:** The cancer has spread to distant sites in the body.

Sometimes additional letters and numerical suffixes are used to subdivide cancer stages. For example, a stage IIIE+S tumor indicates extralymphatic spread (as marked by the *E*) and splenic involvement (as marked by the *S*).

Now the bad news. Because the fundamental concepts behind tumor staging haven't changed substantially since the process was developed many decades ago, certain assumptions considered reasonable at that time don't appear to be appropriate today. Perhaps the most important fact is that formal staging is only done at the initial diagnosis. The drawback of this system is that it doesn't account for recurrence or metastasis, which may occur sometime after a tumor is initially staged.

With the exception of blood-related malignancies (leukemia, myeloma, lymphoma), most cancers are staged based on findings at the time of initial surgery. Additional information to define the cancer stage may come from imaging studies (such as a CT scan of the lungs or abdomen) and specific blood tumor marker studies.

Patients who experience a cancer recurrence in a distant site commonly say that they have "stage IV cancer," but this isn't technically correct. A cancer that initially presents as a localized process ("stage I") will always be labeled as stage I. Clearly, this situation can be quite confusing.

What cancer staging truly means

The stage of a cancer provides very general information about the extent of its spread and observed location within the body. In most cases, this information is essential in defining the best initial treatment plan. For example, if you have a lung cancer that appears to be entirely localized without involvement of regional lymph nodes, it will be treated with surgery (assuming you're medically able to tolerate it); on the other hand, if you have extensive lymph node involvement, you probably won't undergo surgery, and you'll have radiation plus chemotherapy instead.

The relevance of staging varies based on the specific tumor type in question and the available treatment options to be considered in that particular setting. For example, surgery may be used to treat one tumor type (such as ovarian cancer) even in the presence of documented stage IV cancer, while documented regional lymph node involvement (stage II) for other tumor types may modify the therapeutic strategy away from surgery and toward radiation. These decisions are largely based on the results of large-scale clinical trials that have been conducted over the past several decades and have helped to define optimal disease management in particular clinical settings.

Blood tumors are all essentially "stage IV" at diagnosis, and treatment will be with anticancer drugs (possibly with external radiation to large masses) rather than surgery.

Unfortunately, despite improvements in diagnostics, it's impossible to precisely know if an individual cancer truly remains localized at the time of diagnosis, despite negative imaging or tumor marker studies. Therefore, although you may have stage I breast cancer, you may, in fact, have *microscopic* (unable to be seen on imaging studies) metastatic cancer. This is why adjuvant chemotherapy is given for certain cancer types.

Despite the drawbacks and challenges of cancer staging, in general, prognosis is excellent when you're found to have an early-stage cancer, rather than more advanced disease. However, with the increasing effectiveness of treatment options for multiple tumor types — even advanced cancers — you can experience genuinely meaningful benefits associated with treatment, including substantial improvement in cancer-related symptoms, improved quality of life, and prolonged survival.

Chapter 2

Meeting Your Team and Identifying Possible Treatments

• •

▶ Familiarizing yourself with your care team

▶ Grasping the treatment classifications

▶ Understanding your treatment options

▶ Knowing when to get a second opinion

▶ Considering clinical trials

▶ Finding treatment support resources

• •

*O*n your cancer journey, you'll traverse a whole new landscape, meeting many new people along the way. Some of the key people belong to your treatment team, and knowing how they fit into the cancer equation can help you better navigate and understand the terrain. So, this chapter acquaints you with the healthcare providers you're likely to encounter during treatment. Depending on your cancer type and its stage when you're diagnosed, not all providers may be involved in your care, whereas others may become more relevant down the road.

After you understand who you'll be dealing with, you also need to understand some of the new language you'll be hearing: the common terms used to describe a variety of treatment approaches in the oncology area. It would be impossible to define every term, so if you hear one you haven't heard before or if you're uncertain of the meaning of something you're told regarding your cancer and its management, ask a member of your cancer team to provide an explanation. That's what they're there for. And don't stop asking questions until you fully understand what you've been told. As they say, knowledge is power, and you want all the benefits that come with being well informed.

Sometimes you may not like what your cancer team has to say or you may feel uncomfortable with an approach they're recommending. In some cases, there truly are no other options, but other times, there may be additional approaches to explore. When you and your treatment team don't see eye to eye, getting a second opinion may be worthwhile, even if it's just to feel reassured in a decision. So, we also look at when you might consider obtaining a second opinion.

Finally, we take a look at the potential role of clinical trials and how and where you may be able to obtain useful information related to cancer treatments.

Knowing Your Cancer Care Team

Many people can make up the cancer care team. If you're treated at a small practice in a community setting, there may be fewer players, and you may be sent to other outside practices for services that can't be handled at your facility. In contrast, if you're treated at a large cancer center, you may regularly meet with additional cancer care team members and receive all or most of your services under one roof. This doesn't necessarily mean that one setting provides better care than the other. It's simply a matter of the resources that are available.

And even if you're treated at a large cancer center, you still may not meet everyone we talk about here, but knowing who's out there is always useful.

Oncologists

Oncologists are physicians who have received special training in the area of cancer management. In general, this includes cancer surgeons, radiation oncologists, pediatric oncologists, and medical oncologists. In the treatment of cancers involving the blood or lymph nodes, *hematologists* (specialists in conditions involving the blood) may play a primary role in management.

Sometimes people use the term *oncologist* to refer to medical oncologists (or possibly hematologists in the case of blood cancers). These physicians' primary role is to administer anti-cancer drug therapies, including chemotherapy and *biotherapy* (treatments that stimulate the immune system to fight the cancer), and they often assume an added responsibility of coordinating the care among the other physician members of the cancer treatment team.

Oncology nurses

Oncology nurses include several groups of highly trained individuals who are involved in multiple components of cancer care. This includes inpatient care (for example, hospitalization for complications of cancer or its treatment), outpatient care (for example, for the administration of chemotherapy), home care, and hospice care.

In addition, nurses may serve a vital role in responding to your telephone or online requests for general information regarding cancer management or dealing with concerns you may have about a particular problem (for example, if you develop a rash after receiving chemotherapy).

A relatively new subset of nurses is known as *oncology nurse navigators.* These nurses serve as care coordinators. They have both clinical knowledge and administrative knowledge, enabling them to answer clinical questions (such as what to do about that aforementioned rash) and figure out how to identify and eliminate barriers to timely and appropriate cancer treatment.

Radiation oncologists and therapists

Radiation oncologists are physicians who have received special training in administering several types of radiation therapy to manage cancer. This includes both external radiation (delivered from a machine outside the body) and internal radiation (for example, implanted radioactive sources; this is also known as *brachytherapy*).

Radiation oncologists work directly with cancer surgeons and medical oncologists to coordinate efforts to give you the best possible outcome. These highly trained physicians are involved in both curative treatment approaches and alleviating the distressing symptoms of more advanced cancers (known as *palliative care*).

Although your radiation oncologist develops your regimen, radiation therapists are the healthcare professionals who deliver the doses prescribed by your radiation oncologist and who monitor your condition and the effectiveness of your treatment. Radiation therapists aren't physicians, but they receive special training. Your radiation therapist is the radiation therapy team member you'll have the most interaction with.

Surgeons

A variety of surgeons can be involved in your care. In fact, surgery is the oldest and most established strategy for cancer management, including approaches to cure the illness or to improve symptoms when there is more advanced disease.

The term *surgical oncologist* can pertain to a number of types of surgeons who have been trained in surgical cancer management in particular areas. This includes general surgeons, urologists, gynecologic oncologists, head and neck cancer surgeons, neurosurgeons, plastic surgeons, and thoracic surgeons. In addition, some surgeons who participate in more general surgical training programs subsequently develop particular expertise in a specific area of cancer management (for example, breast cancer or colorectal cancer).

Radiologists and pathologists

We've grouped radiologists and pathologists together because they're both essential in diagnosing cancer, but they generally play behind-the scenes roles, so you're unlikely to ever meet them. Radiologists review your imaging studies to make a diagnosis, whereas pathologists make a diagnosis based on the appearance of your biopsy specimens. Both radiologists and pathologists are highly trained medical doctors. You may meet with an interventional radiologist if you require placement of a feeding tube for specialized nutrition, although this procedure may also be performed by a gastroenterologist.

Social workers

Social workers have training and expertise in the often complex social and psychological issues surrounding cancer and its management. You may have seen or experienced firsthand how cancer can disrupt normal daily activities and cause difficulties with family members. For example, you may have serious concerns regarding employment, how to arrange transportation to appointments, and insurance matters. A social worker can play a truly critical role in helping you and your family successfully navigate such issues.

Psychiatrists and psychologists

The terms *psychiatrist* and *psychologist* are often used synonymously, but there are some key differences between these professions. Psychiatrists are medical doctors; they have to receive an MD before they complete an additional four years of training in mental health. In contrast, psychologists have a doctoral-level degree in psychology (either a PhD or a PsyD), so they aren't medical doctors and often can't dispense medications. Both are able to provide talk therapy, though.

Just because you have cancer doesn't mean you require psychological care. Cancers can have vastly different anticipated prognoses and required management plans, both of which can affect your sense of well-being. After all, if you have a superficial skin cancer that can be easily removed and there is no associated risk of reduced life expectancy, you probably won't experience much psychological distress. In contrast, if your disease is widespread and you're given a poor prognosis, you may have significant psychological distress. Everyone has different internal coping mechanisms and available emotional and psychological support resources. So, even if you have advanced disease, you may not need psychological support from a psychiatrist or psychologist if you have enough other support and your diagnosis is not impacting your ability to be treated and engage in activities of daily living.

But in some cases, the support and direct intervention of a psychiatrist or psychologist may be helpful or even essential in permitting you to deal with your particular circumstances. This is particularly true if you develop depression, because depression reduces quality of life and can lead to worse outcomes.

Rehabilitation specialists

Both cancer and its treatment can make it difficult to carry out normal activities of daily living. For example, if you're undergoing curative surgery for a large breast cancer, you may experience problems using your arm after surgery, or while you're receiving chemotherapy, you may develop numbness and tingling in your feet, making it difficult to walk unaided.

Now, we're not saying these things will happen to you, but if such issues arise, a rehabilitation specialist can be invaluable in helping find solutions for the physical limitations you're facing. Not having to struggle through such issues can profoundly improve your overall quality of life.

Dietitians

Dietitians are essential members of the cancer care team. These professionals focus on all aspects of nutrition that have the potential to optimize treatment outcomes while also reducing the risk of side effects and managing cancer- and treatment-related symptoms as they occur, improving quality of life.

Dietitians assess for any nutritional deficiencies at diagnosis that may interfere with successful cancer treatment. When severe malnourishment is present, either due to the cancer (for example, an inability to eat for the past two months due to a growth in the stomach) or an unrelated issue (for example, vitamin deficiency from chronic alcoholism), you're at a major disadvantage when dealing with the anticipated side effects associated with an intensive treatment program.

Dietitians are also responsible for monitoring your care throughout your cancer treatment journey. Depending on your specific circumstances, your dietitian may recommend nutritional supplements or other strategies in an effort to maintain your weight and prevent malnutrition. A dietitian can also counsel and educate you about how to move toward a more nutrient-dense diet to manage conditions like diabetes and high cholesterol, while maintaining a healthy body weight and reducing the risk of a recurrence or a secondary cancer after treatment.

Home health aides

Sometimes having someone in the home to provide assistance during cancer treatment may be helpful, particularly if you don't have family or friends who are able to provide the care you require. This assistance may be temporary (for example, helping with daily activities after a major surgery) or prolonged (for example, ongoing assistance because of pain and debility from advanced disease). Home health aides can assist with tasks like bathing, cooking, shopping, and cleaning, or perform nursing functions like drawing blood, caring for wounds, providing pain medications and other meds, or checking vital signs (heartbeat, breathing rate, temperature, and blood pressure).

Identifying the Treatment Classifications

The treatments you receive will fall under a particular classification based on the intent of the intervention. To help you better understand the purpose of your treatments, this section gives you a look at the various classifications.

Conventional

Conventional cancer care generally refers to the traditional cancer management strategies of surgery, radiation treatment, and anti-cancer drug therapy (chemotherapy, biotherapy, and targeted agents), which are intended to cure or manage cancer. This term may also be extended to include standard medications used routinely in cancer care, such as pain medications and anti-nausea drugs.

Complementary

Complementary cancer care generally refers to a group of interventions that *complement,* or are added to, conventional cancer care. An example of complementary care may be acupuncture to reduce the side effects of treatment. The basic goal with complementary care is to optimize quality of life by addressing physical and emotional well-being.

Neoadjuvant

Neoadjuvant therapy refers to the administration of an anti-cancer therapy program (generally chemotherapy) before curative treatment like surgery is undertaken. Neoadjuvant treatment may be considered if the size of the cancer prohibits complete surgical removal of the mass or renders surgery too invasive. Following several cycles of chemotherapy, it may be possible to accomplish surgical removal with fewer side effects and a more favorable outcome, including easier recovery with fewer complications and improved appearance because less tissue is removed. The use of neoadjuvant chemotherapy is now routinely used in a number of clinical settings, including in cancers of the breast, ovaries, and head and neck region. This approach may also permit more patients to have a chance at a cure by making surgery accessible to them.

Adjuvant

Adjuvant therapy refers to a strategy employed after curative treatment is undertaken and is currently a routine component of cancer care in multiple settings, including in cancers of the breast, colon, and lungs. The basic goal of adjuvant therapy (generally chemotherapy) is to kill any remaining cancer cells that are unable to be seen after the tumor has been removed. There's no way of knowing if you actually have any residual cancer cells in your body after you complete treatment, but extensive clinical evidence has indicated that there is a reasonable risk of this being the case. Therefore, the intent of adjuvant treatment is to kill these microscopic cancer deposits before they have the opportunity to grow and spread to other regions of your body.

Integrative

Integrative cancer care refers to an approach to cancer management that includes, or *integrates,* both conventional and complementary cancer care.

Alternative

Alternative cancer care refers to approaches that are unproven and used instead of conventional medical treatment. An example would be a special diet to treat or manage cancer in place of a method recommended by a medical oncologist. Such approaches aren't recommended, because there's no evidence to support them. In fact, delaying conventional treatment to pursue an alternative therapy may allow your cancer to become more advanced and more difficult to treat or manage. Current knowledge indicates that the best outcomes occur when conventional and complementary medicine are brought together to develop an integrative strategy.

Palliative

Palliative cancer care refers to approaches that focus on alleviating the symptoms of cancer instead of on treating the cancer itself. This may include a variety of strategies. For example, if you have pain from a large cancer, you may undergo surgery to remove that mass to improve the pain, or the symptoms may be alleviated by radiating the mass to shrink it enough to reduce pain, or you may receive pain medications to dull the pain.

 Receiving palliative care doesn't mean you can't at the same time receive active treatment; palliative care doesn't mean hospice care. Recent research has shown that, in some cases, palliative treatment may not only improve quality of life, but also favorably influence survival.

Hospice

Hospice care refers to treatments and measures taken when therapy directed at treating the cancer has been determined to be of no further value. At this point, the focus of care shifts to providing symptom relief and ensuring comfort. *Hospice care* can also refer to certain governmental and private insurance plans that provide specific benefits when it's determined that further treatment is no longer desired or indicated.

Understanding the Treatment Options

Numerous types of treatment are used to target cancer, whether in an attempt to cure it, keep it from *metastasizing* (spreading), or alleviate the distressing symptoms that it causes. You may not receive all these treatments, or you may receive different combinations of these treatments at different times on your cancer journey. Every cancer is unique — there's no one-size-fits-all approach when dealing with this disease, but your cancer team will apply evidence-based and consensus-driven standards when deciding on the best course of action for you.

Chemotherapy

Chemotherapy is the delivery of drugs specifically designed to kill cancer cells by inhibiting their ability to replicate. It can be given before undertaking a treatment intended to be curative (referred to as *neoadjuvant chemotherapy*), after such treatment (called *adjuvant chemotherapy*), or when the cancer has spread to other parts of the body (called *chemotherapy for metastatic disease*). Regardless of when it's administered, chemotherapy is a systemic therapy.

Numerous chemotherapeutic agents are available, and they produce their desired effect on cancer cells in a variety of ways. Some damage parts of cancer cells after they're copied and ready to divide, others damage the part of cancer cells that help them divide, and still others inhibit cancer cells' ability to duplicate themselves (a process that needs to occur before a cancer cell can divide to create more cancer cells). Although chemotherapy is commonly administered through intravenous infusion, it can be given in many ways, including *orally* (through pills, capsules, and liquids), *topically* (by rubbing creams on the skin), by injection into muscle or directly under the skin, *intra-arterially* (directly into an artery feeding the tumor), and *intraperitoneally* (directly into the peritoneal cavity, which is where the intestines are).

Because chemotherapeutic agents target cancer cells in different ways, it's common for several of these agents to be given together. This strategy increases the potent killing effect of these drugs while reducing the risk that some cells will develop resistance to the drugs.

Radiation therapy

Radiation kills living cells by damaging their DNA. The successful use of radiation in cancer is based on the ability to direct the radiation dose to the tumor, sparing the surrounding normal tissue. To ensure that the treatments stay focused on their target, various imaging systems, computer software, and body stabilization mechanisms (like molds and masks) may be used.

Radiation can be delivered externally or internally.

External radiation

When radiation is delivered externally, photon or electron beams are typically used. These beams go through the cancer and destroy both healthy and cancerous tissue along the beam's path. More recently, radiation therapy with proton beams has become available, but only select treatment centers across the country currently offer it. An advantage of proton beams is that they can be directed to deposit most of their energy at the target site, so they tend to cause less damage to healthy tissue than photon beams. However, technological advances continue to improve the administration of photon beams, reducing their impact on healthy tissue.

Internal radiation

A common form of internal radiation therapy is called *brachytherapy*. When this treatment is used, radioactive seeds, ribbons, or capsules are placed in or near the cancer cells. This enables a high dose of radiation to be delivered directly to the cancer, sparing healthy tissue. This treatment may be used for breast, head and neck, uterine, cervical, prostate, gallbladder, esophageal, eye, and lung cancers.

You can also receive internal radiation in a liquid form (such as radioactive iodine or chemotherapy agents with radioactive materials attached), which may be taken orally or received intravenously. When the liquid form is used, the radiation travels throughout the body to seek out and kill cancer cells. This treatment is often used for thyroid cancer and non-Hodgkin's lymphoma.

Surgery

Surgery is the oldest type of cancer care. This treatment is instrumental in curing most malignant conditions. Surgical removal of cancer may be undertaken in all areas of the body. And even if a cure isn't possible, surgery may be used to alleviate distressing symptoms or to avoid complications (for example, placing a rod into the bone of a cancerous lower limb to prevent a fracture and inability to walk), even when survival is unlikely to be improved.

Hormone therapy

Hormone therapy refers to the administration of anti-cancer therapy that favorably impacts growth factors that under normal circumstances control the growth pattern of particular tissues within the body. Hormone therapy may be administered when there is evidence that inhibiting these factors will cause regression of the cancer or prevent its spread.

For example, estrogen is the normal hormone that strongly influences the normal growth of breast tissue. Some malignant breast cancers continue to be strongly influenced by the presence of estrogen, and drugs that act as "anti-estrogens" (such as tamoxifen) can interfere with the spread of metastatic breast cancer or actually prevent its development (when used as an adjuvant therapy). For similar reasons, the administration of anti-androgen drugs can be highly effective in managing prostate cancer.

Hematopoietic stem cell transplantation

Hematopoietic stem cell transplantation is the transplantation of *hematopoietic stem cells* (blood cells that can develop into any other blood cells) to treat certain blood and bone marrow cancers. The stem cells are usually extracted from the bone marrow, peripheral blood, or umbilical cord blood. When the stem cells come from your own blood or bone marrow, the transplantation is referred to as *autologous;* when they come from a donor, it's referred to as *allogeneic.* In addition to treating your cancer, hematopoietic stem cell transplantation may be used to enable you to receive higher doses of chemotherapy than your bone marrow could otherwise tolerate.

Biotherapy

Biotherapy, also referred to as *immunotherapy,* is a very broad category of anti-cancer treatment that relies, at least in part, on a patient's normal immune system to destroy the malignant cells. Biotherapy includes a variety of cancer vaccines, monoclonal antibodies (man-made versions of immune system proteins), and nonspecific immunotherapies (these provide a general boost to the immune system). In recent years, biotherapy has gained increasing acceptance as a valid treatment strategy in a number of clinical settings, and it has been used to treat bladder, breast, colon, kidney, lung, and prostate cancers, as well as melanoma and many blood cancers.

Molecularly targeted drugs

The delivery of molecularly targeted drugs is a truly exciting new approach to cancer management. Every cancer has unique molecular abnormalities. With this therapy, these abnormalities are identified via laboratory assessments; then specific treatments that are known to be active in the presence of these abnormalities are administered.

Getting a Second Opinion

A cancer diagnosis raises many questions. Two of the most crucial questions that you may contemplate during your cancer journey is whether the diagnosis is correct and whether a particular management strategy truly is the best one for you. When such questions arise, having a second set of experienced eyes reviewing your case can help you feel comfortable with what you've been told and enable you to decide on a treatment route with greater confidence.

A second opinion should always be considered an option, but second opinions tend to be most useful when you're facing an unusual cancer, because management options in such cases are not as well defined. Of course, if you or your family ever feels any level of discomfort with the recommendations of your oncology team, a second opinion may help.

You may feel a natural reluctance to ask your cancer provider to help you organize a second opinion, especially if you plan on continuing to receive care from her. But the best doctors don't discourage or frown upon second opinions — in fact, they frequently encourage patients to obtain them, particularly if they suspect the patient wants one. They recognize that patients who have their questions fully answered during this process will likely return feeling more confident and secure.

If your doctor appears threatened when you mention a second opinion, is unwilling to let others assist in developing an optimal treatment plan for you, or appears insecure with regard to his recommendations, it may be time to find another oncologist.

Considering Clinical Trials

Patients often ask about the wisdom of participating in clinical trials. They aren't right for everyone, but if no one participated in them, treatments for cancer and for the side effects caused by its treatments wouldn't advance. Before you can participate in a trial, you'll have to carefully consider many variables, which is best done in collaboration with your healthcare team. Some of the factors you'll be weighing in your deliberations include

- **Specific eligibility requirements:** All trials have *inclusion criteria* (criteria you need to meet to be included in a trial) and *exclusion criteria* (criteria that prevent you from being eligible to participate in a trial). Study investigators use inclusion and exclusion criteria to find their desired patient population, and they may include things like specific cancer type, amount and types of prior therapy, and the presence of any additional medical illnesses.

- **Where the trial is being conducted:** Some trials include thousands of patients and hundreds of cancer centers throughout the world, but many are small and may only be conducted at one or two facilities.

- **Time required for participation in the trial compared with treatment outside the trial:** Studies are generally conducted for a set period of time, as established by the researchers, and you may have to make yourself available for a certain number of appointments. In fact, there may be considerably more appointments to go to than if you were treated by your regular oncologist outside the trial, particularly because there is closer monitoring that may require more assessments.

- **Risks (if any) associated with participation in the trial:** You'll have to weigh the risks of participating in the trial versus receiving treatment outside the trial. If additional risks are identified, you'll have to decide whether the potential payoff is worth assuming those risks.

- **Costs:** Sometimes participating in trials costs money, even if you're not paying for the treatments themselves. For instance, transportation expenses may not be covered, and complications from treatments may result in out-of-pocket expenses, because some insurance companies won't pay for any medical expenses when you're receiving treatment as part of a clinical trial. Before agreeing to participate in a trial, you'll need to carefully research what expenses the trial sponsor covers and how your health insurance factors into the cost equation.

Dispelling clinical trial myths

A number of common myths are out there regarding participation in cancer clinical trials. The most prevalent is that trial participants may receive a placebo, receive no treatment, or receive subpar treatment even when an effective therapy exists. But clinical trials compare a standard therapy for a particular condition with a new therapy that is thought to be more effective or to have fewer side effects based on early study results. So, at the very least, you'll be getting the standard treatment, and you may be one of the first people to get something better. In addition, you'll be advancing medicine. Without clinical trials, doctors wouldn't know nearly as much about cancer as they do today or have as many treatments at their disposal.

Another misconception is that you may become a human guinea pig. But trials conducted in the United States have to meet strict criteria before they can be undertaken. In addition, the clinical investigators and the ethical review committees (called *institutional review boards*) are required to carefully evaluate and monitor how all cancer trials are conducted, ensuring that human rights are always maintained.

If you're asked to participate in a clinical trial and ever have any concerns about the requirements associated with the study or how it's conducted, you should discuss these concerns directly with your own oncologist. You can also speak with the researchers conducting the trial or contact a representative of the trial's ethical review committee. The number-one priority of this committee is to prevent you from experiencing any physical or psychological harm. When you enroll in a trial, you should be given contact information for these resources. If not, ask for it.

Finding clinical trials

If you're interested in participating in a clinical trial, first speak with your cancer team. They may know of appropriate trials within their own institution/organization or in the surrounding region, such as at a cancer program at a local university.

A number of cancer advocacy groups maintain listings of clinical trials relevant to a particular malignancy. The National Cancer Institute also maintains a listing of clinical trials for different tumor types at www.cancer.gov/clinical trials, or you can visit www.clinicaltrials.gov to browse listings.

Keep in mind that any clinical trial listings, regardless of their source, are likely to provide an incomplete outline of the specific eligibility requirements and time commitments associated with trial participation. In addition, some trials may no longer be open for enrollment despite indicating that they're still accepting patients.

Treatment support resources

When looking for treatment support resources, ask your oncologist or healthcare team to point you in the right direction. They may have information readily available to give you, can answer your questions in a meaningful way because they know your history and have access to your records, and know how to find individuals or organizations that can provide you with the information you need.

In addition, numerous cancer-focused organizations offer abundant, well written, easy-to-understand educational materials regarding cancer diagnosis and management. Many of these are available online. Organizations to look into include national not-for-profit organizations like the American Cancer Society (www.cancer.org) and the American Society of Clinical Oncology (www.asco.org); governmental agencies like the National Cancer Institute (www.cancer.gov); hospitals; universities; and pharmaceutical/biotech/device companies.

Chapter 3

Tackling the Side Effects of Cancer and Its Treatments

· ·

In This Chapter

▶ Finding out about side effects

▶ Preserving fertility

▶ Managing physical side effects

▶ Coping with emotional side effects

· ·

You may be concerned that your cancer treatment could be worse than the disease. But as a result of impressive cancer research efforts around the world, we now have a far better understanding of how cancer treatment impacts both physical and emotional well-being. As a result, we can take steps to lessen the impact of cancer and its treatments by preventing and better managing its side effects.

This chapter reviews some of the side effects you *may* face during treatment. The key word here is *may*. The listing of a particular adverse event in this chapter doesn't indicate that it's necessarily a risk for you, even if it's associated with a treatment you're receiving or you're otherwise at high risk of the event. Everyone is different, and you may even experience a side effect we don't discuss.

 Communicating with your healthcare team is essential. Don't assume that side effects are just a normal part of treatment and that nothing can be done about them. Often, numerous steps can be taken to help alleviate or eliminate side effects. This chapter is intended to provide you with the information you need to improve the line of communication with your healthcare team as far as potential side effects are concerned. You also discover some things you can do to prevent or reduce these effects.

All About Side Effects

When linking the term *side effects* with *cancer,* horrific visions pop into most people's heads. If you haven't started the treatment leg of your journey yet, you may be imagining yourself bald, frail, and tired, with your face glued to the toilet bowl. But while some treatment-related side effects may be serious or debilitating, many of them are minor and only minimally impact a person's quality of life. In addition, very few side effects persist for long periods of time, like months or years. Most last only days or weeks.

In this section, we talk a bit about coming to terms with side effects and look at some factors that can increase the risk of these effects. With a proper mind set and some knowledge, you can better prepare yourself for the road ahead.

Putting side effects in perspective

The goal of cancer treatment is to remove or kill cancer cells while sparing the healthy organs and tissues throughout the body. To achieve this, you may receive any number of treatments, from surgery, to radiation, to chemotherapy, to an array of different medications. All these treatments are associated with their own set of side effects, some major and some minor.

Although the list of related side effects can be scary, you're unlikely to experience the vast majority of them, and you may even experience none of them. Everyone is different.

Also, keep in mind that when clinical trials are conducted to test new drugs and treatment regimens, medical professionals are required to report all adverse effects attributable to the treatment being evaluated. In some cases, however, it can be very difficult to determine if a correlation may actually exist between an adverse event and the drug being evaluated. But to err on the side of caution, the adverse event will still be included in the drug labeling information when the drug gets approved. Therefore, despite the list of side effects looking long and scary, you really should just think of them as *potential* effects, not definitive ones.

Focusing on factors that may increase the risk of side effects

Numerous factors can increase your risk of experiencing certain side effects during treatment. By understanding what these risk factors are, you can take steps to mitigate them and prevent complications.

For example, one of the potential side effects of many chemotherapy drugs is a reduction in a type of bone marrow cells known as *platelets*. These cells are responsible for preventing and stopping bleeding. Certain medications, including aspirin, are known to interfere with platelet function. This effect may be favorable in certain non-cancer settings, such as for various cardiovascular problems, but it can lead to major bleeding and other serious consequences when receiving chemotherapy. As a result, your doctor will likely advise you to avoid taking aspirin and similar medications while you're receiving chemo. Be sure to closely follow your oncologist's recommendations.

Also, avoid drinking alcohol while receiving treatment. Alcohol can cause many adverse reaction, depending on which medications it's paired with. For example, drinking alcohol at the same time that you're taking *antiemetics* (medications to prevent nausea and vomiting) may cause short-term drowsiness and lead to dry mouth and dry eyes.

Whatever you do, be honest with your doctor about your history and what medications and dietary and herbal supplements you're taking. Because numerous factors can increase the risk of certain side effects, only your doctor and cancer-care team will be able to properly assess your risk and explain in detail what you can do to reduce your specific risks. But they can only do this if they have a clear picture of your history and situation.

Considerations for Young Adults

If you're of child-bearing age and think you'd like to start a family or expand your family, a cancer diagnosis may make this objective seem out of reach. But cancer doesn't have to crush these dreams. Today, there are many ways to preserve fertility and options that can be pursued to give you the family you always wanted.

Cancer treatment and fertility

Depending on your specific cancer and treatment regimen, the impact on your future fertility may be minor or substantial. Regardless of your gender, the cells within your reproductive organs are highly sensitive to the effects of radiation and chemotherapy, but the degree to which these cells will ultimately be impacted by these treatments depends on numerous factors. If you're receiving radiation, it'll depend on the amount of radiation delivered to the cancer site and the location of that site. If you're receiving chemotherapy, it may depend on the specific drugs used. Your age may also influence the risk of temporary or permanent infertility.

Fortunately, one of the most important developments in cancer management has been the recognition that in addition to controlling the cancer, equal efforts must be made to ensure patients are able to return to as normal a life as possible after treatment. And there is no more important consideration for an adolescent or young adult facing cancer treatment than the potential impact of the treatment on the opportunity to have a family in the future. So, if you're of reproductive age, your oncologist or healthcare team will likely discuss fertility concerns with you and provide you with resources to address those concerns and help you preserve your fertility. If not, it's important for you to initiate such discussions with your oncologist, preferably before treatment starts.

While you're receiving therapy, take every step possible to avoid becoming pregnant or fathering a child, particularly if you're receiving cytotoxic therapy. The last thing you want is to risk your health or put a prospective child at risk of birth defects. Your oncologist and healthcare team can provide guidance on appropriate contraceptive measures and on when it's safe for you to start or expand your family.

Consulting with a reproductive endocrinologist

Unless it's urgent that cancer treatment be started immediately, as may occur with certain types of leukemia and other aggressive cancers, you may want to consider fertility preservation options before initiating chemotherapy, radiation therapy, or other cancer treatments. A reproductive endocrinologist is the specialist you'll consult with to discuss your options. Your oncologist should be able to recommend someone who has expertise working with people who have cancer. This is important, particularly for women seeking treatment and people who have not yet gone through puberty, because hormonal therapies or more invasive procedures may be required, and certain treatments can increase the risk of cancer acceleration. A reproductive endocrinologist with cancer experience will know which treatments are feasible and safest for you, enabling you to better determine which risks you're willing to take. Other considerations when looking for a reproductive endocrinologist or fertility center include pregnancy success rates, cost, convenience, and reputation.

During your fertility consultation, many factors will be considered, such as marital status, tumor type, cancer stage, any other health issues, the planned cancer treatment regimen, and your preferences. If any of these factors prohibits efforts to pursue fertility preservation, the reproductive endocrinologist will likely discuss other options with you, such as adoption, use of a donor egg when you're ready, and surrogacy. Your reproductive endocrinologist can provide you with the resources you need to investigate and pursue such options.

Fertility resources for young patients with cancer

Your oncologist and healthcare team is your best resource for finding a cancer fertility specialist in your area. But there are numerous wonderful online resources that can give you a good idea of what to expect. The American Cancer Society provides the most comprehensive article we've seen on the various options that can be used to preserve fertility. The article is available at www. cancer.org/acs/groups/cid/documents/webcontent/002854-pdf. pdf. (Because URLs sometimes change, particularly for individual articles, if you can't locate the article using the URL we've provided, type "Fertility Concerns and Cancer: What Are My Options" into your favorite search engine, and you should be able to access it.)

Other great online sources include Fertile Hope (www.fertilehope.org), an organization dedicated solely to "providing reproductive information, support, and hope to cancer patients and survivors whose medical treatments present the risk of infertility." In addition to its numerous helpful articles, Fertility Hope offers a database of doctors and services; a helpful glossary of terms; risk calculators that consider your sex, cancer type, and treatment; and a calculator that helps you determine which option may be the best choice to help you build your family.

Another great resource worth checking out is MyOncofertility.org (www. myoncofertility.org), which features a timeline outlining fertility considerations at all cancer stages, from diagnosis to after treatment. Whether you're an adult in your reproductive years or the parent of a child with cancer, the site provides a wealth of information.

Dealing with Common Physical Side Effects

When people think of cancer, the side effects that cause physical changes to the body typically provoke the most fear. But not everyone experiences these effects, and even if you experience one or more of them, they're often short-lived. In this section, we look at some of the most commonly experienced physical effects of cancer treatment and what can be done to manage them or make you more comfortable if any of them happens to you.

Anemia

The term *anemia* stems from a similarly spelled ancient Greek term that means "lack of blood." When you have anemia, you either don't have enough red blood cells or don't have enough hemoglobin (the oxygen-carrying pigment of red blood cells) in your blood to adequately carry oxygen to the cells throughout your body. Symptoms of anemia may include fatigue, weakness, dizziness, shortness of breath, an unusually rapid heartbeat, *pallor* (paleness), leg cramps, difficulty concentrating, and insomnia. If you experience any of these symptoms, be sure to mention them to your oncologist.

Anemia has numerous causes, including current or past uncorrected bleeding; inadequate nutrition; excessive alcohol intake; cancer affecting the bone marrow, which is where the red blood cells are produced; and suppression of bone marrow function by chemotherapy. Anemia is also a common complication of advanced progressive cancer, and, in this circumstance, a specific correctable cause of the anemia may not be identified. To manage the anemia in these cases, recurrent blood transfusions may be necessary.

How your anemia is treated depends on its cause. If it's caused by blood loss, you may need to undergo surgery to correct the bleeding; if it's caused by nutritional deficiencies, you may need to correcting these deficits with supplements or infusion. In certain situations, drugs that are known to stimulate red blood cell production may be prescribed.

Anorexia

Anorexia is a sensation of not wanting to eat or even feeling repulsed by the thought of eating. This event may have many possible causes, including the administration of chemotherapy and other cancer drugs, nausea and vomiting, infection, persistent pain, emotional distress, excessive fatigue, and the effects of progressive cancer.

If you experience anorexia, you should discuss this with your physician as soon as possible. When anorexia remains unaddressed, it can lead to malnutrition, weight loss, muscle wasting, and an increased risk of death. In many cases, once a specific cause is identified (such as pain) and measures are taken to correct the problem, anorexia resolves. Turn to Chapter 19 for tips on how you can revive your appetite when facing anorexia.

Constipation

Constipation is an inability to empty your bowels, or difficulty doing so. When constipated, your stomach may feel bloated and full of gas, you may feel like you need to defecate even after you've passed stool, and you may even experience some leakage of watery stool. If you're unable to have a bowel movement after three days, be sure to consult with your physician, particularly if you see blood in your stool, laxatives are not helping, you have abdominal cramps, and/or you're experiencing severe vomiting.

Like diarrhea, constipation can have many causes. It can be a complication of the cancer itself (for example, the cancer may have caused a bowel obstruction) or of cancer treatment. One of the most common treatments that can lead to constipation is narcotic analgesics (such as opioids), which are used to control cancer-related pain.

In general, because it's far easier to prevent severe constipation before it occurs than to manage the problem after it develops, if you observe a change in your normal bowel habits, you should talk to your healthcare team. You can also find some food strategies for dealing with constipation in Chapter 5.

Diarrhea

Some people think that diarrhea is one watery bowel movement. But from a medical standpoint, you're not considered to have diarrhea until you have four or more such bowel movements in a 24-hour period. If this occurs, you should see your oncologist or primary-care provider as soon as possible, especially if you have any other associated symptoms, such as vomiting, abdominal cramping, fever, chills, an inability to eat or drink, weight loss, blood in your stool, or an inability to urinate.

Like pain, diarrhea may have a variety of causes. It can be a complication of radiation to the bowel, occur after gastrointestinal surgery to remove a tumor, result from certain chemotherapy drugs, or occur after taking various other medications used to treat cancer. Diarrhea can also signify a potentially serious infection within the gastrointestinal system, such as may occur from a foodborne illness; stem from stress and anxiety; or be attributable to the cancer itself. For certain cancers, like those of the colon or pancreas, diarrhea may be the first indication of cancer.

Because the causes of diarrhea are so varied, your physician will need to carefully consider its potential causes before deciding on a particular course of action. However, even if you experience just one bout of diarrhea or are given a certain medication to help with your diarrhea, there are food strategies you can employ that might be helpful (see Chapter 5). And if your diarrhea persists despite prescribed treatments, be sure to notify your oncologist so that other treatments can be tried.

Dry mouth

Dry mouth, which your oncologist may refer to as *xerostomia,* occurs when the salivary glands stop producing enough saliva to keep your mouth moist. As a result, your mouth may feel sticky and dry, your lips may crack, and your tongue may feel leathery and have a burning sensation. In addition, because saliva is essential for chewing, swallowing, tasting, and talking, these activities may become impaired. You may also be at risk of dental problems, such as cavities, gum disease, and mouth sores, because saliva keeps the bacteria in your mouth in check. Therefore, good oral care is essential when facing dry mouth, and a consultation with a dentist may be warranted.

Dry mouth is a potential side effect of a number of anticancer therapies, including local radiation to the oral cavity, which may result in a more serious and sometimes permanent sensation of dryness. In other cases, dry mouth may suggest dehydration, which can occur after bouts of diarrhea or vomiting or as result of prescription pain medications.

A variety of treatments are available to improve the sensation of dry mouth. If radiation therapy is the cause, using radioprotectant medication, which helps lessen the side effects of radiation treatment, may be helpful. Then there are more general medications, such as those that stimulate the salivary glands, serve as saliva substitutes, or moisten the mouth.

But medications aren't the only option. You can try to stimulate the salivary glands by sucking on sugar-free candy or chewing sugarless gum. In the case of dehydration, adequate fluid intake should improve the situation. Using a cool-mist humidifier at night may also prevent your mouth from drying up.

Fatigue

Fatigue (a feeling of tiredness) is a common complication of many cancer treatments. It's also one of the most difficult side effects to effectively manage. This is likely because fatigue has multiple causes, even in the same individual. For example, cancer-related tiredness may result from *anemia* (a reduced amount of available red blood cells to carry oxygen to your tissues), inadequate sleep, low-grade nausea, emotional distress, pain, and inadequate nutrition. And this is only a partial list of possible causes.

If you're experiencing fatigue, be sure to talk with your oncologist and health-care team, because they can work to identify its possible causes and develop strategies to improve your symptoms. For example, if you're found to be anemic, blood transfusions or pharmaceutical agents may be prescribed to help your body to restore more normal red blood cell, hemoglobin, and/or iron levels, boosting energy.

Regardless of the cause of your fatigue, nutrition can play an important role in remedying this symptom and in preventing its associated complications, like malnutrition because you can't muster the energy to prepare food or eat. For useful food strategies when facing fatigue, turn to Chapter 5.

Fluid retention

Cancer and its treatments may cause an abnormal buildup of fluid in the body, a condition your oncologist may refer to as *edema* when the fluid collects in the extremities (legs, arms, feet, hands) or face; *ascites* when it collects in the abdomen; and *pleural effusion* when it collects around the lungs. Other causes of fluid retention may include nutritional deficiencies (such as low protein levels); inactivity; cancer-related vein or lymph system blockages; removal of the lymph nodes; and problems with the kidneys, liver, or heart. Symptoms may include swelling, a feeling of heaviness or tightness, rapid weight gain, decreased urination, difficulty breathing, and stiffness of the joints.

Treatment of fluid retention depends on identifying its underlying cause. If the edema is caused by a treatment, an alternative may be sought or the symptoms may be managed until treatment ends. If it's caused by malnutrition, nutritional strategies may be employed, such as increasing protein intake. Fluid retention from medications or malnutrition is generally reversible, but when it's caused by cancer or by other health problems, the swelling may be more difficult to treat and may be permanent. Nevertheless, in such cases, certain management strategies may be helpful, such as wearing compression socks and stockings, improving nutrition, reducing salt intake, elevating swollen areas when sitting or lying down, and avoiding standing for long periods of time. Your oncologist may also prescribe a *diuretic* (which increases the production of urine).

If you notice you're retaining fluid, it's important to speak with your healthcare team as soon as possible before you initiate any of these suggestions, particularly if you become short of breath, you've gained 5 pounds or more in a week, your hands or feet are cold to the touch, or you're rarely urinating.

Hair loss

Hair loss is probably one of the most feared side effects among people receiving chemotherapy, particularly among women who may struggle with perceptions of being less feminine without hair. Hair loss can also occur in areas exposed to radiation treatments, particularly when administered at higher doses. Although not all chemotherapeutic agents cause hair loss, many do. But even though hair loss is an undesirable side effect of many chemotherapeutic agents, it isn't a serious complication. After all, it doesn't result in the loss of normal body function or pose a risk of death, and hair starts to grow back usually within weeks after treatment ends. At the same time, it can have a profound emotional impact. You may feel anxiety about how you'll be perceived by the outside world and whether you'll be gawked at, particularly because bald heads have become the hallmark of cancer, at least for women.

Today, many options are available to enable you to feel comfortable in your skin when facing hair loss, including impressively stylish wigs made with real hair or synthetic hair that look nothing at all like a Halloween costume topper. Many cancer providers have services available on-site to assist you with this endeavor or can refer you to local establishments that can help. You can also check out www.wigsforcancerpatients.org and www.lookgoodfeelbetter.org. Through these sites, you can order wigs and find articles that contain lots of helpful tips for wearing wigs and scarves and applying makeup to make you feel better.

If you don't like the idea of a wig, many other options are at your disposal, including caps, scarves, and hats. Of course, there is no shame in going out just as you are! You shouldn't feel like you have to cover up. What you decide to do should depend entirely on what you're comfortable with.

Mouth and throat sores

Potentially more serious than dry mouth is the development of open sores in the mouth and throat (your oncologist may refer to this as *stomatitis* or *mucositis*), which can cause moderate to severe pain and an inability to eat, and increase your risk of oral infections because of the multitude of germs found in the oral cavity.

Mouth and throat sores may develop from certain chemotherapy drugs or from local radiation, because these treatments affect the sensitive normal cells that line the digestive tract, which starts with the mouth. If you have a very low white blood cell count and develop mouth and throat sores, they may be caused by an infection in this area. If mouth and throat sores develop during treatment, they can be difficult to treat and lead to complications. As a result, good oral care is absolutely essential before and during cancer treatment.

If your oncologist thinks you can wait a few weeks before starting anticancer treatment, consult with a dentist to get a cleaning and address any dental problems. After that, make every effort to maintain good oral hygiene. Turn to Chapter 5 for some oral care recommendations, food strategies you can use to ensure adequate nutrition, and ways to alleviate the pain. If these strategies don't help you enough, you can ask your doctor about prescribing a medication, such as Carafate, which is generally used to treat ulcers, or Kepivance, which is specifically approved for cancer-related mouth sores. In general, despite the severity of the discomfort, the pain tends to quickly improve as the sores begin to heal.

Nausea and vomiting

Nausea and vomiting can result from a variety of treatments, including chemotherapy and radiation therapy to the abdomen, stomach, spine, or brain. You may even become nauseated from anxiety before you begin treatment. When chemotherapy is the cause of nausea and vomiting, it's referred to as *chemotherapy-induced nausea and vomiting* (CINV). Regardless of the cause of nausea and vomiting, this is a much more serious concern than hair loss or some of the other potential side effects of cancer treatments. This is because nausea and vomiting can affect your ability to perform your daily activities and lead to nutritional deficits, thereby hindering your quality of life. But whether you'll develop nausea and/or vomiting will depend on a variety of factors, including the treatment you're receiving and your tolerance threshold.

But even if you do experience nausea, vomiting, or CINV as a result of treatment, don't despair. A number of highly effective medications can be used to prevent these side effects from occurring and to sustain the response even while treatment is exerting its most taxing effects on your body. In fact, because it's now commonly recognized that the most successful approach to dealing with nausea, vomiting, and CINV is to prevent these effects from happening in the first place, your oncologists may administer preventive medications. And you may continue to receive such medications even if you experience no nausea or vomiting during your treatment. But if you continue to feel nauseated despite such treatments, you should talk to your oncologist so that she can prescribe another medication regimen.

The foods you eat during treatment can be another way to prevent and alleviate this side effect. For information on useful food strategies, turn to Chapter 5.

Pain

Reports indicate that approximately 33 percent to 50 percent of people with cancer will experience pain at some point during their cancer journey. Cancer-related pain can take a variety of forms. It may be mild, moderate, or severe and feel dull, sharp, or achy. It may come and go or be constant, and it may occur at the primary cancer site or at distant sites if the cancer has spread.

Pain takes so many different forms because it can result from a variety of situations. The cancer may be putting pressure on adjacent nerves, bones, or organs, or it may grow into, destroy, or displace surrounding tissue. In addition, cancer cells or immune cells targeting the cancer may secrete compounds that contribute to pain.

Cancer treatments can also contribute to the pain picture. Recovery from major surgery to remove a tumor can be painful, whereas radiation and chemotherapy may cause painful side effects, such as skin irritation and mouth sores. Generally, treatment-associated pain is short-lived — when the treatment ends, the pain usually resolves not too long thereafter. And if you felt pain before you started treatment, cancer treatments may decrease or eliminate this pain. When this occurs, it can serve as an important indicator that the treatment is working as intended. But even if your pain doesn't improve or worsens during treatment, this doesn't indicate that your treatment isn't working.

People with cancer that has spread to their bones may experience more severe pain. But this doesn't mean there's no relief in sight. Numerous medications are available that can effectively manage pain (your oncologist may refer to these as *analgesics*) and permit normal function. These may range from very mild over-the-counter analgesics like acetaminophen (Tylenol) to powerful pain-controlling prescription medicines like morphine.

No matter what's causing your cancer pain, your oncologist and healthcare team can provide you with medications to alleviate pain and the side effects that directly cause pain. They may also suggest complementary treatments and strategies that may be helpful, such as acupuncture or aromatherapy.

Skin reactions

Skin reactions are quite common and may consist of any of the following symptoms: rashes, itching, dryness, *flushing* (redness and warmth of an area of the skin), inflammation, or blistering. They may occur with any drugs, but are a side effect of many chemotherapy agents.

Although most skin reactions are mild, some can be life threatening, so it's always a good idea to mention any skin changes to your oncologist as soon as possible.

Mild skin reactions are simply observed until they improve without a need for specific interventions. For more severe skin reactions, your oncologist will have to consider whether to continue with your treatment. To reach a decision, your doctor will consider the severity of your skin reaction, the documented risk associated with continuing treatment after observing this side effect, and the availability of alternative anticancer treatments. Regardless of the decision made, more serious events will require careful local skin care, including efforts to prevent secondary infections because the normal skin barrier has been breached.

Taste changes

Changes in taste are very common after chemotherapy, and these changes may take a variety of forms. Some familiar foods may taste unusual, others may taste bland, everything may taste the same, or you may develop a metallic taste upon eating. Regardless of your taste-change experience, it can lead to food aversions, anorexia, and weight loss. And although the sensation is generally limited in duration, it can sometimes persist for several weeks after each treatment. If taste changes continue for prolonged periods of time and prevent you from eating, you can become malnourished, which is a serious problem that needs to be addressed as soon as possible.

Turn to Chapter 5 for some nutritional strategies on how to eat your way through taste and smell changes. ***Remember:*** Taste largely hinges on smell, so if your sense of smell is impacted, your taste is likely to be altered as well. And even if you experience taste or smell changes but feel they aren't impacting your nutritional status, discuss them with your healthcare team. If an underlying cause like dry mouth is identified, it can be addressed, which may improve your symptoms.

Weight gain

Weight gain during treatment may be a favorable event, particularly if you were previously malnourished. But it may also be an undesirable effect of treatment, including certain chemotherapeutic agents, steroids, and hormone therapy, or may result from fluid retention or be caused by a lack of activity and/or excessive food intake.

A short-term gain in weight may not pose a problem, especially because nutritional demands are higher during intensive anticancer treatments. But excessive weight gain may pose a problem. Studies have shown that weight gain during cancer treatment can lead to a poor prognosis, particularly if you're already overweight. Gaining weight can also make it difficult to keep other conditions, such as diabetes, under control, which can further increase your risk of unfavorable outcomes.

If you're experiencing unintentional weight gain, see Chapter 4 to learn how to estimate your caloric needs to lose weight. While watching your calorie intake, also try to make sure you're getting at least two and a half hours of moderate activity (like walking) on a weekly basis (see Chapter 17 for more on this). Finally, the clean eating recommendations in Chapter 6 and throughout this book are meant for you. They'll help you nourish your body without all the excess and empty calories from a diet high in processed foods. And don't forget to eat breakfast! Breakfast eaters tend to have an easier time losing weight. The recipes in Chapter 10 will help you jump-start your metabolism when you get up in the morning.

Weight loss

Weight loss may result from your treatment program, such as during recovery from surgery or from nausea and vomiting after chemotherapy. In these cases, weight loss generally isn't considered a problem, unless it becomes pronounced. But weight loss can also point to more serious issues, such as inadequate nutrition or cancer progression. As a result, it's a good idea to keep tabs on your weight during and after treatment. Although your oncologist is likely to monitor your weight, you'll be able to notice any weight loss more quickly if you weigh yourself at the same time daily or every few days.

If you're struggling with unintentional weight loss, see Chapter 4 to learn how to calculate your daily calorie and protein needs. If side effects from treatment are causing you to lose weight, some of the suggestions in Chapter 5 may help you meet your calorie and protein goals. Finally, if the main reason you're having a hard time maintaining your weight is a lack of appetite, try some of the suggestions in Chapter 19 to revive your appetite.

You may also want to make an appointment with a dietitian for an evaluation. If your treatment facility doesn't have one, your oncologist should be able to make a recommendation, or you can visit the Academy of Nutrition and Dietetics Find a Registered Dietitian database at `www.eatright.org/ programs/rdfinder`, where you can search for dietitians in your area and by area of expertise. You can also visit the Academy of Nutrition and Dietetics Oncology Nutrition Dietetic Practice Group website at `www. oncologynutrition.org/members/locator` to find an oncology registered dietitian (RD) and RDs that are board certified in oncology nutrition.

Coping With Typical Emotional Side Effects

In addition to its numerous physical effects, cancer and its treatments can invoke many emotions. Being upset by your diagnosis and afraid of what's going to happen to you and your future is normal, but if any emotion debilitates you and you're unable to function, you need to seek help. In this section, we review the emotional and mental toll that cancer can take and tell you what you can do about these effects if you experience them.

There are numerous sources of emotional support at your disposal, so you should never feel alone. In addition to friends and family, there are psychologists, psychiatrists, social workers, counselors, chaplains, and support groups (online and in-person). Some of these professionals may be accessible directly at your cancer center, but if not, your oncology office can point you in the right direction.

Depression

You may feel very sad after a cancer diagnosis. This response is completely normal. Feeling sad doesn't mean you have depression. It's only when feelings of sadness become unrelenting and affect your ability to function normally that depression may be the underlying problem. Additional symptoms to look for include a lack of desire to engage in activities that previously interested you, pronounced fatigue, altered sleep and eating habits, distractedness, nervousness, and frequent thoughts of death or suicide.

 If you have any of these symptoms, particularly thoughts of suicide, talk to your healthcare team. They'll be able to determine if you need additional support resources and direct you accordingly. Also, discussing how you feel with your family and other loved ones may be therapeutic. Many studies have shown talk therapy to be very effective in treating depression.

 There are also things you can do to help prevent or improve depression. Food can play a key role in how you feel. Several vitamins and nutrients have shown benefit in helping improve mood, including vitamin D, folic acid, vitamin B12, vitamin B6, and omega-3 fatty acids. Make sure you get enough of these nutrients daily. Turn to Chapter 4 to learn more about these nutrients and how to get them through a wholesome diet.

 Another key dietary strategy is to keep blood glucose levels stable. Having them drop too low or get too high can cause your mood to worsen. When blood glucose levels get too low, the stress hormones cortisol and adrenalin are released, and when there are frequent blood glucose spikes, your body's insulin response may become compromised. Keeping blood glucose levels stable keeps insulin and glucagon levels stable, which in turn helps keep your serotonin levels stable. Serotonin is thought to contribute to feelings of happiness and well-being.

 Finally, although depression may keep you from getting up, activity has been shown to be a potent weapon to fight depression. Taking a walk, going swimming, doing yoga, gardening, and anything that gets your heart rate up can release endorphins, elevating your mood. See Chapter 17 to learn more.

Stress

Stress can be physical, mental, or emotional and is your body's normal response to demanding stimuli. Because a cancer diagnosis can rock your world and place considerable demands on your time and emotional reserves, you may experience a variety of different stresses. During these times, your body may release stress hormones like epinephrine, norepinephrine, and adrenaline, which not only help you react to these situations, but also increase your blood pressure, heart rate, and blood glucose levels.

Chronic stress (stress that doesn't go away) can lead to a variety of health issues, including digestive problems like diarrhea, cardiovascular issues like high blood pressure (also known as *hypertension*), and a weakened immune system, increasing your risk of viral infections. Chronic stress also can lead to headaches, insomnia, and anxiety, which ultimately can lead to depression.

Although the feelings invoked by stress are quite natural, you can do things to help alleviate your body's stress response and prevent your stress from becoming chronic. Eating a healthy diet, exercising, and getting enough sleep are all essential. Turn to Chapter 6 for strategies on how to optimize your eating. Of course, if you're experiencing treatment-related side effects that make eating difficult, turn to Chapter 5 to see how you can optimize your nutrition when facing these challenges. For exercise and sleep strategies, turn to Chapter 17.

Anxiety

The terms *anxiety* and *stress* are often used synonymously. Although they may be related, they're actually quite different. Stress may lead to anxiety, which can best be described as a feeling of fear. Because cancer invokes more fear than almost any other disease, it's to be expected that you'll feel quite a bit of anxiety during your cancer journey, particularly when you're waiting for test results.

Although fleeting anxiety isn't a problem, if anxiety becomes paralyzing and leads to an inability to function, your anxiety may have developed into an anxiety disorder and you should discuss your symptoms with your healthcare team to see if additional interventions are warranted.

You can do things to help with your anxiety. First, be sure to talk to your oncologist about your cancer and ask questions if you have concerns or something is unclear. If you have any particular fears over your diagnosis, treatments, or prognosis, don't be afraid to express them. Fears are often far worse than the reality, and having open, frank discussion can be a critical first step to achieving relief or at least substantially diminishing your fears. We also recommend that you follow all the same eating, sleeping, and activity recommendations we outline for stress (see the preceding section), because all those strategies can help alleviate anxiety, too.

Chemo brain

Chemo brain is a term often used to describe an unsettling feeling after chemotherapy of not being fully normal, either with regard to thought processes or the ability to effectively carry out normal daily activities. Some people say it's like being in a fog, and these fog-like feelings have been reported to last for days, weeks, or even months after chemotherapy.

If you experience symptoms that seem to fill the "chemo brain" bill, it's important to discuss this with your healthcare team. They may be able to identify a cause for these symptoms and make changes to your regimen to eliminate or at least improve these negative effects.

Chapter 4

The Role and Power of Nutrition in Fighting Cancer

• •

In This Chapter

▶ Understanding the relationship between cancer and nutrition

▶ Getting a handle on macronutrients and micronutrients

▶ Scoping out fiber

▶ Staying hydrated

▶ Determining body composition concepts and monitoring

▶ Grasping the role of supplements

• •

*W*e've all been told since we were kids that we should eat our fruits and vegetables to prevent illness. After all, as the old adage says, "An apple a day keeps the doctor away." This is because what you eat and drink affects every cell in your body, but although many organizations have published nutrition guidelines for people looking to reduce their risk of developing cancer and other chronic illnesses, finding information on what to consume when you have cancer can be daunting. Yet what you eat and drink during this time is exceedingly important, because it can help you with your recovery and improve your quality of life.

Now, when you're going through cancer treatment, there are two distinct two nutrition goals you'll strive to achieve. The first goal is to eat enough to maintain your body weight/composition and body function. The second goal is to eat the most nutrient-dense foods possible. You may find yourself competing between these goals at various points during your treatment, and that's okay.

In this chapter, we provide you with guidance on how to determine your nutrition goals and how to achieve them. We outline the optimum quantities of macronutrients, micronutrients, fiber, and fluids and where you can get these nutrients, with the focus being on healthy food sources. We also look at how cancer and its treatments may alter individual needs for some of these nutrients and examine how to manage such situations. Then we turn our attention to calories and body composition measures, which are important for you to understand to meet your quantity and quality goals, while ensuring you also achieve a healthy weight. Finally, we turn our attention to dietary supplements. Although many people use supplements during their cancer treatment, they should be used only under very specific conditions because of their potential to interact with cancer treatments.

Grasping Your Nutrition Goals

When you want to eat healthier, your goals may include eating more fruits and vegetables, drinking more water, and cutting out processed foods. But when you're going through cancer treatment, eating the healthiest foods may not always be possible. You may be dealing with gastrointestinal issues, experiencing uncomfortable mouth sores, or feeling so fatigued that you simply don't have the energy to prepare any meal, let alone a healthy one.

That's why when you're going through cancer treatment, you'll have two somewhat competing high-level nutrition goals:

✔ **Quantity:** First and foremost, you need to consume the right quantity of macronutrients to provide the right amount of calories, or energy, to achieve and maintain a healthy body weight and composition, while also fueling your normal daily activities. Studies have shown that as little as a 5 percent loss of body weight can lead to poor outcomes during chemotherapy, including increased side effects and a decreased quality of life.

When you're going through treatment, your body may need more "fuel" in the form of calories and protein to repair itself more rapidly from the effects of surgery, radiation, chemotherapy, and other treatments.

✔ **Quality:** Because eating high-quality, nutrient-dense foods protects against malnourishment, strengthens your immune system, and provides your body with a great source of energy, you need to eat such foods as much as possible when you're able. This may not always be possible when you're undergoing treatment, but after you've completed treatment, this goal is a good one to strive for, along with achieving and maintaining a healthy body weight. Some studies indicate that a healthy diet paired with a healthy weight can help protect against cancer recurrence and secondary cancers.

In summation, if you're struggling with a poor appetite or the side effects of treatment, your focus should be on getting the right quantity of calories and protein to maintain your weight. If this means turning to a box of macaroni and cheese in your pantry, that's fine. But if your appetite is good, you should focus on trying to improve your diet by focusing on eating clean. Turn to Chapter 6 for more information.

As we offer our advice on how to meet your quantity and quality goals, we draw on the most recent guidelines from the American Institute for Cancer Research (AICR) and the American Cancer Society (ACS). In general, these guidelines focus on eating clean and engaging in regular physical activity to help achieve and maintain a healthy body weight. They recommend eating more plant-based foods, like whole grains, vegetables, fruits, and legumes. They also recommend eating less calorie-dense foods, fast foods, and processed foods, as well as consuming fewer sugary drinks. In addition, they recommend limiting red meat, processed meats, alcohol, and salt. Throughout this book, we review how to put these guidelines into action.

Understanding the Importance of Nutrition

Nutrients are needed to maintain life — without them, your body just wouldn't function. Nutrients come from food and provide energy or help with growth and repair in your body. Carbohydrates, protein, fat, vitamins, minerals, and water are all nutrients.

When cancer is present, both it and its many treatments can have a considerable impact on your ability to take in nutrients and on your body's ability to metabolize them, which can lead to malnutrition. When you become malnourished, your body's ability to function properly declines and your immune function decreases, which may make it difficult to fight off an infection during cancer treatment.

Not surprisingly, malnourishment is common in the cancer setting. Studies have shown that 80 percent to 90 percent of people with cancer have signs and symptoms of malnutrition, and the National Cancer Institute (NCI) indicates that as many as 20 percent to 40 percent of people with cancer may die from malnutrition or its associated complications. Scary, right? But we're not telling you these stats to frighten you. We just want you to understand why nutrition is so important, and the objective of this chapter is to give you the knowledge you need to ensure you get the right quantity of nutrients, enabling you to prevent malnourishment while strengthening your immune system and keeping your healthy cells functioning at their best.

By definition, *nutrition* is the science of how the body ingests, digests, absorbs, and metabolizes nutrients. Cancer and its treatments can impact one or all of these steps that food must go through to nourish the cells of your body. This can be caused by a physical issue, such as the location of the cancer, or by a biological or metabolic change, such as loss of appetite from a treatment or increased production of *cytokines* (proteins that carry messages between cells, regulating cellular function).

Here are some examples of how cancer and its treatments can impede ingestion, digestion, and absorption of nutrients and cause metabolic challenges:

- **Ingestion challenges:** Cancer and its treatment can affect your ability to consume nutrients in a number of ways. Depending on the site of cancer, it can be difficult for food or liquids to get from the mouth to the digestive tract. For example, the location of a head and neck cancer may make it difficult to chew and swallow foods; surgery, chemotherapy, and radiation for cancer may make it difficult to get food and liquid from the mouth to the digestive tract.

  Cancer may also cause the body to produce cytokines to try to fight the cancer. When these compounds are produced in very high amounts, they may cause a loss of appetite. Cancer treatments can also lead to anorexia and cause a loss of appetite, making it difficult to consume enough food to get adequate nourishment. In addition, cancer and its treatments may cause a host of other issues that can affect eating, such as a sore mouth or throat, taste and/or smell changes, and fatigue. We talk more about what to do when eating is a challenge in Chapter 5.

- **Digestion and absorption challenges:** *Digestion* is the process by which food is physically and chemically broken down and converted into a substance suitable for absorption and assimilation into the body. Many cancer-related factors can make it difficult to digest and absorb nutrients. For instance, cancer can cause the gastrointestinal tract to become obstructed or blocked so that food and liquids can't be digested or absorbed. In such cases, nutrition may need to be provided intravenously or through a feeding tube until the obstruction is remedied.

  Various cancer treatments, particularly chemotherapy and/or radiation to the abdomen, can sometimes cause lactose intolerance, even if there were no previous issues digesting milk and milk products. This is because chemotherapy and radiation, in addition to malnutrition, can cause changes to the cells lining the digestive tract, making normal digestion difficult. *Lactose,* the sugar naturally found in milk, must be digested by the enzyme lactase in the small intestine. If lactase production is affected by cancer treatment, you may need to limit your intake of milk and milk products for a period of time. Milk that has the enzyme lactase added to it is available, and you may be able to tolerate it as an alternative.

  Cancer of the gastrointestinal tract may make it difficult to digest and absorb nutrients from food, a condition known as *malabsorption.* This can result from the location of the cancer, or it can be a side effect of the surgery used to treat it. Cancer of the stomach, pancreas, gallbladder, bile duct, and small bowel increases the risk of developing malabsorption of fat after surgery. Fat malabsorption may cause severe diarrhea and weight loss from the amount of calories that are not absorbed into the bloodstream but are instead lost in the stool. In such cases, pancreatic digestive enzymes may need to be prescribed to enable the digestion and absorption of fat.

✔ **Metabolic challenges:** *Metabolism* is the chemical process by which living cells make energy available. The same cytokines that can decrease appetite may also cause changes in metabolism. These changes can affect the way the body metabolizes protein, carbohydrates, and fats, resulting in an increase in nutrient needs at a time when eating may be difficult. We look at nutrient needs a little later in this chapter.

As you can see, there are many ways that cancer affects your ability to eat and use nutrients. But don't let this leave you feeling defeated. There are also many ways to bypass and manage these issues, which we examine throughout this book. Of course, if you experience a nutrition-related issue or a side effect that is impeding your ability to eat, be sure to discuss this with your oncologist and treatment team.

Nutrition in a Nutshell

Because nutrition is a science, the more research that's done in the area of nutrition and cancer, the more we learn about the needs of people with cancer. This may be why, at times, it seems that even nutrition professionals can't agree on what to recommend.

Despite constant changes to nutrition recommendations based on new research, some recommendations remain fairly constant, such as your body's needs for macronutrients and micronutrients.

Macronutrients

Macronutrients are nutrients that provide calories or energy to fuel the body's activities. They include protein, carbohydrates, and fats. What follows is a summary of some of the ways cancer changes macronutrient metabolism and how you can meet your macronutrient needs.

Protein

Proteins, which are made up of strands of amino acids, are necessary for maintaining muscle and immune function. Some proteins function as enzymes and hormones, whereas others carry nutrients or oxygen (hemoglobin) where they need to go in your body. During cancer treatments like chemotherapy and radiation, you need to consume enough protein to enable your body to produce new blood cells and intestinal cells between your treatments. Adequate protein levels are also important for healing after surgery and for maintaining proper fluid balance. If your protein levels are low during cancer treatment, you may develop *edema* (swelling from fluid leaking into areas of your body where it isn't normally found, such as your arms, legs, and abdomen).

Although the body can also use protein for energy, this is something you'll want to avoid to ensure the protein you consume is used for maintaining all the aforementioned functions. To do this, you'll need to consume enough carbohydrates and calories along with protein to satisfy your body's energy needs.

In some cases, cancer can trigger your body to make a compound known as proteolysis-inducing factor (PIF). PIF can cause an increase in protein breakdown and a decrease in your body's ability to make protein, resulting in muscle breakdown. For this reason, you may need to eat more protein when undergoing cancer treatment than you're accustomed to. You'll need about 1 to 1.5 g of protein per kilogram of body weight daily to adequately recover from treatment. You can convert your body weight to kilograms from pounds by dividing your weight in pounds by 2.2. Or you can just multiply your weight in pounds by 0.5 to 0.7 to estimate your protein needs.

There is an exception to this rule. If your cancer or cancer treatment has affected your kidneys or liver, it may not be appropriate for you to increase your protein intake. Consult with your oncologist and/or a registered dietitian for specific protein recommendations.

The best sources of protein include lean, unprocessed meats, poultry, or fish; eggs; low-fat milk or yogurt; and cooked beans.

Carbohydrates

Carbohydrates provide energy and are an important means of sparing protein so that it can be used for more vital functions. For this reason, approximately, 45 percent to 65 percent of your calories should come from carbohydrates.

Not all carbohydrates are created equal. Complex carbohydrates from starch and fiber are better than most simple carbohydrates or sugars. Most sources of complex carbohydrates are high in nutrient density, containing fiber, vitamins, minerals, and phytochemicals, whereas refined sugars are low in nutrient density and provide very little, if any, nutrients other than energy.

Does sugar fuel cancer?

You may have heard that "sugar feeds cancer." This is a very oversimplified and potentially dangerous explanation for very complex changes that can happen to carbohydrate metabolism in people with cancer. Glucose is the main energy source for tumors, just as it's the main source of energy for healthy cells. The tumor will get the glucose it needs even at the expense of healthy cells. So, even if you avoid all carbohydrates and refined sugars, your liver will convert the amino acids from the protein you eat into sugar or, worse, obtain it by breaking down your muscles.

In addition, avoiding sugar from fruits, dairy products, and other wholesome foods may lead to malnutrition. Therefore, it's better to reduce your intake of refined sugars, because these don't add any nutrient density to your diet. There is an exception to this rule, however: If you're losing weight because of a poor appetite or symptoms from your cancer or cancer treatment, you need to eat anything that sounds good to you and that you can tolerate. *Remember:* Your body can break down your muscle to free up amino acids to make sugar, so you're better off eating a little refined sugar during these times than forcing your body to break down your muscles to obtain it.

That said, some studies suggest that having increased amounts of insulin circulating in the body may promote tumor growth. *Insulin* is an anabolic hormone that controls blood glucose levels. Because ingestion of refined sugars can cause an increased amount of insulin to be released from the pancreas to metabolize the sugar, avoiding these foods may be preferable. You can also consider pairing sweet with a little protein or fiber, like a few nuts or some fresh fruit, which may lower the insulin response.

Some cancers, such as pancreatic cancer, and some medications used during cancer treatment, such as corticosteroids, can cause high blood glucose levels and sometimes diabetes. If you develop high blood glucose levels or diabetes during cancer treatment, you'll need to follow a diabetes diet plan, which includes eating a consistent amount of carbohydrates at each meal.

Examples of foods high in carbohydrates include whole grains, starchy vegetables (like sweet potatoes, peas, beans, corn), non-starchy vegetables (like carrots and leafy greens), fruits, and low-fat dairy (like milk and yogurt).

Fats

Fats provide energy and slow digestion. We need some fat in our diet. About 20 percent to 35 percent of your calories should come from healthy fats. Fats are a source of and a carrier of the fat-soluble vitamins: vitamins A, D, E, and K. We also get essential fatty acids from fats, which our bodies need to regulate inflammation and perform many other cellular functions, but can't make in the amounts needed. The essential fatty acids are linoleic and linolenic, which can be found in plant oils and cold-water fish. Linoleic acid comes from the omega-6 family of fats, while linolenic comes from the omega-3 family of fats.

Almost everyone gets enough omega-6 fatty acids in the diet from corn, safflower, and sunflower oils; fried foods; and processed foods that contain trans fatty acids. Omega-6s are inflammatory in nature. But we need more omega-3 fatty acids in our diet from cold-water fish, such as sardines, herring, and salmon. There are two essential omega-3 fatty acids in fish: eicosapentaenoic acid (EPA) and docosahexaenoic acid (DHA). Some studies suggest that adults should consume between 1,100 mg and 1,600 mg of omega-3 fatty acids per day. Some studies have also shown that 1,500 mg of EPA may help combat some of the metabolic changes caused by cancer.

There are not many food sources of omega-3 fatty acids, but some foods contain alpha-linolenic acid, which our bodies can convert to EPA. Conversion varies depending on how much omega-6 fat is in the diet. The more omega-6s in the diet, the poorer the conversion. Eating fish two to three times per week is the best way to consume more omega-3 fatty acids. Other good sources of omega-3 fatty acids include ground flaxseeds, canola oil, walnuts, soy nuts, and wheat germ.

Cancer may cause your body to produce a compound called *lipid-mobilizing factor,* which may contribute to weight loss from stored adipose or fat tissue. If you're struggling with weight loss, in addition to consuming nutrient-dense carbohydrates, plenty of protein, and omega-3 fatty acids, it's important for you to consume some additional healthy fats like canola or olive oil, olives, avocados, nuts, seeds, and nut butters. Try to limit saturated fats and trans fats from fatty meats, the skin of poultry, full-fat dairy products, and processed foods made with hydrogenated oils. These fats may increase your risk of developing heart disease during and after cancer treatment.

Micronutrients

Micronutrients are nutrients that can be obtained from food that the body needs in small but very specific quantities to carry out certain functions. They include vitamins, minerals, and phytochemicals. Because taking these micronutrients in excess can cause toxicity, but not getting enough can cause deficiencies, the U.S. government has set various dietary reference intakes (DRIs) for these nutrients for healthy people. The nutrient-related numbers tied to these DRIs are based on recommendations from the Institute of Medicine. The DRI comprises the following four numbers:

✔ **Recommended dietary allowance (RDA):** The amount of nutrients that 97.5 percent of the healthy population needs to meet its dietary needs.

✔ **Adequate intake (AI):** The average intake for a nutrient as observed in a group of healthy people. These are nutrients that do not yet have enough scientific data for an official RDA to be established.

✔ **Tolerable upper level (UL):** The highest amount of a nutrient that can be consumed without toxicity and that is likely safe for almost all people, based on available studies. This is not necessarily an ideal or recommended amount.

✔ **Estimated average requirement (EAR):** The amount of nutrients that 50 percent of the healthy population requires to meet its dietary needs.

The DRIs are based on the needs of healthy people. Because cancer can cause micronutrient deficiencies from poor oral intake, poor digestion, and poor absorption, you may need different amounts of some micronutrients. You can also lose minerals as a side effect of treatment, such as through vomiting or diarrhea, or as result of gastrointestinal surgery.

No blood test can assess for levels of *all* vitamins and minerals. Each nutrient requires a very specific test, and some of these tests are very expensive and are used almost exclusively for research purposes. But in this section, we describe some of the signs and symptoms of vitamin and mineral deficiencies that you and your oncologist can be on the lookout for. We also try to simplify the DRI for someone with cancer.

Vitamins

Vitamins are compounds that are essential in small amounts for almost all cell processes, making them vital for life. They don't provide energy, but in some cases they're important for releasing energy from food. Vitamins fall into two categories: fat soluble (which include vitamins A, D, E, and K) and water soluble (which include the B vitamins and vitamin C).

The fat-soluble vitamins are absorbed into your lymph system and travel in the blood with protein carriers. They can be stored in your liver and fatty tissues and, for this reason, can become toxic if excessive amounts are taken. The water-soluble vitamins are absorbed into the bloodstream and are not stored in the liver and fatty tissues, which means that excess amounts are lost in the urine. They're generally not considered to be toxic, except in rare cases when they're taken in very high amounts. The DRI and good food sources for vitamins appear in Table 4-1.

If you review the food sources for each of the vitamins, you'll see that dark green, leafy vegetables are a good source of at least half the vitamins you need on a daily basis. So, if you can, be sure to eat your greens!

Table 4-1	Daily Adult Vitamin Needs, Upper Limits, and Food Sources		
Vitamin	**Recommended Dietary Allowance or Adequate Intake**	**Tolerable Upper Level**	**Food Sources**
Vitamin A*	Women: 700 mcg Men: 900 mcg	3,000 mcg	Fish oils, milk, eggs, fortified breakfast cereals, bright orange and deep green vegetables and fruits
Vitamin D	Until age 70: 15 mcg (600 IU) After age 70: 20 mcg (800 IU)	100 mcg (4,000 IU)	Egg yolks, liver, fatty fish like salmon, and fortified milk
Vitamin E	15 mg (22.4 IU)	1,000 mg (1,490 IU)	Vegetable oils and seeds
Vitamin K	Women: 90 mcg Men: 120 mcg	Not established	Dark green, leafy vegetables; liver; milk; eggs; and beans
Vitamin B1 (thiamine)	Women: 1.1 mg Men: 1.2 mg	Not established	Pork; green, leafy vegetables; whole grains; legumes; and beans
Vitamin B2 (riboflavin)	Women: 1.1 mg Men: 1.3 mg	Not established	Milk; dairy products; green, leafy vegetables; and whole grains
Vitamin B3 (niacin)	Women: 14 mg Men: 16 mg	35 mg	Lean meats, fish, and poultry
Vitamin B5 (pantothenic acid)	5 mg	Not established	Eggs, legumes, beans, and milk
Vitamin B6 (pyridoxine)	Until age 50: 1.3 mg Women after age 50: 1.5 mg Men after age 50: 1.7 mg	100 mg	Lean meats; fish; poultry; potatoes; green, leafy vegetables; beans; and bananas
Vitamin B7 (biotin)	30 mg	Not established	Eggs, legumes, beans, and milk

Vitamin	Recommended Dietary Allowance or Adequate Intake	Tolerable Upper Level	Food Sources
Vitamin B9 (folate)	400 mcg	1,000 mcg	Green, leafy vegetables; eggs; cantaloupe; beans; beets; and orange juice
Vitamin B12 (hydroxoco-balamin)	2.4 mcg	Not established	Lean meats, animal products
Vitamin C	Women: 75 mg Men: 90 mg	2,000 mg	Broccoli, sweet peppers, strawberries, citrus fruit, and Brussels sprouts

*The requirement for vitamin A is provided in retinol activity equivalents (RAEs) to account for the variability in activity between the active form of vitamin A and beta carotene. Food labels can be confusing because they list vitamin A in international units (IU), but if you consumed all your vitamin A as retinol from food and/or supplements, the RDA in IUs would be 2,333 IU for women and 3,000 IU for men. If you consumed only beta carotene from plant foods and/or supplements, the RDA would be 14,000 IU for women and 18,000 IU for men.

If you've undergone gastrointestinal surgery and have signs and symptoms of fat malabsorption, such as diarrhea, weight loss, oily or foul-smelling stools, and/or abdominal pain and bloating, you may need pancreatic enzymes to help you absorb fat and fat-soluble vitamins. You may also need to take a supplement containing fat-soluble vitamins. There are other causes of diarrhea after surgery, which may require other medications, so be sure to tell your oncologist if you're experiencing diarrhea.

In the following sections, we give you a closer look at each vitamin's function and any cancer considerations.

Vitamin A

This fat-soluble vitamin is needed for proper vision, immune function, maintenance of skin, and normal cell development and growth. The active form of vitamin A that we get from our diets is retinol. It largely comes from animal sources, such as eggs, milk, and butter. This is the form that can be stored in the liver and become toxic if consumed in high amounts without medical supervision. Beta carotene from bright orange and dark green vegetables and fruits can be converted to vitamin A in the body, but it doesn't become toxic.

Vitamin D

This fat-soluble vitamin is needed to absorb calcium and maintain calcium levels in the blood, making it crucial for bone health. Vitamin D is also important for the development of cells, including those of the immune system.

There aren't many food sources of vitamin D, but one of the best sources of vitamin D is sunlight. That's why it's also sometimes called the "sunshine vitamin." Our skin can make vitamin D from sunlight, provided we aren't wearing sunscreen or covered up. Because most of us are indoors during the daylight or live in areas where we can't get enough sunlight from October through May, vitamin D deficiency or insufficiency is becoming more common.

If your cancer is causing you to spend a lot of time indoors, you wear sunscreen when going out, or you're experiencing any symptoms of fat malabsorption, talk with your doctor about your vitamin D status. This is a vitamin for which a simple blood test is available, so ask your oncologist or primary care provider to check your vitamin D level. If it's low, you may need to take a supplement. You may also need a vitamin D and calcium supplement if you're on medications like Zometa or Xgeva to help prevent fractures because your cancer has spread to your bones. In addition, there is some evidence to suggest that having an adequate vitamin D level in the blood may help reduce the musculoskeletal symptoms associated with aromatase inhibitors such as Arimidex, Femara, and Aromasin, which are often given to breast cancer survivors.

Vitamin E

This fat-soluble vitamin is one of the body's main antioxidants. It protects our cells from oxidative damage. Vitamin E deficiency is rare, because it's prevalent in oils and foods containing oils. Toxicity is also rare, but very high intakes of vitamin E may interfere with blood-thinning medications. Also, some studies have suggested that vitamin E supplements may increase the risk of stroke. If you have any signs of fat malabsorption or if you've been following an extremely low-fat diet for a long period of time, you may need to speak to your oncologist about taking a vitamin E supplement.

Vitamin K

This fat-soluble vitamin is needed to make proteins that help the blood clot. You also need it to make an important protein for bone formation. The three types of vitamin K include K1, K2, and K3. Vitamins K1 and K2 are naturally occurring and can be obtained from plant and animal sources, whereas vitamin K3 is man-made and sometimes used in supplements. Our bodies can also make vitamin K2 from friendly bacteria in the intestines.

As with any fat-soluble vitamins, in cases of fat malabsorption, use of pancreatic enzymes and vitamin supplementation may be necessary. Also, if you're on certain blood-thinning medications, you need to keep your vitamin K intake consistent on a daily basis and avoid taking dietary supplements containing vitamin K.

B-complex vitamins

This group of water-soluble vitamins was once thought to be a single vitamin, referred to as *vitamin B,* but it's now known to be eight distinct vitamins: B1 (thiamine), B2 (riboflavin), B3 (niacin), B5 (pantothenic acid), B6 (pyridoxine), B7 (biotin), B9 (folic acid or folate), and B12 (cobalamin). Collectively, the

B vitamins enable your body to metabolize carbohydrates, proteins, and fats, ensuring that your organs and nervous system function properly. They're especially important for heart, brain, liver, and kidney health. Folic acid is also necessary to make the DNA, or genetic material, for all new cells. This is why it's essential in pregnancy. But it's also crucial for the production of red blood cells, which is especially important when you have cancer, because cancer and its treatments can put you at risk for anemia.

Numerous factors can affect your risk of a B-complex vitamin deficiency. If you eat a lot of low-nutrient foods, have a poor food intake due to low appetite, or have gastrointestinal symptoms, such as prolonged periods of vomiting, you may not be getting enough B-complex vitamins. Following a strict vegetarian diet also may make it more difficult to consume enough vitamin B12. Age may be another factor. It's estimated that as many as 50 percent of people older than 50 may not absorb enough vitamin B12. Medications that block the production of acid in the stomach and heavy consumption of alcohol can also decrease absorption of these vitamins from the digestive tract and increase losses in the urine. If you've had gastric bypass surgery in the past to help you lose weight, your cancer has caused you to lose a part of your stomach or digestive tract, or you've had surgery for pancreatic cancer that has affected your small intestine or terminal ileum, you may also be at risk of deficiency.

Some studies suggest that vitamin B6 supplementation may help prevent nerve damage from platinum-based chemotherapies. Like all nutrients, there is a specific window for maximum effectiveness. Supplementation with the right dose of vitamin B6 may help with *neuropathy* (damage to the nerves that can cause numbness, tingling, pain, and sometimes weakness), but if you take too much, it can *cause* neuropathy. Vitamin B6 supplementation may also help with *hand-foot syndrome,* which is a redness, swelling, and numbness of the hands and feet from various treatments, such as 5-FU, Xeloda, or Adriamycin. In addition, because chemotherapy affects rapidly dividing cells, it's important to get adequate amounts of folic acid and vitamin B12, in addition to iron, during treatment.

All supplementation should be done under clinical supervision. Your oncologist needs to know about every dietary supplement you're taking.

Vitamin C

This water-soluble vitamin, also known as *ascorbic acid,* is an important antioxidant, protecting your body from free radicals. It plays a role in the production and maintenance of collagen, which is essential for wound healing. It also facilitates the immune response and enhances the absorption of iron from the digestive tract. If you smoke, you need to increase your vitamin C intake so that you get at least 100 mg per day.

Minerals

Now that you have an understanding of all the vitamins, it's time to turn your attention to the minerals. We're not taking about stuff that's dug out of the dirt, either, like quartz or chunks of iron, but the minerals found in your body. Some major minerals *are* found in large amounts in your body. These include calcium, phosphorus, magnesium, sulfur, sodium, potassium, and chloride. Others are found in much smaller amounts; these are known as *trace minerals,* and they include iron, zinc, iodine, selenium, copper, manganese, molybdenum, fluoride, and chromium.

All minerals play an important role in supporting the biochemical processes of life. They may facilitate metabolic, enzymatic, and hormonal activity; maintain fluid balance; and enable cell production. Minerals also help maintain acid-base balance, or the pH in your body, and have many other specialized functions. As you can see, minerals are very important. You can find the DRIs and food sources for these minerals in Table 4-2.

Table 4-2	Daily Adult Mineral Needs, Upper Limits, and Food Sources		
Mineral	*Recommended Dietary Allowance or Adequate Intake*	*Tolerable Upper Level*	*Food Sources*
Calcium	Until age 50: 1,000 mg Women after age 50: 1,200 mg Men after age 70: 1,200 mg	2,000 mg to 2,500 mg (depending on age)	Low-fat dairy products, sardines and salmon with the bones, beans, broccoli, figs, and almonds
Phosphorus	700 mg	Until age 70: 4,000 mg After age 70: 3,000 mg	Lean meats, salmon, dairy products, and beans
Magnesium	Women: 310 mg to 320 mg Men: 400 mg to 420 mg	350 mg	Whole grains, leafy greens, dried beans and peas, potatoes, sunflower seeds, and dried figs
Sodium	Until age 50: 1,500 mg Ages 51–70: 1,300 mg After age 70: 1,200 mg	2,300 mg	Salt, bread, processed and snack foods, cheeses, lean meats, low-fat dairy products

Mineral	Recommended Dietary Allowance or Adequate Intake	Tolerable Upper Level	Food Sources
Potassium	4,700 mg	None	Vegetables and fruits (most green and orange produce, bananas, and potatoes), dried fruits, low-fat milk, fish, dried beans
Chloride	1,800 mg to 2,300 mg (depending on age)	3,600 mg	Salt
Iodine	150 mcg	1,100 mcg	Seafood, iodized salt, dairy, meat, poultry, eggs, and bread
Iron	Adults: 8 mg Menstruating women: 18 mg	45 mg	Lean meat, poultry, and fish; legumes; dried beans; dried fruits (figs, raisins, apricots, and peaches); and leafy greens
Zinc	Women: 8 mg Men: 11 mg	40 mg	Lean meats, shellfish, poultry, black beans, green peas, whole grains, and yogurt
Chromium	Women until age 51: 25 mcg Women after age 51: 20 mcg Men until age 51: 35 mcg Men after age 51: 30 mcg	Not determined	Whole grains, nuts, and cheeses
Selenium	55 mcg	400 mcg	Lean meats, shellfish, vegetables, and grains
Fluoride	Women: 3 mg Men: 4 mg	10 mg	Fluoridated drinking water
Copper	900 mcg	10,000 mcg	Seafood, nuts, and seeds

In the following sections, we offer a closer look at some of the specific things that the major and trace minerals do and the factors that affect your needs.

Calcium

This mineral is responsible for the development and maintenance of bones. It can also be released from the bones to maintain normal levels of calcium in the blood when intake or absorption is poor. If the body is constantly having to release calcium from the bones to maintain normal blood levels, osteoporosis may eventually develop. A dual-energy X-ray absorptiometry (DEXA) scan is a test that can be done to assess your risk of osteoporosis. Calcium in your blood is also important for nerve function and for maintaining normal blood pressure and muscle contraction, including your heartbeat.

Surgeries involving the gastrointestinal tract may make it difficult for you to absorb calcium. If you're on medications like Zometa or Xgeva to help prevent bone fractures due to metastatic disease, you need to make sure you get the RDA for calcium from food and/or supplements. This is also true if you have low estrogen levels because you've entered menopause naturally or as a result of cancer surgery or treatment.

Sometimes cancer that has spread to the bones can cause calcium to be released into the blood, causing *hypercalcemia* (high calcium levels in the blood). This is when medications like Zometa are used to help lower calcium levels. You don't need to avoid calcium in your diet, but hold off taking any calcium supplements until your calcium levels come down to normal. Also, if you normally take a vitamin D supplement, you should hold off on taking it as well, until your calcium levels come down to normal levels.

Phosphorus

This mineral is important for bone formation and maintenance. It is involved in acid-base balance, is part of the genetic material in our cells, and also helps release energy from food. Phosphorus also makes up part of the membranes that surround your cells. Being part of your DNA, you can see why this mineral is so essential.

If you end up not being able to eat for an extended period of time and are then fed intravenously, refeeding syndrome becomes a concern. *Refeeding syndrome* is a metabolic disturbance that occurs as a result of nutrition being reinstituted when you're in a malnourished state. In such cases, you'll be given more phosphorus in your intravenous (IV) feeding for a period of time.

Magnesium

This mineral is important for the function of hundreds of enzymes, and it affects the metabolism of potassium, calcium, and vitamin D. Magnesium also plays a role in the release of energy from food and facilitates muscle relaxation. As a result, magnesium levels can affect the heart and have an impact on blood pressure.

Numerous factors can affect you magnesium needs, including inadequate intake, vomiting, and diarrhea. Chemotherapy with Paraplatin or Erbitux may also contribute to low levels of magnesium in the blood. If you're on these treatments, your oncologist may monitor your blood levels and recommend an oral magnesium supplement or give you magnesium in IV fluid.

Sodium

This mineral is important for maintaining fluid and acid-base balance. It also plays a role in muscle contraction and nerve function. Because salt is the primary source of sodium in our diets, most people get more than they need. High salt intake in the Asian diet has been implicated in many studies as a potential cause of the high rates of stomach cancer in this population.

Factors that affect your sodium needs include vomiting and diarrhea. If you have these symptoms, you may need to consume a little more sodium than normal to prevent dehydration.

Potassium

Important for maintaining fluid and electrolyte balance, this mineral is also critical for maintaining your heartbeat, thereby helping to control your blood pressure. In addition, it helps with acid-base balance, and by consuming more potassium, you can counteract the effects of too much sodium.

Several factors can impact your potassium needs, including vomiting and diarrhea. The chemotherapeutic agent Paraplatin can also cause lower potassium levels in your blood. If you're taking diuretics to help get rid of excess fluid accumulation, some of these drugs will deplete the potassium in your blood. If you're found to have low levels, your oncologist may recommend that you take potassium pills or receive it intravenously.

Chloride

Like sodium and potassium, this mineral is essential for maintaining fluid and acid-base balance. Your body also needs this mineral to produce hydrochloric acid, which is the acid in your stomach that helps digest food. Finally, cells use chloride to obtain energy from the macronutrients you consume.

Factors that affect your chloride needs are losses from the gastrointestinal tract, such as occurs with vomiting, or if you have a tube draining your stomach contents following surgery. In such cases, you'll need more chloride, and in the latter case, chloride will be added to your IV if you have one.

Iodine

This mineral is needed for your body to make thyroxine, which is the hormone responsible for regulating your *basal metabolic rate,* or the amount of calories you need at rest to maintain your body's function. Although your thyroid gland contains the most iodine, it can also be found in other organs, including the salivary glands, pituitary glands, breasts, and ovaries.

If you're going to undergo radioactive iodine to treat thyroid cancer, you'll need to follow a low-iodine diet for a period of time before your treatment.

Iron

This mineral, which is a component of hemoglobin and myoglobin, has two sources: heme (from animals) and non-heme (from plants). Hemoglobin carries oxygen from the lungs to the rest of the body, whereas myoglobin carries and stores oxygen for use by your muscles. When you're iron deficient, you can develop iron-deficiency anemia and fatigue and have an increased susceptibility to infections. But if you get too much iron, it can be toxic.

Factors that affect your iron needs include poor oral intake of iron from foods, blood loss, and poor absorption of iron from the digestive tract. Vitamin C increases iron absorption, while caffeine, calcium, and fiber can decrease iron absorption. If you have a blood transfusion, that will replace iron. If your intake of iron is poor or if you have a history of surgery for pancreatic or gastric cancer or gastric bypass surgery, you may need an iron supplement. You should only take an iron supplement if recommended by your oncologist or another member of your healthcare team.

Because iron is an oxidant, you shouldn't take iron supplements without having the iron levels in your blood checked. If you've been told that your hemoglobin level is less than 11 gm/dL, you may want to talk with your oncologist about checking your iron levels. You also shouldn't take iron or large doses of vitamin C if you have an iron overload condition, such as hemochromatosis.

Zinc

This mineral enables your body to make enzymes that help your body process and digest carbohydrates and alcohol. It also helps your body make the "heme" in hemoglobin and assists with immune function, wound healing, and the sense of taste. A zinc deficiency can cause diarrhea, impaired immune function, and taste changes.

Factors that affect your zinc needs include poor intake or poor absorption, the latter of which can be a side effect of surgery involving the gastrointestinal tract. Also, losses of zinc from the gastrointestinal tract, such as through diarrhea, can increase zinc needs. Studies suggest that supplementations with 45 mg of zinc sulfate tablets or lozenges may help with taste changes that occur during cancer treatment, especially if intake is poor or losses are high, as with diarrhea. If taste changes persist while taking zinc, the cause of your taste changes is most likely not a deficiency of zinc but may be a side effect of your medications.

Zinc can be toxic in high amounts, decreasing copper absorption and causing changes to your heart. High amounts of zinc can also block iron absorption and impair immune function. Like most nutrients, it's critical not to get too little or too much zinc! Therefore, you should take a zinc supplement only under the direction of your oncologist or healthcare team.

Chromium

Your body needs this mineral to metabolize carbohydrates, fats, and protein. It also works with insulin to help control blood glucose levels. A chromium deficiency can result in *hyperglycemia* (high blood glucose levels). Although chromium can't correct diabetes, it can improve your blood glucose levels if your diet is low in chromium. Factors that may affect your chromium needs are poor intake of chromium-rich foods and a high intake of processed foods.

Selenium

Selenium works with vitamin E as an antioxidant. Some small studies have suggested that selenium may protect against some cancers, however large clinical trials using selenium supplements have not shown benefit.

Fluoride

This mineral stabilizes bones and helps prevent tooth decay. Although fluoride naturally exists in many water sources, many municipalities in the United States add fluoride to the drinking water. It's also included in many toothpastes as a preventive measure against cavities. There is controversy about the fluoridation of water and risk of some cancers, but a causal association hasn't been identified, whereas the benefit to bone and dental health has been established.

Copper

Copper is needed to make hemoglobin, collagen, elastic tissue, adrenalin, and nerve fibers. It also regulates blood pressure and heart rhythm and plays a role in the functioning of the prostate gland and oil glands. High zinc intake interferes with copper absorption.

Consuming more than 10 mg of copper daily can cause serious side effects, including liver damage, nausea, and muscle pain.

Manganese and molybdenum

Manganese is found in your body's glands and bones. It helps metabolize carbohydrates and synthesize fats, including cholesterol. It's also sometimes called the "brain mineral" because it's essential for normal brain and nerve function.

Molybdenum helps with many important biological processes, including waste processing in the kidneys and energy production in the cells.

Deficiencies in these trace minerals are rare, but like all minerals, they can become toxic if ingested in high amounts. If you're on long-term IV nutrition, known as *parenteral nutrition,* you need to be monitored to make sure you don't get too much of these nutrients.

Phytochemicals

Phytochemicals are naturally occurring compounds in fruits and vegetables. Although they aren't considered essential like macronutrients and micronutrients, they have important biological activity in the body. Scientists are still discovering phytochemicals in foods that may reduce the risk of developing some types of cancers. This is a huge task, because a single piece of fruit may have upwards of 100 phytochemicals, and these phytochemicals work together to produce their biological effects.

Many phytochemicals have antioxidant properties. Some of them have very long, hard-to-pronounce names, but you may have heard of some of them, like beta carotene and bioflavonoids. Certain phytochemicals are thought to help the body excrete *carcinogens* (cancer-causing substances) or encourage a process known as *apoptosis* (programmed cell death or suicide). Other phytochemicals, like indoles and lignans, may make estrogen less harmful. These are just a few examples, and as previously mentioned, scientists are still learning how the combination of phytochemicals in food reduces the risk of developing cancer and can potentially fight cancer.

Phytochemicals come from plant-based sources. Vegetables, fruits, legumes, beans, whole grains, herbs, and spices are all good sources of phytochemicals, and this nutrient is what gives vegetables and fruits their deep rich colors. So, richly colored produce like dark orange and deep green produce are good sources. Garlic, hot peppers, oregano, chives, leeks, and onions, which are great natural flavor enhancers, also serve as a good source of phytochemicals. The number of phytochemicals in plant-based food is one of the primary reasons that many nutritionists believe a plant-based diet is the best diet to follow for anyone concerned about cancer.

Fiber

Fiber is a complex carbohydrate that isn't broken down by digestive enzymes. As a result, it doesn't contribute significant calories or energy to your diet, but it's still important. Fiber keeps your digestive system in top working order, adds bulk to your stools, and helps lower cholesterol levels.

For some time, a high-fiber diet was thought to protect against cancer, particularly colon cancer, but studies have been inconclusive. This could be, however, because some of the trials assessing the impact of fiber haven't tested amounts that most nutrition experts would classify as being "high-fiber." Nevertheless, studies have shown fiber to provide a consistent protective effect with regard to cardiovascular health.

The types of fiber

Fiber is classified into two types, depending upon how well it dissolves in water:

- ✔ **Soluble:** Soluble fiber dissolves in water and can help slow the movement of food through the digestive tract, enabling you to feel full longer. It can also hold moisture in stools (making them easier to pass), lower cholesterol levels, stabilize blood glucose levels, and reduce inflammation and blood pressure. One type of soluble fiber is pectin, which is used to thicken jelly.

- ✔ **Insoluble:** Insoluble fiber, which doesn't dissolve in water, facilitates the passage of food through the gastrointestinal tract, making it easier to have a bowel movement. It also slows absorption of sugar into your bloodstream, stabilizing blood glucose levels.

Most foods have both types of fiber in them. Even psyllium, which is a used as a laxative, has both insoluble and soluble fiber. However, there are major food sources for each type of fiber. Wheat bran and the skins and seeds of vegetables and fruits are major sources of insoluble fiber. The flesh of apples and oranges, barley, oats, and oat bran are major sources of soluble fiber. We talk more about how to balance these types of fiber to manage side effects like constipation and diarrhea in Chapter 5.

How to get more fiber

Studies suggest that most people get about half the fiber they need on a daily basis. The AI for fiber is 21 g to 25 g per day for women, and 30 g to 38 g per day for men. The higher end of the range for both sexes is recommended up until age 50, while the lower end of the range is recommended after age 50. Because fiber can cause bloating, fiber intake should be gradually increased over several weeks, and you should consume plenty of water or other fluids. Most people need 8 or more cups of fluid daily.

Considering water safety issues

Choosing the safest source of drinking water requires you to do a little homework. Water can be contaminated with bacteria, which can increase your risk of an illness if your immune system is compromised during cancer treatments. Drinking water can also be contaminated with nitrates from fertilizers, which are known carcinogens. High levels of metals like lead can also be found in drinking water. If you get your drinking water from a public source, you can get a report on your drinking water from the website of the Environmental Protections Agency (EPA; www.epa.gov). The EPA is responsible for the safety of the public water supply.

Also, pay attention to water boil alerts where you live. Occasionally, bacteria will pass through filters and get into the water supply. This bacteria can be killed by boiling your water at a rolling boil for one minute. After boiling, refrigerate in a clean container and use within 72 hours. Keep in mind that boiling water does not eliminate other contaminants like nitrates or lead if they're in your water. A reverse osmosis water treatment unit can remove some bacteria and other contaminants, but there are no known units that can remove all levels of potential contaminants.

If you get your drinking water from a private source like a well, you should have your well tested every year for the aforementioned contaminants. Your local health department or the EPA can give you reputable information on testing your well. If you drink bottled water, you can find information on the safety of your water at www.nsf.org; NSF International is an organization that does voluntary testing and certification of bottled water. The Food and Drug Administration (FDA) regulates bottled water and has established Good Manufacturing Practice regulations for how bottled water is to be handled and bottled; this includes testing of the water for contaminants.

Here are a few ways you can add more fiber to your diet:

- ✔ Eat three servings of whole grains daily, like oats, brown rice, barley, and quinoa.
- ✔ Eat a vegetarian meal at least once a week, using beans for protein.
- ✔ Eat five to nine servings of whole vegetables and fruits daily.

There are times during cancer treatment when eating high amounts of fiber may not be a good idea. For example, if you had a colostomy or ileostomy, you'll need to follow a low-fiber diet for four to eight weeks to avoid having foods block or obstruct the new opening that has been made to enable the passage of stool. In these cases, fiber will need to be increased gradually after eight weeks based on tolerance. Particularly if you've had an ileostomy, fiber may continue to be adjusted to help form your stools. Soluble fiber may be better tolerated than insoluble fiber. You may also have to follow a low-fiber diet if you had an intestinal or bowel obstruction or blockage from your cancer, because this diet may prevent another obstruction.

Staying Hydrated

Water makes up about 60 percent of your body weight. If you don't drink enough water or other fluids, you may become dehydrated. Fever, vomiting, and diarrhea increase your water needs. Thirst is not always a good indicator of your hydration status — in fact, thirst is the first sign of dehydration. Dehydration can lead to a headache, fatigue, confusion, and an elevated heart rate. If you become severely dehydrated, you may need to go to the hospital for intravenous fluids.

Knowing what to drink and what not to drink

Water is the best beverage to drink to stay hydrated. Almost all foods contain water as well. Herbal teas, milk, and juices are also hydrating fluids. If you're experiencing vomiting or diarrhea, fluids with some sodium and/or potassium may help prevent dehydration. Broths and sports drinks may be helpful for this purpose. Look for broths with less sodium and sports drinks with less added sugars.

Alcohol is not a good source for hydration, and, in fact, is a diuretic, meaning it will contribute to water losses. It used to be thought that caffeine-containing beverages like coffee and regular tea were dehydrating, but newer studies suggest that they may not be as dehydrating as once thought. However, they may only provide about 75 percent of the hydration that an equal amount of water or other caffeine-free liquid would provide. In addition, non-caffeinated beverages may be better tolerated when you're not feeling well.

Getting enough liquids

The adequate intake for water set by the Institute of Medicine is 2.7 liters (91 ounces) for women and 3.7 liters (125 ounces) for men. This is a general guideline; needs will vary based on how much you weigh, how much you sweat, and if you have a fever or are losing fluid from vomiting or diarrhea.

One of the easiest ways to estimate your water requirements is to try to drink half of your body weight in ounces. For someone who weighs 150 pounds that would be 75 ounces or almost 9½ cups.

A good way to monitor your fluid intake during times when you don't feel well is to weigh yourself on a daily basis. For every pound lost, you're almost 2 cups of fluid behind. You'll need to add the amount you're behind to your normal intake to catch up.

Following the New American Plate and MyPlate

The New American Plate by the AICR (www.aicr.org) is a good example of how to design your meals to help you achieve and maintain a healthy body weight and transition to a more plant-based diet. Quite simply, it encourages you to visualize your plate when you plan and prepare meals. As you can see from the following illustration, your plate should be two-thirds full with vegetables, fruits, whole grains, or beans. Only one-third of the plate should be animal protein. This is pretty much the opposite of the typical American plate.

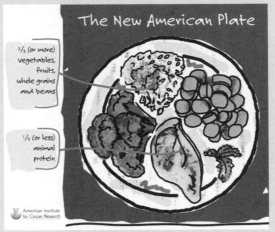

Illustration courtesy of the American Institute for Cancer Research

The U.S. Department of Agriculture (USDA) has adopted a similar eating guide through MyPlate, shown here. MyPlate has replaced the old Food Guide Pyramid as a means to help encourage a diet made up of grains, vegetables, and fruits, with much smaller amounts of protein.

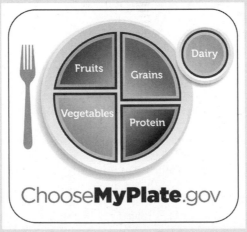

Illustration courtesy of the U.S. Department of Agriculture

One of the most effective ways to ensure adequate hydration is to use the new water bottles that are available almost everywhere these days and hold close to a liter of water. Start the day with a full bottle, and make sure you empty that bottle three to four times a day. Be sure to properly wash the bottle at the end of the day before using it again the next day. If these types of bottles aren't your cup of tea, try to get in the habit of drinking about a cup (or 8 ounces) of water or other hydrating fluids every hour while you're awake.

 Still having issues getting hydrated? Italian water ices and frozen fruit bars can be helpful for hydration. Fruits and vegetables are also good sources of hydration, containing anywhere from 60 percent to 95 percent water.

Concentrating on Calories

Calories are your body's source of energy or fuel. As we note at the beginning of this chapter, during cancer treatment, you need to get enough calories to maintain a healthy body weight (the quantity goal). After meeting this goal, you can move onto the quality goal, or improving your diet by increasing your intake of clean, nutrient-dense foods.

But what if you have excess weight to lose? If you're able to meet the quality goal and eat nutrient-dense foods and engage in physical activity, it may be okay to lose weight during treatment if it's something you feel strongly about or if it's recommended by your oncologist. But you'll want to make sure you do it under the close supervision of your oncologist or a registered dietitian and that you monitor your body composition to ensure that you're losing only excess body fat and not muscle mass. Don't let anyone convince you that losing weight because you're having difficulty eating during cancer treatment is okay. This can lead to complications from nutrient deficiencies and must be addressed right away.

In this section, we take a closer look at calories, including how to recognize empty calories and how to determine your caloric needs.

Recognizing empty calories

Empty calories don't look anything like a vegetable or fruit, but they come from foods that provide calories without providing other important nutrients, like protein, vitamins, minerals, and phytochemicals. Empty-calorie foods still require vitamins to be metabolized, so eating a diet full of empty calories can actually deplete your body's vitamin levels.

Monitoring your diet with a food log

Many people can't remember what they had for breakfast by the time lunch comes around. For this reason, it's often hard to know at the end of the day if you met your nutrition goals. If you're underweight, did you eat enough calories to gain weight? If your weight is stable, did you eat enough calories to maintain your weight? If you're overweight, did you eat the right amount of calories to help you lose weight? And regardless of what you weigh, did you eat enough vegetables and fruits?

Most studies of people who need to lose weight show that keeping a food log is critical to success. This isn't surprising. After all, a food log makes you conscious of what you're eating, while helping you monitor your progress toward your nutrition goals. For instance, you'll be able to clearly see that you still need two servings of vegetables for dinner to reach the ideal quota of five to nine servings of produce.

A good food log requires you to record what you eat, the portion, and how you feel at the time. For example, are you hungry, under stress, or feeling nauseated? Logging all this information can help you see favorable and unfavorable patterns in your eating, while also helping you identify foods that may exacerbate the side effects of certain treatments.

A food log can be done the old-fashioned way — using a pen and notebook — or you can go the high-tech route and use one of the many food diary or food log apps available today. Some examples include My Fitness Pal (www.myfitnesspal.com), Weight Watchers (www.weightwatchers.com), and SparkPeople (www.sparkpeople.com), but there are many others. If you want to go with an electronic food journal, be sure to research the options, because each service has different features and some are free, whereas others may have a one-time or monthly charge.

To determine if a food is an empty-calorie food, read food labels. We provide in-depth information on how to do this in Chapter 7, but if you see added sugars among the first few ingredients or if you can't pronounce most of the ingredients, you may have a food full of empty calories and chemicals. Also, if the food doesn't provide at least 10 percent of the daily value for protein or fiber or contain at least one vitamin or mineral, you're probably choosing a source of empty calories. Common examples of such foods and beverages include sodas, candies, cakes, cookies, and chips, which are items commonly referred to as *junk food*.

Determining your caloric needs

Your weight is a good indicator of whether you're meeting your caloric needs. If you're losing weight, you need more calories, and if you're gaining weight, you need fewer calories, unless this loss or gain is desired. To determine what your caloric needs are based on your current weight, use the following formulas:

✔ If you're trying to maintain your weight, multiply your weight in pounds by 14.

✔ If you're trying to lose weight, multiply your weight in pounds by 9 to 11.

✔ If you're trying to gain weight, multiply your weight in pounds by 16 to 18.

Based on the number you get, you can adjust your caloric intake accordingly. If you're dealing with cancer-related weight loss, for instance, you'll want to increase the amount of calories you're consuming. If you're trying to lose weight, you may need to decrease by a couple hundred calories at a time until you see results. To help determine your specific caloric needs, ask to speak with the registered dietitian at your cancer center or ask to be referred to a registered dietitian in your community.

Keeping an Eye on Your Body Composition

At a very basic level, your body is composed of lean body mass and fat. Lean body mass includes muscle, organ tissue, fluid, and bone, all of which are required to sustain life. A certain amount of fat is needed to protect your organs and to keep you warm, but many people have more fat than they need to be healthy. Maintaining a healthy body composition is important to help minimize side effects and maintain quality of life during cancer treatment. In addition, achieving and maintaining a healthy body weight is one of the most important things a cancer survivor can do to reduce the risk of a cancer recurrence.

In this section, we look at a few body composition measures, including weight, body mass index, body fat percentage, and blood work. Each of these measures has certain limitations, which we review. Using multiple measures generally provides a more accurate representation of your body composition than relying on just one.

Weight

During cancer treatment, you should be weighed on a calibrated scale every time you go in for treatment. As little as a 5 percent loss of body weight has been associated with increased side effects and a less desirable quality of life during treatment. In a 140-pound person, that's a 7-pound weight loss. If you're losing weight because you're having difficulty eating, ask for help as soon as possible. If you don't already have a registered dietitian, ask to see or be referred to one.

If you're overweight or obese, ask your oncologist if it's okay for you to lose small amounts of weight (no more than 2 pounds per week). If your oncologist approves, make sure you're eating healthy and staying active. You may also want to have your body composition monitored to ensure that you're losing extra fat and not lean body mass. A regular scale won't be able to give you any indication of this, so if you don't already have one, you may want to invest in a scale that gives you an estimate of your body fat. These scales are a little more expensive, but they can help you monitor what kind of weight you're losing. Although not perfect, they're reported to be pretty accurate as long as you're not dehydrated or overhydrated when weighing yourself. You'll also want to weigh yourself roughly the same time of the day, because weight fluctuates throughout the day, sometimes by as much as 5 pounds. So, by weighing yourself at the same time every time you check your weight, you'll get a more accurate picture of where you stand.

Body mass index

Body mass index (BMI) defines weight in relation to height. It's a crude estimate of the amount of body fat you have. BMI is used as an indicator of overweight or obesity status. You can find a BMI calculator at `www.nhl bisupport.com/bmi`. A normal BMI is between 18.5 and 24.9. A BMI below 18.5 may be an indicator of malnutrition, whereas a BMI between 25 and 29.9 puts you in the overweight category and a BMI of 30 or more puts you in the obese category. Both low and high BMIs have been associated with an increased risk of developing many cancers.

A drawback of BMI is that it can't take muscle mass into consideration. For example, two people may weigh 170 pounds and be the same height, but one person may be very muscular and the other person may be flabby. Even though they both have the same BMI, the muscular person has a much lower level of body fat. Still, for most people, BMI serves as a good starting point, and if you find that you have a low BMI or a BMI that puts you in the overweight or obese category, you should have your body composition checked to further evaluate your health risks.

Body fat percentage

Knowing your *body fat percentage* (the percentage of your total body weight that is made up of fat) is important. Scientists used to think that body fat protected the organs, kept people warm, and didn't do much else. Today we now know that fat acts like a hormone pump, increasing the amount of hormones like estrogen, insulin, and insulin-like growth factor in the blood. These hormones can promote the growth of abnormal cells and inhibit a process known as *apoptosis,* which tells bad cells to die when they should. This is the process by which being overweight or obese may increase the risk of many cancers.

Numerous methods can be used to assess your body fat percentage. Some can be done at home. For example, you can use a scale that assesses body fat or a fat caliper to perform skinfold tests, but the latter can be challenging to perform and has a high rate of user error, so it isn't recommended. Other methods require special and sometimes expensive equipment, such as ultrasonography, DEXA, and underwater weighing, none of which is likely to be available to you. If you really want to know your body fat percentage, talk to your oncologist about it to get some recommendations. You can also consider seeking an evaluation at a local health club, which may have calipers or a bioelectrical impedance unit or scale available, or find a registered dietitian who is able to do these assessments or refer you to someone who can.

If you're a male with more than 20 percent body fat or a female with more than 30 percent body fat, you have more body fat than is considered healthy. If you're undergoing cancer treatment, talk with your oncologist about whether it's safe for you to lose weight during treatment. If you're finished with cancer treatment, talk with your primary-care physician about a weight-loss program.

Blood work

Your oncologist will most likely do quite a bit of blood work to monitor your response to cancer treatment. A couple of these tests may shed some light on your body composition and nutritional status, including your blood urea nitrogen (BUN) and serum albumin levels. If your BUN is high, you may be underhydrated and need more fluid to maintain a normal percentage of your weight as water. As for your serum albumin, it can be used as a very crude indicator of your body's protein status. If your serum albumin is low, it could mean a lot of things because it's not specific to protein intake, but it could also be an indication that you need to eat more protein.

Being Smart about Supplements

Whole foods are generally the best way for you to meet your nutrient needs. Studies that try to use dietary supplements to reproduce the beneficial effects observed from nutrients contained in foods often don't produce the same effects. It's also very difficult to reach toxic levels of nutrients through food sources. That said, during cancer treatment, there may be times when supplements are needed.

Supplement contamination

You may be wondering how dietary supplements can be contaminated. Well, the Dietary Supplement Health and Education Act (DSHEA) of 1994 created new regulation for the safety of dietary supplements, including vitamins, minerals, herbs, and amino acids. This act made it so that supplements were not regulated the same as foods and pharmaceuticals. After the passage of this act, manufacturers of supplements were responsible for the safety of their product(s) and didn't have to prove to the FDA that they were safe before going to market. For many years, it has been "buyer beware" when it comes to supplements.

After many years of adverse reports about dietary supplements, in 2007 the FDA published Current Good Manufacturing Practices (CGMPs) to be followed by manufacturers to try to ensure safety and quality of supplements. The manufacturer is still responsible for making sure that what's on the label of a supplement is what's in the bottle and that it's free of unwanted contaminants. But because the FDA has limited resources, it doesn't test supplements for quality and purity. Some companies will test products that are sent to them or independently test products off of shelves. Not surprisingly, these companies have found that what's on the label isn't always what's in the bottle.

If you're considering taking dietary supplements, in addition to getting professional advice, do your homework. Some companies do independent testing and will test products sent to them for quality. ConsumerLab.com (www.consumerlab.com) offers reviews of supplements and an encyclopedia that reviews studies that have been done on various supplements. NSF International (www.nsf.org) and U.S. Pharmacopeial Convention (www.usp.org) also test products for quality. Finally, the FDA provides tips for making informed decisions, as well as warnings and safety information, including reporting on adverse effects from supplements; this information can be found at www.fda.gov/food/dietary supplements.

It's up to your oncologist to determine whether you should be taking supplements. Studies have shown that a high percentage of people with cancer use supplements during cancer treatment, but in some cases, it's done without the oncologist or healthcare team knowing about it, which can be a dangerous practice. Dietary supplements can be expensive, their quality can be questionable, and they can interact with medications, reducing the efficacy of cancer treatments.

In this section, we take a closer look at supplements, including why most supplements should be avoided. We also examine cases in which they may be beneficial. Even if we cover a scenario that applies to you, it's important to first discuss any supplementation with your oncologist.

Why you should avoid most supplements

Many supplements are metabolized by the same pathways as cancer drugs. Therefore, they can interact with these drugs, interfering with treatments like chemotherapy, anesthesia during surgery, and even radiation therapy. Much more research is needed to understand these interactions, but because this risk exists, you shouldn't use them without the supervision of your oncologist. Unfortunately, we often only learn about interactions after someone has experienced an adverse response after taking a supplement.

There is promise that some supplements may help make cancer treatments more effective and minimize the side effects of treatment, but many studies are still needed. In addition, quality control is a problem in the supplement industry. Dietary supplements have been removed from the market as a result of being contaminated with other drugs, such as blood thinners and antidepressants (see the nearby sidebar).

Supplements worth discussing with your oncologist

We cover a lot in this chapter about nutrient needs and individual circumstances that may lead to the need for supplementation. There are a few supplements worth discussing with your oncologist that may help you maintain your nutritional status and immune health during treatment. Here are the ones to consider:

- **Eicosapentaenoic acid (EPA):** This is a fatty acid found in cold-water fish. Some studies suggest a dose of 1,500 mg per day may help with weight and muscle maintenance, while also strengthening your immune system.

- **Vitamin D:** Like EPA, vitamin D is important for immune function. Many people do not get enough for good bone health.

- **Calcium:** If you don't consume several servings of the food sources of calcium that we list in Table 4-2, earlier in this chapter, supplementation to meet the RDA may be beneficial.

- **Multivitamin/mineral and/or B-complex supplement:** If you're not eating well and relying more on comfort foods than on nutrient-dense foods, you may need these supplements to help cover your basic micronutrient needs and help release energy from the foods you're eating so that your body doesn't deplete your vitamin stores. Try to find supplements that do *not* contain more than 100 percent of the DRI, unless directed by your physician or healthcare team.

Chapter 5

Dealing with Side Effects That Impact Nutrition

In This Chapter
▶ Understanding how side effects impact nutrition
▶ Seeing how food can ease side effects
▶ Coping when eating is a challenge

Cancer treatment can affect people in different ways, but a common concern is that it will impact the ability to eat and thereby reduce quality of life. Despite cancer treatments becoming increasingly targeted, the risk of side effects hasn't been eliminated. Now, this doesn't mean side effects are inevitable, and it's highly unlikely that you'll experience every side effect you're ever informed of, but you may at times contend with symptoms that impede your ability to eat. During these times, you may think that achieving the quantity and quality nutrition goals we discuss in Chapter 4 are out of reach. But malnutrition and its associated risks, such as impaired immunity and poorer outcomes, aren't inevitable. You can do many things during treatment to help your body get the nutrients it needs.

In this chapter, you get a general overview of how side effects can impact your ability to take in and use nutrients properly. We examine foods that can worsen symptoms and food strategies that can ease side effects and improve nutrient intake. The side effects we look at include fatigue, nausea, diarrhea, constipation, sore mouth or throat, and taste and smell changes, because these are the most common symptoms that impede the ability to get enough nourishment.

Anorexia (loss of appetite) is another common side effect that can lead to malnutrition, but we don't cover it in this chapter. If this is the main symptom you're struggling with, turn to Chapter 19 for tips on how you can revive your appetite.

Throughout this chapter, you find many tips that you can use to guide your eating so that you can meet your quantity and quality goals. Some of the recommendations are beneficial for several side effects, so use as many of the tips as possible to find what works for you. You can even try them for side effects we don't specifically cover if you think it'll help.

How Side Effects Can Affect Nutrition

Cancer treatments often come with a long list of potential side effects. These effects may make it challenging to eat, alter your body's ability to digest and use nutrients properly, and/or affect your body's nutrient needs. Difficulty taking in nutrients is the most prevalent problem, because almost all symptoms can make it hard to consume nutrients. When you have an upset stomach or a sore mouth or throat, or when food doesn't taste right, eating is no longer enjoyable and you may not feel like eating.

There are also the potential digestive challenges caused by treatments. Chemotherapy and radiation treatments, for instance, can cause lactose intolerance, temporarily impairing your ability to digest milk products. This can lead to various gastrointestinal issues, including gas, bloating, and diarrhea. If you experience diarrhea, there's a good chance you'll absorb less water, electrolytes like sodium and potassium, and other nutrients like zinc. This can lead to dehydration and electrolyte imbalances; proper electrolyte levels are essential for maintaining normal cellular function, muscle action, and blood chemistry. So, as you can see, there's a cascade of effects.

How Food Can Ease Certain Side Effects

As you read this chapter, you may notice a common theme or two: Some foods will aggravate many of the side effects that can be experienced during cancer treatment, while others can ease many of the side effects. For example, foods containing or prepared with a high amount of fat can be difficult to digest or absorb, making an upset stomach, nausea, and diarrhea worse. On the other hand, low-fat, high-protein foods can help alleviate nausea and enable you to maintain lean muscle mass and strength.

We hope that as you read this chapter, you come to appreciate that food can be used as medicine to help relieve side effects. For example, ginger can be used to settle an upset stomach. Honey may help heal a sore mouth or throat. *Glutamine* (an amino acid found in high-protein foods) and *probiotics* (the healthy bacteria in yogurt and kefir) may help nourish the body and reduce side effects that affect the digestive tract. These are just a few examples of how food can help ease side effects. The following section is filled with suggestions on how to modify or add foods to your diet when facing a specific nutrient hindrance.

What to Do When Eating Is a Challenge

When symptoms make it difficult to eat, you may need to focus more on the quantity nutrition goal outlined in Chapter 4 to ensure you get enough calories, protein, vitamins, minerals, and fluid to maintain your nutritional status and immune function. But this doesn't mean the quality goal just goes out the window. Eating high-quality, clean foods may also help ease side effects so you can meet your quantity goal. See Chapter 6 for more on clean eating. So, if you can tolerate these foods, you should give them preferential treatment.

In addition, try to avoid foods that may aggravate your symptoms and increase your intake of foods that may ease your symptoms. We outline these foods in the following sections, but you may find that your experiences differ slightly. To get a better sense of which foods sit well with you and which don't, consider logging all the foods you eat in a food journal and recording how they make you feel. Many nutrition apps have this functionality built in. (See Chapter 4 for more information and some apps you can consider.)

Whatever you do, don't assume that side effects are par for the course and that you should just accept them. Always discuss the side effects you're experiencing with your healthcare team. Your oncologist can work with you to personalize an intervention to reduce side effects, such as by reducing a drug dosage, trying another drug regimen, or prescribing a medication to help manage the symptoms.

Never discontinue a treatment or try another regimen without consulting your oncologist, because this can have disastrous consequences.

Now, let's see how you can use nutrition to combat some of the most commonly reported side effects of treatment.

When you have nausea or vomiting

When cancer patients are portrayed on TV and in the movies, they're often retching into a toilet bowl. Although this doesn't happen to everyone, radiation therapy to the abdomen and many chemotherapies can cause nausea, vomiting, and/or an upset stomach, which can make eating a challenge. As a result, you may end up eating and drinking less, which may lead to malnutrition and/or dehydration. If you become dehydrated from inadequate fluid and electrolyte intake, your nausea may worsen. Sometimes just having an empty stomach can increase the severity of nausea.

Fortunately, many medications can help manage nausea and vomiting; these are referred to as *anti-nausea* and *antiemetic* drugs, respectively. In addition, there are foods that you can eat to help maintain your nutritional status and hydration while avoiding aggravating your stomach. There are also foods you may want to avoid, such as high-fat foods, which take longer to leave your stomach and can worsen nausea as a result.

Here are some suggestions for managing nausea and vomiting:

- ✔ **Be sure your oncologist is aware that you're nauseated and take any medications for nausea as prescribed.** Don't wait until you're experiencing nausea to take medications that have been prescribed for it. Take these medications as prescribed to try to prevent nausea until you're able to resume your normal diet. If you continue to experience nausea despite taking your anti-nausea medication, contact your oncologist.

- ✔ **Stay well hydrated.** Even if you can't tolerate much solid food, make sure you drink or even sip fluids throughout the day to prevent dehydration. Typically, clear liquids are better tolerated initially. Water is the fluid of choice. Also, try juices, *fruit juice spritzers* (juice with a little seltzer), herbal teas, broths, fruit sorbets, and frozen fruit bars. (If you find that you can tolerate frozen fruit bars well, check out our Triple Antioxidant Yogurt Popsicles in Chapter 15.) When you can tolerate clear liquids, try adding some bland foods based on your tolerance.

- ✔ **Eat small, frequent, bland meals.** Try to avoid an empty stomach, which can make nausea worse. Start the day with some salty crackers or pretzels kept at your bedside table. Other foods that are generally well tolerated are fruit, mashed potatoes, oatmeal, Cream of Wheat, dry toast, and rice. Cottage cheese, yogurt, kefir, tofu, eggs, and low-fat cheese may also work.

- ✔ **Pay attention to what you eat before your treatment.** Research has suggested that the meal you eat before treatment may determine whether you experience nausea. Consume *bland foods* about two hours before treatment. The foods listed in the preceding bullet point would work well.

- ✔ **Try to get 20 to 30 g of protein at each meal.** Some studies suggest that protein, in addition to ginger (discussed in the next bullet point), may help with nausea. This amount of protein taken several times a day has also been shown to help maintain muscle mass, which is critical during cancer treatment. A protein drink, a three-egg omelet, a 3-ounce chicken breast, ¾ cup of cottage cheese, or a smoothie made with 8 ounces of low-fat milk and 8 ounces of yogurt or kefir can help you achieve this goal.

✔ **Try ginger.** Some research suggests that the active compounds in ginger may have anti-nausea properties and may help food move through the digestive tract faster, further alleviating nausea. To reap the benefits of ginger, try drinking an ounce of a natural ginger ale like Ginger Brew, Ginger Beer, or Fresh Ginger before your meals. Because many mass-market ginger ales don't actually contain ginger, be sure to carefully read labels before buying. Other ways to consume ginger include ginger snaps, ginger tea, crystallized ginger, and ginger chews or candies. One company that specializes in ginger products is Reed's (www.reedsinc.com).

High intake of ginger can interact with blood-thinning medications. If you're taking a blood thinner, make sure your doctor is okay with your using ginger.

✔ **Drink liquids between meals.** Sometimes having too much liquid in your stomach in addition to food can worsen nausea. Try drinking your liquids an hour or two before and after meals.

✔ **Avoid your favorite foods.** You or your loved ones may be tempted to prepare your favorite foods to try to provide comfort during times when eating is a challenge. However, if you try to eat your favorite foods when you're experiencing nausea, you may develop an aversion to these foods.

✔ **Limit or avoid spicy, acidic, and caffeinated foods and beverages.** These foods can further irritate your stomach, making nausea worse.

✔ **Limit or avoid greasy, fried, or high-fat foods.** High-fat foods or meals take longer to leave your stomach than low-fat foods do. Having food in your stomach too long can make nausea worse. Avoid obviously high-fat foods like bacon, sausage, full-fat dairy products, doughnuts or other pastries, or any greasy foods.

✔ **Try an acupressure wristband.** Some studies suggest that acupressure wristbands may help alleviate nausea from chemotherapy, radiation, or surgery in some people. These bands work by putting pressure on the acupressure point on the wrist that is used for controlling nausea. The bands are available at most drugstores, are inexpensive, and come with instructions for use. Sea Bands is a common brand that you can look for (www.sea-band.com). The bands should be used in combination with anti-nausea medication prescribed by your oncologist.

✔ **Talk with your doctor about acupuncture.** Some studies show that acupuncture may help with nausea from chemotherapy or surgery. Your doctor may be able to refer you to a licensed acupuncturist.

✔ **Create a relaxing eating atmosphere.** Stress can affect the digestive tract, causing or worsening nausea. Try as many stress management techniques as needed to relax before and after your meals. Deep breathing or a light walk may be helpful. Some people find that playing their favorite music during meals helps. You can also ask a loved one to give you a little massage or try massaging an acupressure point yourself to relieve nausea. One area to target is the soft, fleshy area between your thumb and forefinger.

✔ **Try cold or cool foods.** If you're experiencing nausea, just the smell of food may turn your stomach. During these times, it's okay to make a meal out of a cold sandwich, stuffed tomato, or fruit or vegetable plate with a protein source. If a cold meal isn't an option, this may be a good time to ask someone to do the food preparation for you so you don't have to smell the food while it's cooking.

When your stomach is upset

Nausea and vomiting aren't the only stomach issues caused by cancer treatments. You may also develop indigestion, heartburn, and even gas. If you're experiencing such effects, in addition to taking any medication as prescribed, the following changes to your diet and lifestyle can help manage these symptoms and prevent pain or discomfort:

✔ **Avoid irritants to prevent heartburn.** Irritants will make heartburn symptoms worse. Tobacco and alcohol are the worst offenders; caffeine is also high on the list. Certain foods should also be avoided, including acidic ones like tomato products and citrus products, because they can cause heartburn. Other foods may make it easier for acid to "back up" from your stomach into your esophagus; avoid chocolate and mint for these reasons.

✔ **Reduce gas by limiting or avoiding gas-forming foods.** Many normally desirable foods, including high-fiber fruits and vegetables, can cause gas and pain. Raw salads, raw vegetables, the cabbage family of vegetables, and beans may cause more gas to be produced in your digestive tract. Because these foods are healthy, try adding them back into your diet one at a time when you feel better. Other gas-forming foods to avoid include carbonated beverages and chewing gum. Also, avoid sipping any beverages with straws.

✔ **Limit or avoid high-fat foods to prevent heartburn.** Fatty foods take longer to leave your stomach than other foods, which can cause heartburn. Stay away from fried foods, doughnuts and pastries, fatty meats, and full-fat dairy products.

✔ **Limit or avoid sugar alcohols to prevent gas and bloating.** Sugar alcohols, including sorbitol, mannitol, xylitol, and maltitol, are used to sweeten foods as an alternative to sugar. These sweeteners can contribute to bloating and stomach discomfort.

✔ **Elevate the head of your bed and don't lie down right after eating to prevent heartburn.** This tip relates to the simple rule of gravity. By elevating the head of your bed and avoiding reclining after eating, it's harder for acid to back up into your esophagus and cause heartburn.

✔ **Ask your doctor about over-the-counter remedies.** Over-the-counter antacids like Tums or Rolaids may be helpful for heartburn. These contain calcium, which helps neutralize stomach acid. Like any other nutrient, too much calcium can be harmful, so you shouldn't use more than the recommended dosage. Another potentially beneficial over-the-counter drug is Gas-X, which contains simethicone, a gas-reducing agent. Also, Beano (an enzyme-based dietary supplement) may help when eating gas-forming foods. Again, even though these products don't require a prescription, you should use them only under medical supervision to reduce the risk of introducing new side effects from a drug interaction.

When you have a sore mouth or throat

Chemotherapy and radiation kill rapidly dividing cells like cancer cells, but they also affect the rapidly dividing cells lining your digestive tract, including those lining your mouth and throat. For this reason, you may experience a sore mouth or throat during cancer treatment, which can make eating exceedingly uncomfortable. Some foods and liquids may increase discomfort by irritating your mouth or throat, whereas others may even be soothing and enable you to meet your quantity goal.

When dealing with a sore mouth or throat, be sure to take any medications that have been prescribed to treat this. In addition, try the following nutrition tips to maintain your nutritional intake and ensure adequate hydration:

✔ **Drink smoothies and/or high-calorie, high-protein liquid supplement drinks.** Liquids are likely to be less irritating to the lining of your mouth or throat than solid foods, and you may even find them soothing. Drinkable yogurt or kefir may feel silky going down, and the healthy bacteria they contain may help you heal. Homemade smoothies and shakes also work well. Try the Pomegranate Antioxidant Smoothie recipe in Chapter 10.

Ready-to-drink liquid supplements taken several times a day can help you meet your nutritional needs. Orgain, which is made with organic ingredients, is one of the cleanest meal replacements on the market. It can be found at some drugstores and health-food stores, or you can order it online through various retailers, including Amazon. Other options include Carnation Instant Breakfast drinks, Ensure, Boost,

Muscle Milk, and even some supplemental drinks intended for weight loss, like Slim-Fast shakes. If you drink enough to meet your caloric needs, you won't lose weight, regardless of a drink's intended purpose.

✔ **Eat soft, bland foods.** If liquids are well tolerated, try moving on to soft, bland foods, which are less likely to irritate the lining of your mouth or throat than coarse, acidic, or spicy foods. Focus on soft, high-protein foods like tuna, chicken, eggs, refried beans, and cottage cheese.

✔ **Avoid irritants.** Tobacco, alcohol, and foods and beverages that are hot, spicy, acidic, or hard/coarse (like bread and crackers) will most likely increase pain. Even healthy foods like fruits and fruit juices, because of their acidity, will often increase pain. Try to avoid these foods until your mouth and throat are healed.

✔ **Increase the nutrient density of what you can eat and drink.** Add protein powders or nonfat dry milk to some of the soft, bland foods mentioned earlier. Also, small amounts of healthy fats and oils like canola oil or olive oil, avocado, or soft margarine or butter can be added to foods. Even a little pure maple syrup may be tolerated. Cooked cereals like Cream of Wheat, Cream of Rice, and oatmeal work well with some of these additions.

✔ **Try honey.** Several studies have shown that honey may help reduce pain and speed healing of a sore mouth or throat, especially during radiation therapy, but it may also be worth trying honey if you experience this side effect from chemotherapy. One tablespoon three or four times daily during treatment is generally recommended. For maximum benefit, honey should be taken 15 minutes before treatment, 15 minutes after treatment, and 6 hours after treatment. While using honey, just be sure to practice good oral hygiene (see the next bullet) to prevent cavities. If you have diabetes or high blood glucose, you'll need to count the carbohydrate in honey toward your daily allowance.

✔ **Maintain good oral hygiene.** When you have sores in your mouth or throat, your risk of infection is increased. Good oral hygiene can help prevent an infection and may promote healing. Rinse your mouth before and after meals with some saltwater. Don't use mouthwash containing alcohol. Also, be sure to use a toothbrush with very soft bristles to brush your teeth. Try making a homemade rinse by mixing 4 cups water, 1 teaspoon salt, and 1 teaspoon baking soda. Sip, swish, and spit after every meal. Mix daily.

✔ **Ask your oncologist about using glutamine.** Glutamine is a nonessential amino acid that may become essential during a stressful illness, because the body uses it in higher-than-normal amounts for a variety of functions. Glutamine is also the preferred fuel of the cells lining your digestive tract, including your mouth and throat. Some studies suggest swishing your mouth with and swallowing a glutamine mixture may help with pain and healing. Glutamine is available over the counter. It's usually taken in doses of 10 g three times a day or 15 g twice a day. It can be mixed with smoothies or fruit juices and nectars. The online resource ConsumerLab.com (www.consumerlab.com) can help you find brands of glutamine that have passed quality testing.

There are some concerns that glutamine supplements may interact with some chemotherapies. For this reason, it should only be used if recommended and supervised by your oncologist.

✔ **Try sucking on frozen fruit and ice chips.** Sucking on frozen fruit and ice chips may help numb your mouth or throat, relieving pain or discomfort so you can eat. In addition, sucking on ice chips during chemotherapy infusion has been shown to reduce the likelihood of a sore mouth, particularly with the chemotherapy agent 5-fluorouracil (5-FU).

There are also medications that can help with a sore mouth or throat, so seek help from your healthcare team if you need it.

When food doesn't taste right

Cancer treatments can also cause changes to the way you taste and smell foods, making the thought of eating less appealing. Some foods may not have any flavor, whereas other foods may start to taste bitter or even metallic. In addition, sweet foods may taste significantly sweeter than usual. Other foods may become completely intolerable during treatment. This has sometimes been reported with meat and coffee.

When food doesn't taste right, you'll really need to think of eating as essential to your treatment. Just as you wouldn't miss a dose of your prescribed medications, you shouldn't miss a meal. But don't worry, you won't be struggling with this for the rest of your life. Taste usually returns sometime after treatment ends, so this is by no means a permanent effect. But until that happens, try the following to ensure adequate nutrition:

✔ **Avoid your favorite foods if they don't taste right.** You know what your favorite foods taste like, which is why you like them so much. If your taste buds are off, your favorite foods may not be enjoyable, which may turn you off from eating. You may also develop an aversion to your favorite foods, which won't go away after you're done with treatment and your sense of taste is restored.

✔ **Try new foods and flavors.** Trying new foods may be a way to add some excitement to your eating. In addition, if you don't have an expectation of what a food is supposed to taste or smell like, it's hard for it to taste or smell "off," right? Because some foods may taste almost flavorless to you, consider amplifying their flavors by adding lots of herbs, spices, sauces, and marinades. Citrus and tomato flavors may work well, too, as long as you don't have a sore mouth or throat. Try anything with a tomato-based sauce, such as a chili. Many people report that very spicy Italian or Mexican foods work well.

✔ **Use mouthwash or brush your teeth before meals.** This may help eliminate a bad taste in your mouth, which can make food taste bad or "off." Try the rinse recommended in the preceding section or Biotene or other dry-mouth products.

✔ **Expand and alter your protein sources.** Many times meat will not taste right or it may become unappealing during treatment. Try more poultry, fish, eggs, and vegetarian sources of protein, such as tofu and beans. If your mouth is not sore, fruit- or tomato-based marinades may make your protein foods taste better. Even a soy sauce or teriyaki marinade may go a long way.

✔ **Ask your doctor about zinc supplementation.** Some studies suggest that zinc sulfate taken during radiation therapy to the head and neck may help the sense of taste return sooner after the end of treatment. Also, if you've been experiencing diarrhea, you may lose a lot of zinc in your stool, which can lead to a deficiency that can make taste changes worse. If this is the case, supplementing with 45 mg of zinc may help your sense of taste return sooner.

Too much zinc is not a good thing (see Chapter 4). Prolonged use of zinc is not recommended, and you should take this supplement only under medical supervision.

When food doesn't smell right

How you sense flavors is tied to your sense of taste and smell. So, when cancer treatment affects your sense of smell, foods may not taste right and become unappealing. You may also smell things differently from how you remember them, leading to food aversions. When food stops smelling right, the following recommendations may help:

✔ **Focus on cold or cool foods.** Sometimes just the smell of food will cause a food aversion. Because food odors generally become more pronounced when they're cooked, you may want to avoid eating hot meals. Cold fare during these times is perfectly acceptable, regardless of the time of the day. Eat a sandwich or tomato stuffed with chicken, tuna, or egg salad. A fruit plate with yogurt or cottage cheese, or a raw vegetable plate with a bean dip is also a good choice. You can also drink your meals. Smoothies or meal-replacement shakes are good choices, and consuming them through a covered glass or a straw prevents your nostrils from getting a whiff of what's in your glass.

When we say you should focus on eating cold foods, we aren't directing you to eat foods that have been left out on the kitchen counter for several hours to cool. This is a dangerous practice that could increase your risk of a foodborne illness. You can store foods in the refrigerator to allow them to cool.

✔ **Ask someone else to cook for you.** If you don't have to smell the food while it's cooking, you may be able to tolerate hot foods. See if someone else is willing to prepare a hot meal for you and bring it to you ready to eat. Most likely, your loved ones will be happy to help out.

When you're too tired to eat

One of the most common symptoms experienced by people being treated for cancer is fatigue. If you're tired, you may not feel like grocery shopping or preparing meals or snacks, which may lead you to eat less than normal.

The calories from food are energy, so if you eat less, you'll have less energy and feel more tired. A vicious cycle may develop where the symptom of feeling tired leads to poor nutritional intake, making your fatigue worse.

The following tips are aimed at helping you meet your quantity goal without further compromising your quality goal when you're too tired to eat:

✔ **Drink your meals.** This may be a time to drink your meals by consuming smoothies and high-calorie, high-protein liquid nutritional supplements. If you're very tired, the easiest way to do this is to use ready-made liquid nutritional supplements. When you have a little more energy, you can make your own smoothies and shakes. Numerous liquid supplements are available, including Orgain, Carnation Instant Breakfast drinks, Muscle Milk, Ensure, Boost, and even Slim-Fast. For more information on these, see the smoothies recommendation under "When you have a sore mouth or throat," earlier in this chapter.

✔ **Snack on healthy foods throughout the day.** Some of the snack foods mentioned in Chapter 19 for helping with appetite can also be useful when you're too tired to eat. Guacamole or hummus with baked corn chips, trail mix, and almond or another nut butter on celery sticks or apple slices all make for healthy, high-energy snacks.

In the following sections, we offer some meal ideas for breakfast, lunch, and dinner that don't require a lot of time or energy to prepare.

Breakfast

Breakfast is an important meal and shouldn't be missed. To fully appreciate why this is the case, see Chapter 10. If the recipes in that chapter appear too involved for you, this doesn't mean you should skip breakfast.

Here are some quick and easy meals to get you off to a good start, and if you aren't a "breakfast person," enjoy a lunch or dinner option instead:

- ✔ **Eat whole-grain, high-fiber cereals with your choice of milk and fruit.** Look for cereals that contain at least 3 g of fiber and not more than 5 g of added sugar, if possible. Barbara's, Kashi, and Food for Life brands may have cereals that fit this criteria. Your supermarket may carry these and other wholesome cereals, and your local health-food store is likely to have even more options available.

- ✔ **Try frozen, whole-grain waffles with a fruit topping.** To complete this meal, add a small glass of vegetable or fruit juice and a source of protein, such as peanut butter, yogurt or kefir, or a hard-boiled egg.

- ✔ **Try a cottage cheese and fruit plate.** One-half to three-quarters of a cup of cottage cheese provides an ample dose of protein to start the day, and a cup or two of fruit can meet your fruit goal for the day.

- ✔ **Try whole-grain toast, bagels, or English muffins with almond butter, peanut butter, or hummus.** To complete this meal, add a small glass of vegetable juice or fruit juice, or have a piece of fruit.

Lunch and dinner

Browse Part III of this book for some lunch and dinner ideas. The recipes in Chapters 11 and 12 may be particularly useful. If these recipes look like they require more energy than you have to spare, consider these options:

- ✔ **Try a bean burrito or tostada.** Take a whole-wheat or corn tortilla and add ½ cup low-sodium canned vegetarian, refried, or whole beans that have been heated. Top with lettuce, tomato, shredded low-fat cheese, and a dollop of sour cream, if desired. Still too much effort? Amy's brand frozen burritos are pretty clean and may be a good option for you.

- ✔ **Try a low-fat, low-sodium canned bean soup.** Add some whole-grain crackers or a slice of whole-grain bread and a vegetable or fruit salad for a more complete meal.

- ✔ **Try a tuna or chicken salad sandwich or stuffed tomato.** Three-quarters of a cup of one of these salads can meet your protein needs for a meal, and the tomato will provide a serving of veggies. Although basic tuna and chicken salads are easy to prepare — simply mix these proteins with a touch of mayo and desired seasonings — some supermarkets sell them already prepared. Just be sure to read the labels to find the healthiest ones.

✔ **Try whole-grain pita bread with hummus, carrots, celery, or any other vegetables that you may have ready to eat.** If you use store-bought hummus or hummus that has been prepared in advance (see our hummus recipe in Chapter 14), this is almost a complete meal without any cooking required.

✔ **Try a baked potato with cottage cheese or yogurt, whatever frozen vegetables you can easily heat up, and maybe a little salsa.** On days when you have a little more energy, prepare several baked potatoes that can be reheated and topped with easy ingredients for a complete meal on days you have less energy.

If you don't feel like monitoring potatoes in the oven or only want to make one potato, use your microwave. Simply wash and prick a large potato with a fork in several places, put the potato on a plate, and microwave it for 5 minutes. Turn the potato over and then microwave it for another 5 minutes. If the potato isn't soft, continue microwaving until it's tender. Russets are considered the potato of choice for baked potato recipes.

When you're constipated

Constipation is usually defined as having difficult or less frequent bowel movements than what's normal for you. Cancer treatment, including pain and some anti-nausea medications, can lead to constipation. Other factors that can reduce bowel activity include a decrease in fiber and fluid intake and a decline in activity, such as may occur from fatigue.

Numerous steps can be taken to help get the bowels going, including the following:

✔ **Drinking plenty of fluid:** Fluids help soften the stool and make it easier to pass through your gut. Water is the fluid of choice. On occasion, you can try a senna tea (such as Smooth Moves tea), as long as your oncologist approves.

If you do use senna tea, be sure not to overuse it. In some cases, dependency can occur and you'll require senna to have a bowel movement. Follow the directions on the package label.

✔ **Eating plenty of fiber:** Insoluble fiber has a laxative-like effect and speeds up the passage of food and waste through your digestive tract. Whole grains, especially whole wheat, are good sources of this fiber. Vegetables, beans, fruits, and dried fruit are also great sources. Remember to slowly increase your intake of fiber to decrease the chance of gas and bloating.

✔ **Trying warm prune juice:** Prune juice contains a natural laxative. Try drinking 4 ounces of prune juice at the time of day that you normally have a bowel movement.

✔ **Adding ground flax meal or wheat bran to your foods:** These can be added to cooked cereals, salads, yogurt, and muffins to boost your fiber intake. Start with 1 tablespoon per day, and increase up to 3 tablespoons throughout the day as tolerated. Take any oral medications an hour or two before or after consuming flax meal to avoid interfering with their absorption.

Drink plenty of water and other fluids when you increase your fiber intake, because fiber draws water into your digestive tract.

✔ **Being active:** Physical activity can stimulate bowel movements. If your doctor approves, try getting at least 30 minutes of activity most days of the week. You can achieve this just by taking leisurely walks.

✔ **Eating yogurt and kefir:** The probiotics or good bacteria in these foods can help keep your gut healthy and promote normal bowel movements. Aim for two to three servings per day, if possible.

If you're experiencing constipation, talk with your healthcare team. They may recommend over-the-counter medications such as stool softeners or gentle stimulants.

If constipation persists and you also experience nausea and vomiting, contact your doctor and healthcare team. Some cancers can cause a blockage of the digestive tract. If this happens, you may be advised not to eat too much fiber or foods like flax meal and wheat bran, or you may be told not to eat anything at all for a while.

When you have diarrhea

Diarrhea is typically defined as having three or more bowel movements per day than what is normal for you. Because cancer treatment affects all rapidly dividing cells, it can also cause changes to the rapidly dividing cells of the digestive tract. This can lead to diarrhea and affect the amount of nutrients and fluid that your body absorbs from food. When insufficient quantities are absorbed, dehydration and malnutrition can result.

To prevent diarrhea and its complications, you can try these strategies:

✔ **Avoid foods that are irritants.** Some foods and beverages may worsen diarrhea and should be avoided, including fried foods, fatty foods, caffeine, and alcohol. In addition, *lactose* (the sugar in milk and milk products) may become difficult to digest during treatment, causing diarrhea. Try to limit dairy products, except for yogurt or kefir, which can help improve symptoms. If you enjoy milk, consider buying milk that has the enzyme lactase added or using lactase tablets to help with digestion. You can also try a milk alternative like soy, rice, or almond milk.

✔ **Avoid using sugar alcohols.** Sugar alcohols like sorbitol, mannitol, xylitol, and maltitol are used to sweeten foods in place of sugar to reduce calories. But they can make diarrhea, gas, and bloating worse, so you should avoid using them or consuming foods and drinks that contain them until your symptoms improve.

✔ **Maintain hydration.** When you have diarrhea, you won't absorb as much water from your foods and fluids as you should, which can lead to dehydration if the diarrhea continues. Also, your nutrition intake may decline, which can further increase your risk of dehydration. Sip on clear liquids throughout the day, including sports drinks, broths, decaffeinated teas, coconut water, and water. Room temperature liquids may be better tolerated than chilled liquids. Try to drink at least a cup of liquid after any loose bowel movement.

Weighing yourself can help you monitor your hydration status if you have diarrhea for more than a day. Weigh yourself at the same time every day. For every pound of weight lost, you're almost 2 cups of fluid behind. You'll need to drink that amount in addition to your normal fluid requirements to catch up. Turn to Chapter 4 for more on staying hydrated.

You can easily make your own electrolyte drink, and it's considerably less costly and may even taste better to you than some sports drinks. Plus, it's all natural, with no artificial colorings or flavors. Simply add the following ingredients to a glass, mix, and enjoy: 6 ounces water, 2 ounces apple juice, 1 teaspoon sugar, and a pinch of salt.

✔ **Eat potassium-rich foods.** Potassium is critical for maintaining hydration. When you have diarrhea, you may not absorb enough potassium from your foods and fluids, and you'll be losing this important mineral in your stool. Some potassium-rich foods that may be tolerated when you have diarrhea include bananas, canned or peeled ripe pears or peaches, applesauce, potatoes without skins, pulp-free orange juice, and cooked carrots.

✔ **Eat sodium-rich foods.** Sodium is important for hydration. Although you normally wouldn't want to take in too much sodium, when you have diarrhea, you won't absorb as much of this mineral from your diet and you'll also lose it in your stool. To restore sodium levels, try sipping broths and eating pretzels and salty crackers.

✔ **Balance your fiber intake.** You may remember being told to follow the BRAT (bananas, rice, applesauce, toast) diet when you had diarrhea as a child, or your pediatrician may have recommended it for a sick child of yours. The BRAT diet foods are good sources of soluble fiber, which can help absorb some liquid from and form your stool. Other good sources of soluble fiber are instant oatmeal, white rice, pasta, canned Mandarin oranges, and canned or peeled ripe pears and peaches. Fruit pectin, such as Sure-Jell (which is used to thicken jelly), is also a good source of soluble fiber and can be added to cooked cereals, soups, or smoothies with some of the aforementioned fruits and a little rice milk or lactase-treated milk.

While increasing your soluble fiber intake, you'll also need to decrease your insoluble fiber intake. Insoluble fiber has a laxative effect and speeds up the passage of food and waste through your digestive tract. Therefore, you'll want to avoid eating whole-wheat products, seeds, nuts, dried fruits, and the skin of vegetables and fruits. Gas-forming vegetables like broccoli, cabbage, beans, and onions may also be problematic during this time.

✔ **Eat probiotic-rich foods.** Probiotics are bacteria that help keep your digestive system healthy. Cancer treatments like chemotherapy, radiation to the abdominal area, and even antibiotics used during cancer treatment can decrease the amount of healthy bacteria in your gut or eliminate them altogether. Studies show that consuming foods that contain probiotics, such as kefir or yogurt without seeds, can help manage diarrhea. Try to consume two to three servings of these foods daily.

If you can't tolerate probiotic-rich foods, ask your doctor or health-care team about taking a probiotic capsule that contains *Lactobacillus*. Numerous brands are available, but Culturelle (www.culturelle.com) or Align (www.aligngi.com) are ones that are commonly used and relatively easy to find.

✔ **Ask your doctor about glutamine.** We discuss glutamine earlier in this chapter, under "When you have a sore mouth or throat." With regard to diarrhea, some studies suggest that glutamine taken in 10-g doses up to three times daily may help.

Again, there is concern that glutamine supplements may interact with some chemotherapies, so you should only use glutamine under the supervision of your healthcare team.

Consult your healthcare team if you have diarrhea. They may recommend over-the-counter medications like Imodium or Gas-X.

Part II

The Importance of What You Eat and How You Prepare It

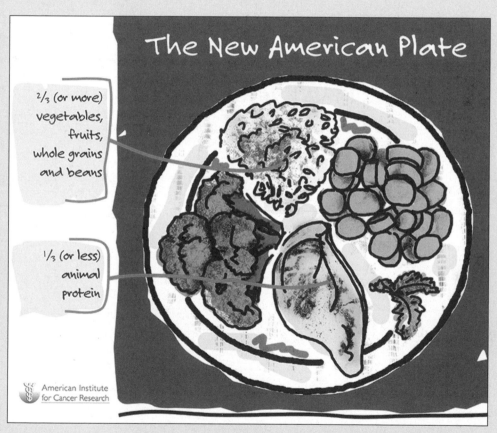

The New American Plate

²/₃ (or more) vegetables, fruits, whole grains and beans

¹/₃ (or less) animal protein

American Institute for Cancer Research

Illustration courtesy of the American Institute for Cancer Research

Find out more about a variety of whole grains you can incorporate into your diet to meet the goals of the New American Plate in an article at www.dummies.com/extras/cancernutritionrecipes.

In this part . . .

- ✔ Get acquainted with the clean-eating lifestyle and how you can use it to meet your food goals, even if you have special dietary considerations.

- ✔ Organize and stock your kitchen for clean, cancer-fighting eating.

- ✔ Discover the superfoods, spices, and herbs you should incorporate into your diet to pack the greatest cancer-fighting punch.

- ✔ See which kitchen tools and gadgets can keep your foods safe from toxins and enable you to cook with ease.

Chapter 6

Embracing and Transitioning to a Clean Eating Lifestyle

*A*wareness of clean eating has increased in recent years, with magazines, books, websites, and other media dedicated to advancing this concept. But what does it mean to eat clean? What foods are "clean" and what are the goals of this method of eating? More important, how do they mesh with your goal of beating and keeping your cancer away? These are likely some of the questions you're contemplating, and we tackle them in this chapter.

We start by looking at what clean eating is so that you get a good idea of the core concept. Then we review how a clean eating plan may help you maintain a good nutritional status during cancer treatment and help you reduce the risk of a cancer recurrence or of a secondary cancer as you enter survivorship.

Because any plan that changes eating habits can cause feelings of hunger, cravings, or deprivation, we look at how you can tackle these feelings in a wholesome way. Then we look at how you can boost your clean eating with foods that are known to bolster the immune system, giving your clean eating an additional cancer-fighting kick. Finally, we examine how you can make adjustments to your clean eating plan to manage any special dietary considerations, from food allergies and sensitivities to cancer-related weight loss.

If you're currently meeting your quantity goals during treatment (read more about these goals in Chapter 4) and want to eat healthier, or if you've completed treatment and want to take every step possible to protect your future health, this chapter is for you. Throughout you'll find suggestions you can use to improve your eating habits. But if you're struggling with a problem that is impeding your ability to nourish yourself, you need to tackle that hurdle before you can jump on the clean eating bandwagon. For more on managing cancer-related side effects that impact nutrition, turn to Chapter 5.

Introducing Clean Eating

When you're given a cancer diagnosis, figuring out what you can do to help beat it and go on to live a healthy life is first and foremost on your mind. You generally can't choose your cancer treatments, but you can take control of what you put into your mouth. This can provide a sense of empowerment when you're otherwise feeling helpless.

But knowing what and how to eat isn't always easy. You may read about new research in magazines or stumble upon websites that seem to have all the answers. Well-meaning friends and family may give you unsolicited nutrition advice. This may leave your head spinning or cause you to adopt a potentially harmful food strategy, which is the last thing you need.

In this section, we look at clean eating and why this is an ideal food strategy, whether you have cancer, have another chronic illness, or just want to be healthy.

What clean eating is

In a nutshell, "eating clean" is simply another way to say "eating healthy." The principal goal is to base your diet on consuming whole, unprocessed foods as much as possible. These foods don't need to be organic, although you can certainly choose organic foods if you can afford them and feel you'd derive additional benefits from them. (For more on organics, see Chapter 7.)

When eating clean, you're avoiding highly processed foods — the so-called _convenience foods_ that tend to be high in refined sugar, sodium, trans fats, and artificial flavors and colorings. Instead, you favor foods that are as close to nature as possible, such as unprocessed fruits and vegetables, whole grains, legumes, lean meats, low-fat dairy, and nuts and seeds. But don't think this means you'll be eating nothing but bland foods or spending hours in the kitchen. Clean eats are just as delicious as they are nutritious, and they don't need to be difficult to prepare, as you see when you peruse the recipes in this book.

If you didn't eat a healthy diet before your cancer diagnosis, don't beat yourself up over it. And don't think that you caused your cancer. Likely a variety of factors contributed to its development. But adopting a clean way of eating after a cancer diagnosis and treatment provides an opportunity to feel better, improve your general health, and protect you from cancer and other diseases down the road.

The benefits of clean eating

Clean eating has numerous benefits. First and foremost, eating foods lower on the food chain automatically improves your diet by putting more cancer-fighting vitamins, minerals, and phytochemicals at your body's disposal. In addition, you're cutting out empty calories from refined sugars and unhealthy fats, making it easier to keep your body in a healthy weight range, while also reducing your exposure to numerous food additives that may be associated with a variety of ill health effects.

At the same time, because clean eating is not a rigid diet plan but a lifestyle choice, it gives you the flexibility you need when you're going through treatment. If you're not able to eat clean foods or you're only able to eat certain clean foods at various points during your cancer journey, that's okay. You can decide at all times how much of your diet is going to be clean, and because clean eating enables you to eat from all food groups, you can always adjust your eating to focus on the foods you tolerate the best. Therefore, whether you're striving to meet the quantity goal or the quality goal we outline in Chapter 4, clean eating can help you get there.

Eating clean also enables you to eat more frequently. Now, this doesn't mean you can stop thinking about calories or portion sizes altogether. Clean foods aren't calorie-free, and they can cause unwanted weight gain if eaten in excess, but they do tend to be lower in calories and more filling in smaller quantities than processed foods, while providing considerably more nutritional bang for the buck. As a result, they can leave you feeling full after eating smaller portions, which also enables you to add two or three daily snacks to your diet. Spreading out your food intake helps keep your body's blood glucose levels stable, minimizing the insulin surges that some studies have associated with accelerated cancer growth or with the development of chronic diseases like diabetes.

How to apply clean eating principles

Diet plans can be difficult to follow. They all have very strict rules for what you can and can't eat and when to eat. This isn't the case for clean eating,

TIP

which promotes healthy eating using common-sense principles that can be easily put into practice.

Here are some points to keep in mind as you move toward a clean diet:

✓ **Focus on eating nutrient-dense foods as close to their natural state as possible.** This means avoiding processed food (in other words, anything in a box, can, or container that has a long shelf life and sells itself as a complete meal or side dish and contains a long list of ingredients, some of which you may not recognize) whenever you can and favoring nutrient-dense foods, such as fresh produce, whole grains, legumes, and lean meats (chicken, turkey, fish) and dairy. Turn to Chapter 7 for the clean eats you'll want to add to your pantry and refrigerator.

✓ **Expand your palate by eating a wide variety of wholesome foods.** If you read a study that says a particular food has shown promise in fighting your specific type of cancer, you may suddenly be tempted to eat that food morning, noon, and night. But it's rarely a good idea to focus on one particular food, because this can lead to an overdose of a vitamin, mineral, or phytochemical; result in a food–drug interaction; or cause a food allergy. It may also prevent you from reaping nutrients from other foods, which may be equally or even more beneficial to your health.

✓ **Plan on eating five or six times daily.** Eating small, frequent meals (often referred to as *grazing*) is healthier than gorging yourself with large meals. Spreading out your meals helps keep your blood glucose levels stable, provides a steady stream of energy, and helps ward off any treatment-related gastrointestinal effects.

✓ **Use the New American Plate to guide your meal ratios.** The American Institute for Cancer Research developed the New American Plate to guide eating to optimize nutrition. This method comprises a plate made up of two-thirds (or more) of vegetables, fruits, and whole grains or beans and one-third (or less) of an animal protein. Turn to Chapter 4 to see how this plate should look. If you're a vegetarian, substitute a plant-based source of protein, such as beans or tofu, for the meat. Alternatively, you can use a whole grain that's high in protein, like quinoa.

✓ **Strive for *more* than five fruits and vegetables, and get colorful!** Fruits and vegetables are the healthiest foods on Earth. They're high in vitamins, minerals, and thousands of phytochemicals, which work together to benefit our bodies in ways we can't even imagine. A considerable amount of disease-fighting power is contained in the very compounds that give produce its pigment. By varying the color of the produce you eat, you'll get a wider array of nutrients. Plus, you'll be creating a beautiful plate — and, as they say, you eat with your eyes first. To see your how many fruits and vegetables you should be consuming every day based on your age, gender, and physical activity level, try the Centers for Disease

> Control & Prevention's fruit and vegetable calculator at www.cdc.gov/ nutrition/everyone/fruitsvegetables/howmany.html.

✔ **Understand that you may have to make allowances.** Clean eating enables flexibility, so if your treatment or cancer is preventing you from focusing on clean foods or you can't eat them in the proper ratio, don't stress over it. It's important for you to nourish yourself however your body will accept nutrition, and if that means turning to canned soup, crackers, and soda for a while, that's fine. As your food tolerance and energy levels improve, reintroduce clean foods to your diet and cut back on the processed ones.

What foods to avoid

Certain foods just aren't clean, often because they contain large quantities of compounds that aren't healthy, but there may be times when you end up eating these things. In some cases, there are ways to clean them up or minimize risk before consumption. Because clean eating isn't meant to be a restrictive diet, but a lifestyle, it affords flexibility. And when you're facing cancer and its treatments, you need all the flexibility you can get. So, don't beat yourself up if you eat any of the foods or compounds we outline here. As long as you avoid them most of the time, you're good.

Many people find the 80-20 rule works well for them: Try to focus on eating clean 80 percent of the time if you can, which means 20 percent of your choices can be a little more relaxed.

Artificial sweeteners

Artificial sweeteners are synthetic sugar substitutes that are often significantly sweeter than sugar. They're sometimes derived from natural substances, including herbs (like Stevia) and even sugar (like Splenda). Although there has been speculation that artificial sweeteners can increase cancer risk, there is no clear evidence of this. Some studies do suggest that they can cause greater weight gain than sugar, and obesity is a known risk factor for cancer.

Having artificial sweeteners once in a while likely doesn't pose any tremendous health risks, and if you need to use them because you also have diabetes, that's fine, too. But because these sweeteners don't provide any nutritive benefits, it's ideal to avoid them whenever possible. If you can, you're better off adding a little honey, succanat, or other natural sweetener to your food or simply going without. The more sweets you cut out of your diet, the less you'll crave them. If you do need to use a sugar-free sweetener, opt for one derived from natural sources (like Stevia), rather than products derived by combining various chemicals (like aspartame).

Fast foods

Traditional fast foods, like burgers, pizza, and fries, are most certainly unhealthy and can contribute to weight gain if eaten frequently. These foods are also highly processed, having many additives to ensure a longer shelf life and better flavor. But many of today's fast food establishments have added more wholesome options to their menus, like salads, plain baked potatoes, grilled chicken sandwiches, and fruit smoothies. You can almost always find healthier options. For more on making better fast food selections, turn to Chapter 16.

Processed foods

Simply put, processed foods are foods that have been altered from their natural state. They may be found in boxes, cans, jars, and bags. As such, even shelled and bagged natural walnuts can be considered processed. But if you were restricted from buying anything in a container, you'd be missing out on a lot of wholesome eats. The processed foods you should strive to avoid are the so-called "convenience foods" that have a long shelf life, lots of additives (like artificial colors and flavors), and little nutritive value. You know, like those boxed dinners that line the middle aisles of the grocery store, or the hot dogs and other nitrate-preserved meats, or the chips in that new flavor.

Some convenience foods can fit into your diet, but try to make the best choices. Take the time to read labels. You may find that even two seemingly similar boxed dinners have very different nutrient stats. Turn to Chapter 7 for more on how to compare labels and make more wholesome selections. And if you do end up indulging in a boxed dinner or having hot dogs, eating foods that are high in vitamin C may help counteract any potential ill effects. Vitamin C can combat the inflammation triggered by certain additives, and some evidence suggests that vitamin C–rich foods can prevent nitrates from being transformed into cancer-causing compounds.

Refined sugar, sodium, and saturated and trans fats

Processed and fast foods generally contain these things in high amounts, and are they're partially what make these foods unclean eats — they have little nutritive value and can cause ill health effects when eaten consistently or in larger quantities. High intake of refined sugar provides nothing but empty calories and can lead to weight gain and diabetes; excess sodium intake can lead to fluid retention and high blood pressure; and saturated and trans fats can clog blood vessels, leading to heart disease. And these are just some of their known ill health effects. When sugar, sodium, and fats are obtained from unprocessed foods, you generally don't have to worry about consuming them in excess.

Transitioning to a Clean Eating Lifestyle

When you start a diet, you pick a day on which to start your new way of eating so that you can achieve a specific goal, such as losing weight, reducing your cholesterol, or keeping your blood glucose under control. The problem with diets is that they can only be maintained for a short period of time due to their restrictive nature. When the diet ends, weight and health status slowly creep back to pre-diet levels. A diet is really a way of life, so a clean eating diet is a lifestyle!

With clean eating, you don't have to pick a day to start. You can start any-time, even if you've just enjoyed fried butter at the state fair. The goal of clean eating is to optimize your nutrient intake and improve your overall health for life, not just for a short period of time.

Moving from french fries to fava beans

Now, if you've been used to indulging in french fries and don't know what a fava bean is, it may be a little challenging at first to get into clean eating mode. You'll have to spend a little time planning your meals and snacks and educating yourself on how to eat wholesomely, but you're already doing that — you're perusing this book, right? And as you'll see when you read on, eating clean is easier than you may think. There are no secret formulas to follow or calculations to perform.

Knowing what to expect

You probably already have a good sense of which foods are healthy eats, even if you're not used to eating them. As you adjust to incorporating more of these foods into your diet, you're likely to experience a whole range of exciting benefits. Here's a taste of some of them:

- **Improved overall health:** Poor diet has been associated with many diseases, including cancer. This is likely because a poor diet contributes to a variety of disease risk factors, including weight gain, nutrient deficiencies, exposure to toxins, and inflammatory responses. Eating wholesome, nutrient-dense foods reduces all these risk factors, leading to improved overall health.

- **More energy:** Cancer treatment can leave you exhausted. And even if you've already completed treatment, the stresses of everyday life can be a real energy drain. When you pair this with an unhealthy diet, just getting through the day may be difficult. By eating nutrient-dense foods, your energy levels go up because you're getting all the macronutrients and micronutrients you need.

✔ **Weight loss and maintenance:** Clean foods tend to be lower in calories and more filling than unclean foods, so even if you're not counting calories, you may lose weight. If you're overweight, this may be a nice perk of eating clean. And because eating clean is a lifestyle, you're more likely to keep the weight off. Just be sure to discuss any weight loss goals with your healthcare team first. On the other hand, if you're underweight or experiencing cancer-related weight loss, you'll want to prevent any additional weight loss. See "Cancer-related weight loss," later in this chapter, for some recommendations.

✔ **Improved overall appearance:** When you eat clean, the nutrients nourish all the cells in your body. As a result, your skin may become clearer and smoother, your hair thicker and shinier, your eyes brighter, and your nails stronger. You'll get better results than any beauty product can provide. Of course, some cancer treatments may have an effect on skin, hair, and nails, which may not improve until treatment is finished.

Of course, eating clean requires a bit more effort than eating whatever you want, at least initially. So here's what you can start to expect with regard to your time:

✔ **More frequent shopping trips:** Clean foods tend to have a shorter shelf-life than preservative-laden convenience foods. To prevent these foods from spoiling before you can eat them, it's better to shop more frequently. This also helps you eat these foods when they're freshest and taste the best.

✔ **Longer shopping trips:** Although you'll be shopping more frequently, these trips may take longer because you'll be spending time reading labels to identify clean eats. Making foods from scratch also requires more time gathering ingredients than placing a container of heat-and-eat fare in your cart, but they'll taste better and be much more nutritious, making them well worth the extra time and effort.

✔ **More time spent planning meals and cooking:** Because you'll be cutting out convenience foods, or at least reducing your intake of them, you'll initially spend more time looking for clean recipes, compiling shopping lists, and cooking. But the more clean meals you prepare, the less demanding this will become. And clean meals don't need to be complex or have countless ingredients. A baked fish filet with a baked sweet potato and a side salad requires very little time or effort to make, so even if you have little energy, a clean, nutritious meal is easily possible. And if you don't have the energy to prepare much of anything, be sure to enlist the help of your loved ones. They'd likely be more than happy to help, and if you encourage them to join you in the clean-eating efforts, meal planning and cooking can even become a fun activity.

Deciding whether to take it slow or jump right in

Because eating clean is a lifestyle, you have the flexibility to ease into it or to jump right in. If you decide to go slow, you simply start replacing some of your unhealthy staples with clean substitutes. For example, having unsweetened iced green tea in place of soda, carrot sticks instead of potato chips, or low-fat plain yogurt with some berries instead of pudding. As you get comfortable with the replacements, you simply keep making more replacements until you're at your goal clean eating level.

Alternatively, you can jump right in, but this is a much more difficult approach, particularly if you have a lot of unhealthy foods in your house. If so, see Chapter 7 for guidance on how to clean up your kitchen before you get started. Also, keep in mind that this approach can lead to more pronounced cravings and feelings of deprivation, which places you at higher risk of reverting back to your old eating habits. So, if you do take this route, be sure you have plenty of support and resources in place to help you stay the course.

If you're undergoing treatment, a slower approach is more prudent. Treatments may already be affecting your ability to nourish yourself and to metabolize nutrients. Radically changing your diet at this time can cause more gastrointestinal issues — from gas, to constipation, to diarrhea — and you don't need to be dealing with these things on top of everything else.

Dealing with hunger, cravings, and feelings of deprivation

When you first start making clean replacements, seeing that chocolate cake in the bakery aisle that was once part of your nightly routine may be enough to set you over the edge. You may crave it, feel deprived that you can't have it, or hunger for it, particularly if you're shopping on an empty stomach.

But don't despair! Although these are all powerful feelings, your brain can be rewired to overcome them so that soon enough you can pass by that cake without batting an eye. In this section, we look at how feelings of hunger, cravings, and deprivation manifest and how to manage them so that they don't get the better of you.

Deciphering hunger cues

Hunger is in your DNA. After all, you need to eat to live, and your body doesn't let you forget it. Your stomach rumbles or aches, you start feeling weak, and a headache may develop, all in response to a drop in blood glucose level, changes in hormone levels, or a depleted stomach and intestines. But sometimes appetite — a physical desire for or an interest in food — can be mistaken for physiological hunger.

When you're not sure your hunger is genuine, try waiting 10 to 15 minutes before giving in to the compulsion to eat. You may also try drinking a glass of water, because thirst cues can sometimes mimic hunger cues. If after these measures you start to feel hunger pangs, then you're likely genuinely hungry. But if not, your hunger was likely spurred on by an emotional trigger, particularly if the desire to eat has passed.

Recognizing when you've had enough

Ever feel horribly sick after overindulging and wish you hadn't taken all those extra helpings? Unfortunately, a common side effect of eating too much isn't tons of energy from all those calories, but fatigue and gastrointestinal issues galore. To avoid these unpleasant effects, you want to eat just enough to achieve *satiety* — a sense of satisfaction with your food intake levels, not regret.

Although your *hypothalamus* (a small gland on top of your brain stem) is responsible for regulating your appetite and letting you know when it's time to put down the fork and leave the table, there are some things you can do to set your hypothalamus up for success:

- **Slow down.** It takes approximately 20 minutes for your stomach to notify your brain that you're full. So, if you scarf down a foot-long sub in less than five minutes, your hypothalamus won't have gotten the message "Hey, cease and desist, at least until further notice." By eating slowly, you're enabling your stomach and brain to communicate as nature intended them to. One way to eat more slowly is by taking the time to really chew your food so that it all has a uniform texture in your mouth. This also helps with digestion, enables you to extract more nutrients from your food, and potentially offers additional protection from foodborne pathogens by exposing more food surface area to your stomach acid. Plus, the additional chewing lets you really savor the flavors, making the eating experience more enjoyable and relaxing.

- **Periodically gauge your hunger level.** As you work through your meal, periodically stop to see if you're still feeling hungry. If you do, keep on eating and slowly chewing your food. If you notice that you feel full before your plate is clean, stop. You don't need to be a member of the clean plate club every time.

- **Learn proper portions.** Super-sized food portions have led to a skewed view of what a proper portion is. A proper serving of meat is no larger than a deck of cards, a serving of a whole grain like brown rice is ½ cup cooked, and a serving of most fruits and vegetables is also ½ cup. But if your fruits and veggies are prepared in a healthy way, you can eat them as desired until you reach satiety. This is particularly beneficial if you need large volumes of food to feel full (although it's better to focus on using veggies to achieve this, because they tend to be lower in calories and have less sugar than fruits).

Managing cravings

Food cravings aren't a sign of weakness, but they may be a sign of addiction, particularly if your diet has largely consisted of processed foods. The salt, sugar, fat, and additives in these foods reward the pleasure centers in your brain, but as they cause you to gain weight over time, your body starts to crave more of them to get its fix. Ever see someone put salt on already salted fries or done this yourself? If so, put down that salt shaker, and rest assured that cravings often go away after a month or so of eating clean.

When you nourish your body with nutrient-dense foods like whole grains, fruits, vegetables, and legumes, you may find that the double-chocolate fudge cake you enjoyed too much is now entirely too sweet for you. And you'll instead start to hunger for healthy bites that do a body good and give you sustained energy to get through the day.

Until you get to this point, you may crave those unwholesome eats and go through a withdrawal period. Try these tips to tackle the craving:

- **Keep unwholesome foods out of the house.** The sight of food alone can be enough to inspire a craving. But out of sight, out of mind. And if you do have a craving, not having the desired food within reach makes it significantly more difficult to give in. Of course, if you're experiencing a lack of appetite or have cancer-related weight loss, it's important to eat whatever is appetizing to you, even if it's junk food.

- **Distract yourself.** Research indicates that cravings generally subside after 20 minutes. To hit this mark, distract yourself with activities that take this length of time to complete. Go for a walk, take a bath, mop your kitchen floor, or do a crossword puzzle. If you select a physical activity, rather than a mental one, you may get an additional rush of *endorphins,* those feel-good chemicals released by your brain. If you still have the craving after you complete the activity, have a wholesome snack in its place.

- **Give a nod to your craving.** If your craving occurs around the time you typically have a snack or meal, be sure to stick with your schedule. In such instances, consider having a wholesome snack that mimics the flavor or texture of the food you're craving. For example, an apple or unsweetened applesauce for a piece of apple pie, a small piece of dark chocolate and some almonds for a slice of fudge cake, and crunchy carrot or celery sticks with a little guacamole instead of crispy chips with a processed onion dip. If you really can't resist your craving, have a small portion of the food you desire.

✔ **Remember why you're doing this.** As difficult as it may be to change your whole manner of eating, think about all the benefits you're reaping by doing so. With each healthy bite you take, think of all the cancer-fighting nutrients you're putting into your body. They're like little soldiers helping your body along as it works toward recovery and keeping you healthy. At the same time, think about any unhealthy bites as enemies harboring an array of health-thwarting weapons. Making such associations can change your food perceptions, making it easier to stay on track.

Handling feelings of deprivation

It's normal to feel a sense of deprivation as you embark on removing foods from your diet that you're accustomed to, or that have brought you comfort, or that are associated with happy memories. But in some cases, the deprivation may be spurred on by factors you can control and remedy without straying from your clean eating plan.

Here are a few factors you should consider if you develop a sense of deprivation:

✔ **Are you eating too bland?** Although clean eating restricts unwholesome nutrients like sugar, sodium, and unhealthy fats, that doesn't mean you should be eating flavorless foods. Season your food well with spices, herbs, and a variety of condiments. (See "Appreciating new foods and flavors: Discovering nature's flavor enhancers," later in this chapter.)

✔ **Are you getting enough calories?** Unless you want to lose weight, clean eating doesn't restrict calories. You just want to get your calories from nutrient-dense sources so you reap the greatest health benefits. (See Chapter 4 to figure out how to calculate your daily energy requirements.)

✔ **Are you being too strict or taking it too quickly?** The goal is to eat as clean as possible as much as possible, *eventually* getting to a goal where the vast majority of your diet is clean (like the 80-20 we mention earlier in this chapter). But if your diet has been mainly processed foods and suddenly you throw them all out and become strict with your eating, you'll feel just like you've been put on a highly restrictive diet. Take a step back and give yourself wiggle room so that your body can better adjust to your new way of eating. For example, instead of completely cutting out that boxed macaroni and cheese, clean it up by adding wholesome ingredients to it, like veggies, beans, tuna, or a combination of these. Eventually, you can strive to replace the boxed mix with clean substitutes most of the time.

✔ **Are you rewarding yourself in other ways?** Food is often treated as a reward, and until clean foods start feeling like rewards to you, you may need to set up more non-food rewards for yourself. Focus on things that make you feel good, whether it's some pampering, a hobby, time with friends and family, or learning a new activity. *Remember:* Although foods are essential to life, there's much more to life than eating.

Making allowances and living with lapses

No matter how well you do with eating clean, you'll fall off the clean eating wagon. It happens for a variety of reasons, not all of which are in your control. No one can maintain a diet that's absolutely perfect 100 percent of the time, but your goal isn't to do that anyway. Remember the 80-20 rule? Even this rule enables allowances and lapses 20 percent of the time.

But if you find that you're exceeding whatever goal you've set for yourself, whether its 80-20 or even 50-50, there are strategies you can use to get back on track:

✔ **Find the obstacles to develop solutions.** Stop and think about what's keeping you from eating clean. If a cancer- or treatment-related side effect is to blame, turn to Chapter 5 for some food strategies you can use to overcome this obstacle so that you can get back to eating clean. If you're on vacation or exceedingly busy, turn to Chapter 16 for some ways you can improve your eating when you're grabbing quick bites or away from your own kitchen. If you simply have too many unwholesome foods in the house, turn to Chapter 7 to find out how to set yourself up for success. Regardless of the cause, there are solutions. But you can't find solutions if you don't identify the cause, right?

✔ **Take advantage of the flexibility and reevaluate your goals as needed.** Regardless of what goal you set for yourself, it's adjustable. If you stress over rigidly sticking to that goal no matter what, you're making it difficult to remain successful. Make sure your clean eating goals always remain realistic. For instance, if you're receiving chemotherapy and spending a great deal of time with your head in the toilet, an 80-20 goal isn't realistic for you, but after you complete your treatments, it may be.

✔ **Don't beat yourself up over lapses.** Even if you spent a week indulging in nothing but junk food or you've fallen back into your old eating habits, don't beat yourself up over it. Just get back into your clean eating plan, and if you need to start slow again, that's fine. Think about what caused the lapse in your clean eating and how you may be able to prevent similar occurrences in the future.

The longer you eat clean and the more clean foods you incorporate into your diet, the less you'll crave junk food. Pair that with the numerous benefits clean foods provide, including increased energy levels and simply feeling and looking better, and the incentive to stay the course also goes up.

Appreciating new foods and flavors: Discovering nature's flavor enhancers

As you adjust to eating clean foods, you may think they taste bland or unappealing compared with the foods you've been used to consuming. This isn't because clean foods aren't flavorful, but because food manufacturers have made significant investments in pumping processed foods with sugar, sodium, and a variety of artificial flavors and other additives to amp up their flavor and increase their shelf life, enhancing manufacturers' bottom line.

Clean foods aren't pumped up with a bunch of additives. The taste sensation they provide is as nature intended. And as you increasingly eat clean foods, your palate will come to appreciate these unique flavors, which often have many more subtle notes than any food manufacturer can achieve. In addition, you'll quickly find eating whole foods to be a more pleasurable experience. After all, eating a ripe banana tastes better and is considerably more satisfying than eating a small cookie made to taste like bananas by using isoamyl acetate. Why go for fake when you can have the real thing?

All that said, you don't have to eat whole foods just as they are to keep them clean. When you combine clean foods, you'll naturally create whole new wonderful taste sensations. In addition, nature has made many awesome flavor enhancers, and there are some minimally processed ingredients that are acceptable to use. Give some of these a try:

- ✔ **Lemon and citrus juices:** These acidic juices can perk up the flavor of everything from chicken and fish, to produce, to whole grains. They can also keep foods like avocados and bananas from turning brown, making them more palatable when added to certain recipes, like guacamole and fruit salad. As a bonus, you get a healthy dose of vitamin C.

- ✔ **Fresh herbs:** Herbs are like little flavor bombs, and they're packed with vitamins, minerals, phytochemicals, and fiber to boot. They can be used in any dish. For some herbs that are known to have a cancer-fighting kick, turn to Chapter 8.

- ✔ **Hot peppers:** Hot peppers like jalapenos or habaneros can add a kick to your foods, whether you're adding them directly to a recipe or you get industrious and make your own hot sauce. If you're dealing with cancer-related taste impairments, hot peppers may be an especially useful tool in your food-flavoring arsenal.

- ✔ **Spices:** If you peruse the baking aisle in any grocery store, you'll see there are a vast number of spices, which can be used to flavor everything from sweet treats to savory dishes. For cancer-fighting spices to add to your spice rack, see Chapter 8.

✔ **Salt:** You can add a little salt to your foods. Salt has gotten a bad rap because convenience foods contain astronomical amounts of sodium, which can have ill health effects, particularly over time. But some sodium is needed for optimum health, so don't feel bad about sprinkling on a little salt, particularly if your diet includes very few processed foods. Just be sure to limit your total sodium intake to less than 2,300 mg daily or to no more than 1,500 mg if you're older than 51 years or have high blood pressure, diabetes, or chronic kidney disease. This means adding less than ¼ teaspoon of salt to any of your foods or recipes daily.

✔ **Condiments:** In the condiment arena, mustard reigns supreme in its ability to impart flavor. It has been reported that adding a dollop of yellow mustard to cooked broccoli helps the body absorb sulforaphane, one of broccoli's cancer-fighting compounds. Other condiments to consider include salsa, guacamole, mayonnaise, and naturally brewed low-sodium soy sauce. Avoid condiments that have artificial flavors and colors added to them, like prepared barbecue sauces.

Enhancing Clean Eating with Immune-Boosting Foods

When you eat clean, you're already naturally boosting your immune system, because you're giving your body the vitamins, minerals, phytochemicals, and other nutrients it needs to keep your cells healthy and to protect your body from cancer-causing agents like environmental toxins and pathogens like cold viruses. Eating clean also reduces inflammation in the body, another condition that has been linked to cancer and other diseases.

But if you want to ensure you're getting enough of the nutrients that are known to keep the immune system functioning optimally, here's what you should focus on:

✔ **Foods rich in vitamin C:** Vitamin C increases the production and activity of white blood cells, strengthening the immune system. Good sources include broccoli, bell peppers, strawberries, citrus fruit, kiwi fruit, and Brussels sprouts.

✔ **Foods high in vitamin E:** Vitamin E neutralizes harmful free radical molecules that cause cell damage, enabling the immune system to focus on healing. Good sources include nuts, seeds, vegetable oil, spinach, and tomato products.

✔ **Foods rich in zinc:** Zinc is essential for proper T cell and natural killer cell function and proper *lymphocyte* (small white blood cells that play a role in the body's immune response) activity, and it may be directly involved in antibody production to help you fight infections. Good sources include lean meats, liver, poultry, shellfish, black beans, green peas, whole grains, yogurt, wheat germ, sesame seeds, pumpkin seeds, dark chocolate, and peanuts.

✔ **Foods rich in beta carotene and other carotenoids:** Beta carotene supports the *thymus gland* (a gland in the upper chest cavity that processes lymphocytes), making it one of your most important sources of immunity. Good sources of beta carotene and other carotenoids include orange fruits and vegetables, including carrots, apricots, nectarines, mangoes, pumpkin, and yams.

✔ **Foods rich in omega-3 fatty acids:** These essential fatty acids fight inflammation and boost the immune system, but when consumed in excess, they may have the opposite effect, suppressing the immune system. If you get your omega-3 fatty acids from food sources, you're unlikely to get too much. Find this nutrient in marine foods, such as salmon, sardines, and herring; seeds and nuts; and canola and flaxseed oils.

✔ **Garlic:** Garlic contains *allicin,* a pungent antioxidant that can fight a variety of pathogens and serves as a natural antibiotic. It also has anti-inflammatory properties. In addition, garlic contains selenium, which has been referred to as the "immune system mineral." Selenium stimulates the development and function of all types of white blood cells and enhances the ability of lymphocytes and natural killer cells to activate and respond to invaders, such as bacteria and viruses. Allicin is best obtained from freshly chopped or crushed garlic. Selenium can be found in garlic, lean meats, shellfish, vegetables, and grains.

For more information on these and other foods you can use to boost your intake of cancer-fighting foods, turn to Chapter 8. You can also learn more about these nutrients in general in Chapter 4.

Dealing with Special Dietary Considerations

Special diets are increasingly permeating the mainstream culture, whether it's to address a food allergy, gluten sensitivity, or another dietary need or desire. But regardless of your dietary needs, you can still eat clean. In fact, it's the optimal way to eat when you have dietary concerns. You just need to tailor the foods you eat to accommodate your special needs.

In the following sections, we cover some common dietary considerations and how you can tailor your eating to address these issues.

Food allergies and sensitivities

If you have a food allergy or sensitivity, you must remain vigilant about what foods you put into your mouth, avoiding the foods you're allergic or sensitive to. But because you're eating fewer processed foods, which generally have long lists of ingredients (many of which may not be clear), it'll be easier for you to ensure you won't inadvertently consume any of the foods you have issues with.

Gluten sensitivities

As with any food allergy, you'll be avoiding this specific allergen, which can be found in barley, bran, bulgur, cereal, couscous, farina, flour, food starches, Kamut, malt, matzo, oat bran, oats, rye, *seitan* (a vegan protein substitute), spelt, triticale, udon, wheat, and any processed food that has a label that indicates it contains gluten. Because clean eating focuses on eating lots of fruits, vegetables, lean meats, and gluten-free grains like rice and corn, it can help you maintain a gluten-free diet.

Vegetarian and vegan diets

Both vegetarian and vegan diets avoid the consumption of animal products, with vegan being the stricter of the two, allowing for no consumption of any animal products whatsoever. It's easy to be either a vegetarian or a vegan and eat clean, because you're already eating lots of clean, wholesome foods through your plant-based diet. Your greatest challenge remains getting enough protein, particularly if you're cutting out processed foods. Natural, vegan sources of protein to consider include amaranth, quinoa, buckwheat, spirulina (an algae), soy protein, legumes, nuts, and seeds. If you're willing to eat some processed foods, you can consider seitan, meat substitutes, and vegan or vegetarian protein powders.

Comorbidities

When you have *comorbidities* (coexisting diseases) like diabetes, high blood pressure, high cholesterol, or some other condition, you need to follow your doctor's dietary recommendations closely. Fortunately, clean eating makes it easier to achieve this task, because it optimizes nutrient intake and cuts out a lot of problem foods already, like those high in sodium, sugar, and saturated and trans fats. You'll also be more in tune with reading labels and knowing which foods can help you meet your doctor's recommendations.

Cancer-related weight loss

Eating clean may help with cancer-related weight loss (called *cachexia*), which is considered an inflammatory process. Focus on anti-inflammatory and antioxidant-rich foods, such as we describe earlier in this chapter under "Enhancing Clean Eating with Immune-Boosting Foods." You also want to add more high-calorie clean foods to your diet, such as nuts and nut butters, smoothies, whole grains, and avocadoes. If your cancer-related weight loss is due to an eating problem, turn to Chapters 5 and 19.

If you continue to lose weight while eating clean, you may need to allow other foods back into your diet. Talk to your oncologist as soon as you notice yourself unintentionally losing weight.

Chapter 7

Stocking Up on Cancer-Fighting Foods

*E*ating when you're dealing with cancer is a real challenge because so many variables come into play, including your cancer type, stage, treatment, and any other medical conditions you may have. However, regardless of your cancer type and where you're at, there are two high-level nutritional goals you should strive to achieve: quantity and quality (see Chapter 4). You want to be getting enough calories, protein, vitamins, and minerals to maintain your weight, lean body mass, and immune function. After you've met the quantity goal, you want to focus on eating the healthiest foods possible — eliminating junk foods.

Preparing your kitchen to meet the quantity or quality goals may sound like a daunting task, but don't despair. This chapter is here to help! First, we review how to read food labels. Because you'll be sorting through items that you already have and shopping for new foods, this is important knowledge that can help you optimize the quality of the foods you consume, even if you're working toward the quantity goal. Next, we provide insights on how to take stock of what you already have, including foods that don't come with labels, and offer guidance on what to keep and toss. Then we look at wholesome, cancer-fighting foods to stock your kitchen with, including pantry, refrigerator, and freezer items. Finally, we help you figure out how you can save money while shopping for this fare.

With the insights you gain in this chapter, you'll be on your way to a well-stocked, organized kitchen that will help you eat optimally during your cancer battle, regardless of which goal you're currently trying to meet. In addition, you'll have a sparkling clean kitchen that others will envy. So, let's get started!

Knowing Your Food

You've probably heard the expression "You are what you eat." Now, this doesn't mean you'll turn into a doughnut if you eat one, but if your diet consists of nothing but lots of doughnuts, you may start looking round like one on the outside and become nutritionally deficient like one on the inside. Many people don't realize that you can be overweight *and* malnourished. This state doesn't arise just by eating nothing but one food type either, like doughnuts or chicken nuggets. If you're consistently eating a variety of foods, but these foods don't offer much nourishment, you risk malnourishment.

Although the practice of making poor food choices creates an unhealthy situation for anyone, when you're facing cancer or another chronic illness, a tremendous burden is placed on the body, so making good choices becomes even more important. To make sure you're eating enough to maintain proper body function and optimizing your nutrient intake, you need to know what's in the foods you're putting in your mouth. You also need to make sure the foods you consume are safe to eat.

An important way to determine food quality and safety is to carefully read food labels, which appear on the outside of packaged and processed foods. If you haven't ever taken the time to really examine these labels, you may feel like you're reading a foreign language. But in this section, we go over everything you need to know about those tricky food labels. We look at the Nutrition Facts label, ingredient lists, and food product dating. We also look at some of the buzzwords on food labels so that you know what they truly mean.

Reading the Nutrition Facts label

The Nutrition Facts label (shown in Figure 7-1) appears on all packaged and processed foods, as mandated by the Food and Drug Administration (FDA). This label serves as a food's table of contents, outlining all the main nutrients it contains and how much each nutrient is contributing toward the recommended daily value. Other important information contained on the Nutrition Facts label includes the food's suggested serving size and calories.

Nutrition Facts

Serving Size 2 crackers (14g)

Servings Per Container About 21

Amount Per Serving

Calories 60	Calories from Fat 15

	% Daily value*
Total Fat 1.5g	2%
Saturated Fat 0g	0%
Trans Fat 0g	
Cholesterol 0mg	0%
Sodium 70mg	3%
Total Carbohydrate 10g	3%
Dietary Fiber Less than 1g	3%
Sugars 0g	
Protein 2g	

Vitamin A 0%	•	Vitamin C 0%
Calcium 0%	•	Iron 2%

*Percent Daily Values are based on a 2,000 calorie diet. Your daily values may be higher or lower depending on your calorie needs

	Calories:	2,000	2,500
Total Fat	Less than	65g	90g
Sat Fat	Less than	20g	25g
Cholesterol	Less than	300mg	300mg
Sodium	Less than	2400mg	2400mg
Total Carbohydrate		300g	375g
Dietary Fiber		25g	30g

Figure 7-1:
A Nutrition
Facts label.

Illustration by Wiley, Composition Services Graphics

By placing nutritional information in a standardized format, the Nutrition Facts label enables you to assess and compare food products. For instance, if you find yourself relying on crackers to cope with the gastrointestinal (GI) side effects of chemotherapy, you can compare the Nutrition Facts labels of different products to find the one with the most favorable nutrient profile. In this case, it would be the crackers with the most calories and the highest protein levels because your goal is to prevent weight loss and maintain lean muscle mass. You can also use the label to find the cracker with the least fiber and fat, especially saturated fat. (Fiber may worsen GI side effects if you have diarrhea. Fat slows down digestion, which can also make the GI side effects worse if you're nauseated.)

Let's look at the various components of the Nutrition Facts label:

✔ **Serving Size and Servings Per Container:** Serving Size and Servings Per Container are the first bits of information you see on a Nutrition Facts label. If you eat more or less than the serving size indicated, you'll be consuming a different number of calories and nutrients than indicated on the label.

✔ **Calories:** Although most people want to cut calories, when you're going through cancer treatment, taking in enough calories is crucial to boosting energy levels and helping many treatments work better. If you can get your calories from clean, nutrient-dense sources, that's certainly ideal because you'll be getting extra support through the added vitamins, minerals, and other nutrients that these foods contain. But no matter what foods you get them from, calories are essential for meeting the quantity goal. (For a more in-depth look at calories, turn to Chapter 4.)

✔ **Nutrients:** The Nutrition Facts label divides the nutrients in two distinct areas:

- The first section appears right below the calories and includes fat, cholesterol, sodium, total carbohydrate (including fiber and sugars), and protein. Except for protein and fiber, these are the nutrients most people should limit because they're often eaten in excess. But with cancer, fat can help you reach your quantity goals while being a good energy source, provided you're getting a healthy fat (you'll know if it's a healthy fat if you see a fairly high percentage of fat listed on the label, but no or very little saturated and trans fats). Many packaged foods have a high sodium content, because sodium is often used to preserve foods.

- The second section of nutrients is the vitamins. Ideally, you'll want to get as close to the 100 percent daily value as you can on a daily basis, so looking at the Nutrition Facts label can help you keep tabs on this. If a food has 20 percent or more of the daily value of a vitamin, mineral, or fiber, it's considered high in that nutrient. In addition, a food that has 20 percent or more of the daily value of iron would be a good choice if you have iron-deficiency anemia.

Deciphering the ingredients list

Another important part of understanding what you're eating is to take a look at the ingredients list, which appears next to the Nutrition Facts label and can shed additional light on a food's quality. The ingredients are listed in order of prominence. So, for instance, if you look at a jar of strawberry jam and the first ingredient is sugar, the quality of that jam is likely not as good as one that lists strawberries as its first ingredient, even if they share the same total sugar content. This is because strawberries have nutritional value and sugar doesn't.

As you get further into an ingredients list, you may start noticing items that you don't recognize and maybe can't pronounce. The longer the list, the more processed the food is and the more such items you'll see. Per the FDA, more than 3,000 ingredients can be added to foods in the United States, and the list continues to grow. Many of these ingredients are food additives, which are used to enhance a food's nutrient profile, increase its shelf life, or improve its texture, taste, or appearance.

Although many additives sound like they belong in test tubes, rather than in something on your pantry shelf, they aren't all bad. For instance, *riboflavin* is a fancy term for vitamin B2 and *guar gum* is a fiber isolated from the seed of the guar plant. At the same time, although every additive in the foods you eat has been approved by the FDA, that doesn't mean you shouldn't care about them. In general, the fewer hard-to-pronounce items in the ingredients list, the better — you just want to strive for foods that are as natural as possible.

Understanding food product dating

Many packaged foods also include food dates, which serve as another important indicator of quality and, in some cases, of safety (for additional food safety strategies, see the nearby sidebar). When you're undergoing cancer treatment, you may be at an increased risk of a foodborne illness due to low white blood cell counts, so you'll need to pay close attention to product dating to make sure you don't eat spoiled foods.

Ensuring food safety

Food safety is important for everyone, but it's especially important when you have cancer. This is because cancer and its treatments can weaken your immune system and lower your white blood cell count, increasing your susceptibility to infections. Although avoiding exposure to every potential pathogen is impossible, there's a lot you can do to reduce your exposure to organisms that cause foodborne illnesses. What follows are some strategies to enhance food safety.

✔ **Maintain cleanliness.** Wash hands in warm soapy water for at least 20 seconds before and after handling food and especially after using the bathroom. Keep all countertops, cutting boards, and utensils clean and sanitized. (You can use a solution made of 1 tablespoon of unscented liquid chlorine bleach per gallon of water.)

✔ **Avoid unpasteurized milk, cheese made with raw milk, raw meat, poultry or fish, lunch meats, deli salads, and raw sprouts.**

✔ **Avoid cross-contamination.** Keep raw meat, poultry, seafood, and eggs, along with their juices, away from ready-to-eat foods, whether in your shopping cart, refrigerator, or countertop.

✔ **Ensure proper food preparation.** Wash all produce under running tap water, including those with skins and rinds that aren't eaten. Cook all animal products to the appropriate temperature: 160 degrees for beef, 165 degrees for poultry and fully cooked hams, 145 degrees for seafood, and 160 degrees for egg dishes.

✔ **Store foods properly.** Refrigerate or freeze meat and other perishables within two hours of cooking or purchasing, or within one hour if the temperature outside is above 90 degrees. Refrigerated foods need to be kept at less than 40 degrees. Use all leftovers within three to four days if stored in the refrigerator.

For more information, check out the Food and Drug Administration publication "Food Safety For People with Cancer," available at www.fda.gov/downloads/Food/ResourcesForYou/Consumers/SelectedHealthTopics/UCM312761.pdf.

Here's a list of some of the dates you'll encounter and what they mean:

- **Sell by:** This date indicates how long a store can display a product for sale. For safety reasons, you shouldn't buy any products after this date has expired. You'll see this label primarily on raw foods that must be stored and prepared a certain way to prevent contamination, such as meat, poultry, eggs, and certain dairy products. These same foods often come with a Safe Handling label, which outlines how a food should be stored and prepared to ensure food safety.

- **Best if used by/before:** This date serves as an indicator of when a product has the best flavor and quality. It doesn't reflect a purchase or safety date. You can continue to use many products beyond this date if they're stored properly (generally, that means stored in a refrigerator at or below 40 degrees).

- **Use by:** This is the last date recommended by the manufacturer for using a product while it's at peak quality. If a product has a use-by date, use the product by that date.

Keep in mind that all dates are just guidelines. Even if you store a product properly, it has been handled by numerous individuals before it has gotten to you, so no matter what date a label gives, trust your senses. If any product smells, looks, or tastes funny, throw it out or return it to the store for a refund. You don't want to risk a foodborne illness. You have enough to contend with.

Looking at buzzwords in food

When food shopping, you'll see all kinds of buzzwords on food packaging. Some of these are clever marketing terms that are intended to get you to buy products by making them sound healthier or better than their competitors, even if they aren't. Use of these terms isn't regulated by the FDA. Other terms can only be included if the product meets certain standards. Confusing, right? We take a look at some of the buzzwords you'll encounter shortly, but remember that a product's Nutrition Facts label and ingredients list will always serve as your best indicators of a food's nutritional quality.

Here's some of the lingo that can paint a misleading picture about a food's quality:

- **All natural:** There's no governmental regulation on what this term signifies, but several manufacturers have faced class-action lawsuits when they've used this label on products that were heavily processed or contained non-natural or genetically modified ingredients, such as added color, artificial flavors, and synthetic substances. You should also keep in mind that even when something is truly "natural," it isn't always healthy. For example, natural potato chips may be made from potatoes, oil, and salt, but it doesn't automatically make them a healthy choice.

✔ **Energy boosting:** This often means that caffeine has been added to a product. These products often are high in sugars or artificial sweeteners and other non-nutritive substances, so you're better off getting an energy boost through other means, such as by taking a quick nap or eating a healthy snack.

✔ **Cage free/free range:** Cage-free chickens are raised outside of cages, whereas free-range chickens spend time outside in the fresh air. Although the latter methods of raising chickens is more humane than keeping the animals locked up in small cages, free-range chickens often still live in less-than-ideal conditions. And these terms do not imply anything about what type of feed the chickens are receiving.

✔ **Grass fed:** Grass is the natural diet for cattle, but they're sometimes fed grain toward the ends of their lives to fatten them up. This applies to conventional beef and even some organic beef. The benefit of eating beef from cattle that has been raised exclusively on grass is that this meat has less saturated fat and more nutrients, particularly omega-3 fatty acids, than conventional beef. The problem is that even if beef is labeled "USDA grass-fed," that doesn't guarantee that the cattle has consumed nothing but grass, because there is no verification of such claims. But if a label indicates "100 percent grass-fed" or "grass-finished" and verification by a third party such as the American Grassfed Association is indicated, then you can be certain that the cattle didn't receive any grains or other feed.

✔ **Organic:** You'll see organic stickers and labeling on everything from produce to meat to ice cream. There's a lot of confusion about what *organic* means. Many people think that it's synonymous with *healthy, natural,* and *pesticide free,* but this isn't necessarily the case. Most crops simply wouldn't grow without the use of pesticides and fertilizers, and organic farmers still use these agents, but they use types derived from natural sources. This means that organic plants must be grown without the use of synthetic pesticides or fertilizers made from synthetic ingredients or sewage sludge. They also may not undergo bioengineering or receive ionizing radiation. When it comes to organic foods from animals, antibiotics or growth hormone may not be administered.

Although the organics industry is heavily regulated and products must meet stringent criteria to be classified as organic, this term doesn't necessarily indicate that a product is a healthier option. For instance, no scientific evidence has conclusively proven organic produce to be safer or healthier than their non-organically grown counterparts. When it comes to organic food products, although the USDA National Organic

Program sets food guidelines, there is no associated regulation of fat, sodium, and other nutrients that are likely to have a greater impact on health than the type of pesticide or fertilizer residue that is left on a product.

There are three different organic claims that can be used on food labels:

- Foods that have the USDA organic logo and indicate being "100 percent certified organic" must be made of only organic ingredients.

- Foods that bear only the USDA organic seal must be made from at least 95 percent organic ingredients.

- Foods that have labels stating "made with organic ingredients" must contain at least 70 percent certified organic ingredients, but they can't use the USDA organic seal.

Bottom line: Buy organic produce if it looks better to you or makes you feel better about what you're eating, and buy organic products if you're comfortable with their nutritional stats.

If you opt to buy non-organic foods, there are numerous things you can do to improve their safety. For example, trim fat from meats, because this is where the majority of pesticide residues are found, and use low-fat dairy products to avoid exposure to unnecessary additives. You can also remove the outside layers of greens and wash all produce well prior to consumption. Whatever you do, make a point to eat a variety of foods to minimize exposure to any one compound.

Now let's look at some of the food labeling that's clearly defined by the FDA. All these terms give a glimpse into a food's nutritive profile:

- **Calorie free:** Contains less than 5 calories per serving. *Remember:* Unless directed by your oncologist, you are not on a diet to lose weight — your goal is to optimize nutrition and maintain your quantity goals. Calories are essential for this.

- **Light/lite:** Means a variety of things. It can indicate that a product contains one-third fewer calories or has half the fat of the regular product. It can also mean that a low-calorie, low-fat food has half the sodium it normally would. Finally, this term can be used to describe the color or texture of a food.

- **Low calorie:** Contains 40 calories or less per serving.

- **Reduced calorie, fat, sodium, sugar, or cholesterol:** Contain 25 percent fewer calories, fat, sodium, sugar, or cholesterol than their original counterparts.

- **Cholesterol free:** Contains less than 2 mg of cholesterol per serving, and 2 g or less of saturated fat per serving. Recently, there has been some genetic evidence to suggest a link between cancer and cholesterol levels, and clinical trials are currently underway to see if cholesterol-lowering drugs may also play a role in the treatment of some cancers. For this and other health reasons, limiting cholesterol intake can be important for optimizing health.

- **Low cholesterol:** Contains 20 mg of cholesterol or less per serving, and 2 g or less of saturated fat per serving.

- **Fat free:** Contains less than 0.5 g of fat per serving. *Remember:* Fat isn't necessarily bad. You just want to limit your intake of saturated and trans fats.

- **Low fat:** Contains less than 3 g of fat per serving.

- **Sodium free:** Contains less than 5 mg of sodium per serving. The American Institute for Cancer Research recommends limiting consumption of salty foods and foods processed with sodium.

- **Low sodium:** Contains 140 mg or less of sodium per serving.

- **Sugar free:** Contains less than 0.5 g of sugars per serving. High intake of refined sugars may increase insulin levels, which may cause changes in cell regulation, an effect that isn't good for people with cancer. And because refined sugars offer no nutritive value, they should be consumed in moderation anyway.

- **Low sugar:** Has not been defined.

- **No salt or sugar added:** Doesn't mean these products are sodium or sugar free. It just means no salt or sugar was added to the product during the manufacturing process.

Getting Your Kitchen Organized

Now that you understand food labels and have a better idea of how to determine a food's quality and safety, it's time to get your kitchen in gear. Does this have you looking at your kitchen thinking, "Wouldn't it be nice if I could just snap my fingers and be done with it?" Unfortunately, getting your space optimized for nutritious, cancer-thwarting eating will require a little bit of elbow grease — you'll have to assess all the food items you have stored in your house and then make decisions as to what to do with them.

Don't feel like you need to do all the organizing yourself! Even if you hate relinquishing control or are afraid of burdening people, remember that your family and friends want nothing more than to see you well again, and we'll wager that they'd be delighted to help! The task will also become much less difficult the more people you recruit. And if you have young children or grandchildren, you can even use it as an educational opportunity (for example, by having them help you sort items by type or expiration date). Just think of all the memories you'll create at your pantry-purging party! Who knows? Maybe you'll even inspire them to purge their own pantries when they get home.

Identifying where everything is

So, where to start? Well, the first thing to do is to consider every place you store food in your house. Writing down these places may be useful, particularly if you have multiple refrigerators, freezers, food-storage cabinets, or pantries.

After you've established all the places that need tending to, you'll systematically go through the items stored there. You'll also want to consider where in your home you may want to set up food stations to meet specific needs, such as if you're experiencing chemotherapy-induced nausea and vomiting. For example, you may want to keep certain nonperishable items like crackers, hard pretzels, or cans of ginger ale near your bedside or in your living room for those times when you're too tired or weak to get up. You can consider keeping these items in baskets so that your space remains tidy and these items stay together, making them more easily accessible.

Taking stock of the foods you have

Now that you know where all your food is stored, you'll tackle each area individually. The kitchen is the place most people go to hunt for or gather food, so addressing this space before all the others will have the most immediate impact on your and (by extension) your family's eating habits. In addition, starting with the kitchen will give you a good sense of how much space you'll ultimately have available to store the food staples you'll consume during your cancer journey.

Your kitchen cabinets or pantry are a great place to start. After that, you can tackle the refrigerator and freezer, because you'll be in a good rhythm and be able to more quickly go through your perishables, which you won't want to keep out too long.

Generally, perishable foods shouldn't be out longer than two hours to prevent them from spoiling. If you're currently undergoing treatment, you'll want to be especially mindful of this because your immune system may be compromised, making you more susceptible to foodborne illnesses.

Get started by grabbing a few boxes, bins, or other sturdy storage containers that you can use to sort items. You'll want to mark some as *keep* and others as *toss*. You can also consider making a *donate* box and a *symptom alleviators* box, the latter of which can contain the non-clean foods that still serve the very important purpose of helping you get through treatment. Items placed in this box can eventually be distributed to your food-station baskets.

To make the task less daunting, empty each shelf individually onto your kitchen counter or table, and then sort through each of these items, placing them into the appropriate storage container. When you're done with this, do the same with the refrigerator. As for what to actually put in each bin, we provide insights on that in later sections of this chapter.

While your cabinet shelves and refrigerator/freezer are empty, take the opportunity to clean these spaces by wiping them down with a nontoxic cleaner. Although many such commercial products exist, some have been shown to contain carcinogens, so to avoid such an exposure, you're better off making your own (turn to Chapter 17 for instructions). You may also consider purchasing new boxes of baking soda to put in your refrigerator and freezer to absorb odors. Baking soda absorbs odors, which may help ward off nausea by preventing a noxious odor from your refrigerator from hitting your nose.

Finding foods to keep

As you no doubt guessed, the box marked *keep* is where the foods that you plan to eat go. What you decide to place in this box is entirely up to you and will depend on whether you're physically capable of going all out from the start or need to make allowances until you can get there. Even if you decide to get radical with your clean eating, you may want to finish off some items before replacing them with healthier versions. If your budget is tight, this is likely your best option.

Here are items you should definitely keep:

- **Raw and unprocessed foods:** These foods are sold in their natural state, having received little intervention beyond being picked and packaged. Examples of raw and unprocessed foods include whole nuts (with the shells intact), raw seeds, raw honey, and fresh fruits and vegetables. However, if you have low white blood cell counts, these foods are not recommended.

- **Minimally processed foods:** These foods have undergone some processing, whether being canned, washed, frozen, dried, pasteurized, or cooked. However, this processing doesn't compromise or has only a minimal impact on their nutritional value. Examples of minimally processed plant products include ready-to-eat fruits and vegetables, such as peeled and bagged baby carrots; whole-wheat flour; almond and other nut butters (provided no additives are present); canned and dried beans; whole grains, such as quinoa, brown rice, oats, and buckwheat; and maple syrup and filtered honey. Examples of minimally processed animal products include eggs; plain low-fat yogurt; cheese; low-fat, hormone-free milk; and fresh and frozen meat, poultry, and fish without added ingredients.

✔ **Monounsaturated and polyunsaturated fats:** Examples of monounsaturated fats include olive oil, canola oil, avocados, and various nuts, such as almonds, macadamias, and cashews. Examples of polyunsaturated fats include corn and safflower oil, sesame seeds, flaxseeds, and walnuts.

✔ **Foods made from whole grains:** Cereals that contain all components of the grain, including the germ, endosperm, and bran, are called *whole grains*. Refined grains contain only the endosperm. Although the endosperm is also nutritious, stripping away the bran and germ removes fiber, protein, vitamins, essential fats, and antioxidants. Examples of whole grains include buckwheat, plain popcorn, steel-cut oats, millet, bulgur wheat, and pearled barley. Whole-grain products can be identified on food packaging labels when the first ingredient listed is "whole wheat," "whole meal," or "whole corn." If the first ingredient is "wheat flour," for instance, the product may not contain whole grains.

✔ **Low-sodium and low-sugar foods:** For information on what qualifies a food as low in sodium and low in sugar, turn to "Looking at buzzwords in food," earlier in this chapter. Foods high in sugar cause insulin spikes, which some research indicates may lead to negative changes in cell growth. Sodium and sugar information is listed on a product's Nutrition Facts label. (See "Reading the Nutrition Facts label," earlier in this chapter, for more information on how to decipher these labels.)

✔ **Preservative- and additive-free foods:** Preservatives and additives are usually put in foods to extend their shelf life or enhance their flavors, textures, and appearances. All the aforementioned keeper foods are free of preservatives. Other foods that meet this criteria include items such as plain oils, vinegar, spices, coffee (not instant), and tea (bags or loose leaves, not iced-tea mixes). Now, just because a food has an additive or preservative doesn't necessarily mean it should be tossed. Some of these come from natural sources and are fine. (See "Deciphering the ingredients list," earlier in this chapter, for more on this.)

Deciding what to dump

Although it may seem wasteful, don't feel bad about tossing your unhealthy fare and being aggressive about it! The healthier you eat, the better you'll ultimately feel.

At the same time, you absolutely need nourishment, so if you can't eat the healthy stuff for a while, don't beat yourself up over it. Your body is an extraordinary machine, and it will extract nourishment from whatever foods you consume, even if the food label reads like something out of a science lab. Just place these items in your *symptom alleviators* box. If you decide to set up food stations for yourself, you can distribute the non-perishables collected in this box between your food stations.

If you can, here's what you should get rid of:

- **Items with safety issues:** Be sure to get rid of any questionable items. These include foods past their sell by or use-by dates; items in damaged packaging or in dented cans; and moldy, foul-smelling, or freezer-burned foods. You'll also want to remove from your spice cabinet any spices or dried herbs that have lost their aroma, because these have lost their potency and are no longer effective flavor enhancers. You may also want to see when you bought your oils. Even the healthy oils can go bad, so if you can't remember when you bought an oil, it may be time to throw it out.

- **Soda and other sweetened beverages:** Soda is extremely high in sugar. One can of cola, for instance, has the equivalent of ten sugar cubes, with each cube providing 4 g of sugar. As you can imagine, this causes a very high insulin response, while providing no nutrients. Diet soda is no replacement either, because it contains a host of artificial sweeteners and food colorings. Sweetened beverages like soda are linked to weight gain and obesity, which has been shown to increase the risk of developing many cancers and of a recurrence of many cancers. Some studies also suggest that diet drinks don't lead to a decrease in calorie consumption. If you don't need these beverages to manage side effects, eliminating them from your kitchen is a good idea.

  On the flip side, when you're receiving chemo, soda may help curb nausea and vomiting. In particular, ginger ale and lemon-lime sodas (like 7UP or Sprite) can be beneficial. When purchasing ginger ale, just look for a brand that actually lists ginger in the ingredients list (some of the big-name brands don't), because ginger has shown some efficacy in alleviating nausea.

- **Processed, high-fat, cured meats:** All meats are processed to a certain extent. After all, you don't see a bunch of pork chops running around, do you? What we mean by processed meats are those that are not just cuts of meat, but products that have been otherwise altered, such as through the addition of various fillers, additives, seasonings, and preservatives. Sausages, hot dogs, fish sticks, and meatballs come to mind. These items not only contain artery-clogging saturated fats, but also contain carcinogens and compounds that potentially have other ill health effects — for example, nitrates.

- **Hard margarine and other processed butter spreads:** In the past, margarine was thought to be a healthier option than butter, but more recent studies have indicated that people who regularly consume hard margarine may have the same risk of heart disease as those who regularly consume the same amount of butter. This could be because many hard margarine products contain trans fats, and even when trace amounts are present, they can accumulate and clog arteries over time. If you use spreads sparingly, butter or soft margarine is a better option. You can also try keeping olive oil in an airtight container in your refrigerator and using that as a spread.

- **High-sodium and high-sugar foods:** Any item that contains more than 480 mg of sodium per serving is high in sodium, but even levels below that may be high. You certainly don't want to hit close to your daily allotment of sodium just by eating one or two servings of a product. Foods high in sodium include snack foods like potato chips; processed, prepared foods like TV dinners; condiments like certain marinades and salad dressings; and canned foods, including vegetables. As for sugar levels, these have not been clearly defined, but any food that contains a lot of refined sugar or is high in simple carbohydrates qualifies. These include items like cakes, candies, cookies, pies, puddings, and foods produced with white flour.

Restocking Your Cancer-Fighting Kitchen

After you finish cleaning out your kitchen and any other food storage areas, it's time to restock. When doing so, you'll have to keep the quantity and quality goals in mind. Think about where you are with your treatment and what you can handle. Are you struggling to eat, experiencing decreased appetite, or losing weight? If so, your shopping list should include high-calorie items that can help you get through these effects. This doesn't mean you should go out and buy a double-chocolate fudge cake or any other high-calorie food with little nutritional value. There are plenty of healthy high-calorie foods you can eat, such as avocados, dried fruits, nuts, seeds, bananas, sweet potatoes, and beans, just to name a few. These foods will help you maintain your weight while giving your body real nourishment and energy.

You'll also have to keep your energy levels in mind. Are you at a stage where you need foods that are quick and easy to prepare, or do you have the energy and interest to spend some time in the kitchen? Again, there are many healthy foods that are easily prepared, so you don't need to resort to TV dinners.

Finally, you have to consider any special nutrition needs and restrictions. Are you dealing with kidney issues and need to restrict your protein intake? Do you have difficulty swallowing because of mouth sores? Or are you dealing with constipation from a medication you're on? Factors like these will factor into your shopping list, so be sure to discuss such issues with your health-care team. They can help you determine which foods are best for managing your situation.

It would be impossible for us to account for every situation, but you can find some good general information on managing the most common physical and emotional side effects of treatment in Chapter 3. The National Cancer Institute also provides some great eating hints at `www.cancer.gov/cancertopics/coping/eatinghints/page7`, which can help you put your shopping list together.

You may already have many things on the lists in the following sections, and you certainly don't have to buy everything we include here. These lists are just meant to serve as a guide on what to look for when you're shopping.

Staples for your fridge

When you're hungry or looking to put a meal together, the refrigerator is generally the first place you look. Now, because the items stored in the refrigerator and freezer are perishables, you need to be mindful about their use-by dates. You also don't want to overdo it with items that have a more limited lifespan, like dairy products, produce, and meats. You need to plan your meals out as best you can and then shop accordingly.

Following is a list of items you can feel good about stocking in your fridge and freezer. Most likely, you're already buying many of these items.

- **Symptom alleviators:** These include items like puddings, custards, sorbets, gelatin snacks, sherbet, frozen yogurt, and popsicles. Try to find versions with the best nutritional stats. Although these foods won't win any awards in the nutrition department, they can help you get through your treatment. Also, some sorbets and fruit pops are made with 100 percent fruit, so they're guilt-free. And, if you have some energy, you can make your own fruit gelatin, which is almost like Jell-O but made with agar, a type of seaweed. You can find a recipe in Chapter 15.

- **Cheeses:** Cheese is a good source of calories and protein. Look for low-fat versions when available. To prevent any foodborne illnesses, avoid any raw milk cheeses, cheeses with mold (such as blue cheese, Roquefort, and stilton), or cheeses with dried vegetables (like pepper jack).

- **Condiments:** May include items like mustard, ketchup (try to buy reduced-sugar or reduced-sodium versions), salsa, soy sauce (buy low-sodium varieties), and hummus, all of which need to be refrigerated upon opening. When deciding between condiments, read labels to find the ones with the best nutrition profile.

✔ **Cottage cheese/ricotta cheese:** Preferably plain, low-fat cottage cheese with no fruit added to reduce sugar content. You can add your own fruit for a more wholesome treat.

✔ **Eggs:** Try to find eggs from free-range chickens. Some studies have indicated that these eggs may be more nutritious than commercially produced eggs. If you can afford to spend a little extra, consider buying omega-3 eggs, which are from chickens fed a higher omega-3 diet.

✔ **Fish and seafood:** Buy fish that are known to be lower in mercury, such as light tuna (often canned) and wild-caught Alaskan salmon. The Monterey Bay Aquarium Seafood Watch program has resources to help you make informed choices when it comes to fish and seafood. Check out www.montereybayaquarium.org/cr/seafoodwatch.aspx for more information.

✔ **Fresh or frozen fruits and vegetables:** If frozen, make sure no sugar or salt has been added. Some good cancer-fighting fruits to consider include apples, avocados, bananas, berries, kiwis, oranges, and papayas. Some good cancer-fighting vegetables include carrots, cruciferous vegetables (broccoli, Brussels sprouts, cabbage, kale), leafy greens, mushrooms, and tomatoes.

✔ **Fresh herbs:** Because these generally last for only a few days, you should only buy them shortly before you need them. See Chapter 8 for more on which ones to pick.

✔ **Fruit and vegetable juices:** Buy varieties that have no added sugar. Check the ingredients list to see if sugar is listed, and if buying cranberry juice, make sure it's 100 percent juice and not "cranberry juice cocktail," which contains only a small amount of juice.

✔ **Lean meats and poultry:** Ideally, beef should be from grass-fed cattle and poultry from free-range chickens. Other good options include bison, ostrich, pork, and turkey.

✔ **Milk, soy milk, rice milk, or almond milk:** Buy plain, low-fat varieties, not flavored versions. With regard to cow's milk, look for hormone-free brands. This is indicated by a label that says "rBST- and rBGH-free." Don't drink raw milk — the risk of contracting a foodborne illness is too high.

✔ **Sour cream:** Buy low-fat versions.

✔ **Yogurt or kefir:** Buy plain and unsweetened varieties. You can add your own flavorings. Many different types of yogurt are on the market, including Greek, skyr (Icelandic), and non-dairy varieties, such as those made from coconut milk or soy milk. Just make sure you choose one that says "contains live and active cultures" on its packaging.

Staples for your pantry

The pantry is generally where you turn when you're looking for a quick snack or meal ingredients. This is also where you may keep some cancer alleviators, like crackers, hard pretzels, and popcorn. When arranging your pantry and introducing items, you'll want to keep the items you use most toward the front.

Because the items stored in your pantry are non-perishables, they'll generally have a longer shelf life than refrigerator items. Still, you'll want to try to be mindful of the use-by dates. For example, if you have five cans of beans, you'll want to make sure you first use the ones that will expire first.

Here are some items to consider adding to your pantry:

- ✔ **Applesauce:** Buy unsweetened and, if you can, versions made with apples that come from the United States.

- ✔ **Baking soda and baking powder:** In addition to having baking soda on hand for baking, you may want to buy a few boxes to freshen your refrigerator and freezer and a few more to use if you're making your own natural cleaning products. (See Chapter 17 for more on this.)

- ✔ **Broths, stocks, and bouillon:** Try to get low-sodium versions in any flavor you like and without trans fats.

- ✔ **Symptom alleviators:** Bland foods like soda crackers, plain popcorn, hard pretzels, plain pita chips, melba toast, and white bread are good to have on hand, because they're easy on the stomach. Soda (particularly ginger ale and lemon-lime varieties) may also be helpful in easing an upset stomach.

- ✔ **Canned goods:** Good items to have on hand include tuna, wild salmon, soups, tomatoes processed without any additives, and water-packed fruits.

- ✔ **Cereal grains:** Consider oats (rolled and steel cut), oat bran, wheat germ, and plain hot wheat cereals (like Cream of Wheat). See the Cranberry Snow recipe in Chapter 15; it's a fluffy Scandinavian dessert made with hot wheat cereal.

- ✔ **Dried fruits:** Consider apricots, blueberries, cranberries, figs, mangoes, and prunes. Whenever possible, try to buy unsulphured versions. They may not look as pretty (for example, apricots will look brown instead of bright orange), but they taste great.

- ✔ **Dried herbs, spices, and salt:** See Chapter 8 for some spice recommendations. As for salt, sea salt and pink salt (like Himalayan) are best because they generally have less additives than table salt.

✔ **Flour:** Consider having whole wheat and unbleached white flour on hand. Whole-wheat flour is healthiest, but it can have a strong flavor and lead to baked goods with a rougher, denser texture. So, until you get used to whole-wheat flour, you may want to use it combined with some white flour in your home-baked goods. And if you have stomach issues, white is likely best until you get over them. You can also experiment with other flours on the market, like barley, coconut, millet, oat, and spelt.

✔ **Garlic and onions:** Any types are fine. Store onions separate from your potatoes to prevent your potatoes from spoiling prematurely.

✔ **Grains:** Whole grains like brown rice, wild rice, quinoa, wheat berries, and bulgur wheat are the most nutritious, but if you're dealing with stomach issues, white rice is best.

✔ **Honey and maple syrup:** These are great natural sweeteners. Whenever you can, buy pure unfiltered honey. Also, buy pure maple syrup, and not the typical pancake syrup containing high-fructose corn syrup. Although it costs much more, pure maple syrup comes from nature and is not a mix of refined sugar and additives. If you have a low white blood cell count, you'll need to use pasteurized honey and maple syrup.

✔ **Jam:** Look for all fruit jams that have no added sugar or high-fructose corn syrup.

✔ **Legumes:** Consider black beans, chickpeas, garbanzo beans, kidney beans, split peas, and lentils. You can buy them dried or canned. If you buy canned, just look for brands that have less sodium.

✔ **Nut butters:** Consider almond and cashew butters. Peanut butter without added fat or sugar is also okay.

✔ **Nuts and seeds:** Consider nuts like almonds, Brazil nuts, cashews, macadamias, and walnuts, and snacking seeds like pumpkin and sunflower seeds. Just look for unsalted versions that have no additives. It's fine if they're roasted. You can also consider buying seeds like sesame and flaxseeds to add a nutritive boost to your foods.

✔ **Oils:** Consider canola, corn, flax, olive, safflower, sesame, and sunflower seed oils.

✔ **Pasta:** Try to buy versions that are whole grain.

✔ **Pasta sauces and marinara sauces:** Look for versions with the least additives and lowest sodium levels.

✔ **Potatoes, sweet potatoes, and yams:** These are filling, packed with nutrition, and gentle on the stomach. They can also be easily prepared in the microwave, making for an easy meal or snack. Just be sure to store them away from light and separate them from your onions to ensure their longevity.

✔ **Salad dressings:** Look for versions with the least additives.

✔ **Tea:** Black tea, chamomile tea, ginger tea, green tea, peppermint tea, and white tea are great to have on hand. Other varieties are fine, too. Just avoid any diet teas or teas with combinations of herbs.

✔ **Vinegar:** Consider keeping apple cider, balsamic, red wine, and plain on hand.

Navigating the Grocery Store

You've probably heard before that you should shop the perimeter of the grocery store first. That's because the perimeter is where the least processed foods are located — it's where you'll find the produce, meat, and dairy, whereas the middle aisles contain a lot of prepackaged foods. The rationale is that by shopping the perimeter first, there will be less space in your cart for junk food. This strategy can be a really useful one if you're trying to eat clean to meet the quality goal, but it may not work if you're simply trying to meet your quantity goals, because a lot of the foods that can help you through this period can be found in those middle aisles.

You may also want to start with the middle aisles if you have a lot of staples to buy to restore your pantry and fridge, particularly if you'll be spending some time comparing labels. This way you minimize the amount of time that your perishables are out of refrigeration, reducing the risk of anything spoiling.

In this section, we examine how to build and stick to your shopping list, which will make your shopping trip more efficient and enjoyable. We also look at how you can save some money when shopping without compromising the quality of the foods you're buying.

Building and sticking to your list

You've probably gone grocery shopping before without a list, simply picking up things that look good. It's something most of us have done, but the problem with this is that it's difficult to plan your meals this way. You may end up coming home with too little or too much, both of which are undesirable. To make sure you always have the foods you need, keep a shopping list.

To get a list going, you can keep a notepad by your refrigerator, adding items as you need them. Although this method may work just fine for you, particularly if you're very organized and you have a designated weekly shopping day, there are some drawbacks: Because the list is on a piece of paper, it's easily lost and the list isn't always with you, making impromptu stops at the grocery store difficult. Also, other people in your household may not have access to the list, so they may not know to stop at the grocery store on their way home to pick up milk and bread, for instance.

These problems can be solved if you have a smartphone, because you can invest in a grocery list app. There are many such apps available, each with its own features. Many apps enable you to maintain a joint list with others and send push notifications when an item is needed, store shopping lists, and check off items as you acquire them. Some apps even enable you to manage your coupons.

Here are a few tricks for maintaining a solid grocery list:

- ✔ At the beginning of the week, plan out your menu for the week, also accounting for snacks.

- ✔ If you're planning on trying out any recipes, add all the ingredients you'll need (along with quantity) to your list.

- ✔ When you're starting to run low on any staples, be sure to add those items to your list to ensure you don't run out.

- ✔ List like items together, and put these groupings in the most efficient order based on your grocery store's layout.

- ✔ When at the grocery store, try your best to stick to your list.

It may take a while for you to get into the rhythm of maintaining a grocery list, particularly if it's not something you've done before. That's okay. If you stick with it, you'll see how this strategy facilitates your eating, whether you're working toward the quality goal or striving to meet the quantity goal.

Cancer on a budget

Cancer can place a considerable strain on your budget. You're spending time and money to get to your appointments, and you're undergoing expensive diagnostic tests and treatments. You'll want to save money where you can, but you shouldn't have to survive on ramen noodles. This is the time your body needs nourishment the most, so food quality is essential.

Here are some of the ways you can save money on your groceries, enabling you to eat like a king or queen:

- ✔ **Maintain a grocery list and stick to it (see the preceding section).** In addition to ensuring that you never run out of a needed food item, a grocery list also helps ensure that you don't overbuy, reducing the potential for food waste. However, if you're not feeling well and something looks appetizing, consider adding it to your grocery cart.

✔ **Clip coupons.** It may be a bit time consuming, but clipping coupons can end up saving you a pretty penny. You can find coupons in the Sunday newspaper, store circulars, and online, and you may be able to stack coupons from different sources to reap maximum savings. Before using any online sites, check their legitimacy at www.cents-off.com.

✔ **Buy generic, when possible.** Many stores have a store-brand equivalent to the name brands. In many cases, the store brand has similar stats but costs considerably less.

✔ **Stock up when there are super sales.** Foods with a long shelf life (like frozen vegetables, canned tuna, and fruit juices) are good to stock up on when there are really good sales. Just be sure not to overbuy. If you end up ultimately not using these foods, you're losing money.

✔ **Store your foods properly to reduce waste.** Make sure to wrap your foods properly or place them in appropriate storage containers to prevent them from spoiling or affecting the flavor of other foods. And when using a food, make sure to close that container properly and put the food away promptly. Even leaving a nonperishable item like a sleeve of soda crackers exposed to the air for a short period of time can cause them to become stale very quickly.

✔ **Keep your refrigerator and pantry as uncluttered as possible.** If your food storage areas are too packed, you won't know what you have, and you may end up spending money on duplicates or having to toss expired items, both of which waste a considerable amount of money.

✔ **Use your leftovers.** You don't simply have to reheat your old eats, but you can reinvent them. For example, your leftover vegetables can find their way into an omelet or soup, making you feel like you're eating a whole new meal. Or you can opt to freeze your leftovers, enabling you to use them at times when you don't have the energy to cook.

✔ **Compare store circulars to find the one with the best deals.** Different stores have different deals, so you may want to vary where you shop on a weekly basis or visit different stores to reap the most savings. You'll just have to consider whether the additional travel and time this takes makes store hopping worthwhile.

✔ **Get rain checks.** Just because a sale item is out of stock doesn't mean you can't ultimately get it. Go to customer service to get a rain check for that item, and be sure to use the rain check when the item is back in stock.

✔ **Watch the register.** When there are sales, these may not always show up at the register. By watching the register, you can catch these mistakes, and they can be corrected before you pay. This practice also helps you ensure that the clerk scans all your coupons, including any instant coupons attached to items.

✓ **Stock up at other places.** The grocery store isn't the only place for you to stock up. Groceries are available at numerous other stores, including chain retail stores, health-food stores, farmer's markets, online retailers, and even your own garden. Chain retail stores and online retailers may be great places to get non-perishables for a good price, whereas farmer's markets and your own garden can be great resources for fresh and affordable produce. Health-food stores may be a good source for getting nuts, dried fruits, honey, and other specialty items for less than you'd pay at the grocery store.

With a little effort and some ingenuity, you can meet your food goals while keeping your expenses down. But don't feel like all the burden should be on you. Enlist others to help. If you have children or grandchildren, get them to help you with the coupon clipping. If you have leftovers to use, see who can come up with the most innovative way to use them. There are many ways to involve family and friends in your money-saving efforts.

Chapter 8

Cancer-Fighting Foods, Spices, and Herbs

*S*uperfoods are foods that should be in everyone's diet to reduce the risk of cancer. They should also be eaten during and after cancer treatment to provide your body with the nutrients it needs to stay strong, fight the cancer, and help to prevent a recurrence or a secondary cancer. But notice that we said "superfoods," rather than "superfood." Although it may be tempting to eat a large volume of one particular food when you read about its beneficial results in a promising cancer-related study, no single food can protect you from cancer or support you during cancer treatment. In fact, most studies support a concept known as *synergy,* which means that combinations of foods and nutrients work together to provide protection against disease.

In this chapter, we cover our top ten recommended superfoods. Not surprisingly, many of them are vegetables and fruits, because they're loaded with vitamins, minerals, and phytochemicals. These foods have been the focus of many studies to see if the phytochemicals in them help protect against cancer. Consider including these foods in your diet on a regular basis, if not a daily basis.

After reviewing superfoods, we talk a little bit about herbs and spices. In addition to adding quite a bit of flavor to your foods and minimizing the need for adding salt, they may have other beneficial effects. We look at some of these benefits for eight herbs and spices, including how they may be used to alleviate symptoms from cancer and its treatments.

Finally, because many foods have the potential to interact with medications, we talk about how to protect yourself from drug–food and drug–herb interactions.

Meeting the Superfoods: How and Why They Differ from the Pack

In this section, we introduce you to our top ten superfood picks. These foods have been studied the most for their potential to protect against and fight cancer, and they've shown good results. This isn't surprising given that these foods score high in nutrient density (see Chapter 4), and they're particularly high in antioxidants and phytochemicals, both of which keep your cells healthy and trigger the bad ones to die off (a process your oncologist may refer to as *apoptosis*).

Tomatoes

Technically speaking, tomatoes are fruits because they have seeds, but we use them as vegetables because of their savory flavor. No matter what you consider them, tomatoes are nutritional powerhouses.

Have you ever wondered why tomatoes are red? The phytochemical lycopene is what gives them their distinctive color. Lycopene is a *carotenoid,* a pigment responsible for the yellow to red color of many foods. Carotenoids are powerful antioxidants, and tomatoes are loaded with antioxidants.

Green tea

Green tea comes from *Camellia sinensis,* the same species of plant that black tea comes from. Both green and black tea contain the powerful antioxidants polyphenols and flavonoids, but unlike black tea, green tea is not fermented. Green tea has received more attention because it appears to have higher levels of *catechins* (an antioxidant) than black tea.

Studies that have shown benefit suggest that drinking three to five cups of green tea a day may offer protection.

Because green tea contains caffeine, you need to be careful about the time of day you drink it, particularly if caffeine keeps you awake at night. Also, if you're sensitive to caffeine or are taking medications like MAO inhibitors, it's important to talk with your doctor before drinking green tea. Green tea leaves also contain vitamin K, which is a nutrient that is known to interfere with blood-thinning mediations like warfarin (Coumadin), so if you're taking these medications, talk with your doctor before consuming green tea.

Nuts (especially Brazil nuts and walnuts)

In Chapter 4, we briefly mention that not so long ago, nuts were too high in fat to be considered part of a healthy diet. Fortunately, after years of research, we now know that nuts contain heart-healthy mono- and polyunsaturated fats. That said, they're still high in calories, so portion control is important. You don't want to outweigh their health benefits by gaining unintentional extra pounds. For example, ⅓ cup of nuts contains an average of about 160 calories. But this nutrient density can be a good thing if you're struggling with cancer-related anorexia and weight loss, because a small amount will provide a decent supply of weight-sustaining calories.

In addition to containing healthy fats, nuts are a good source of potassium, iron, zinc, calcium, phosphorus, magnesium, folate, selenium, and vitamin E. They also contain some protein and fiber. Walnuts are an excellent source of anti-inflammatory omega-3 fatty acids, and some research indicates that this nutrient may be better absorbed from food than from supplements. Brazil nuts can provide 100 percent of the daily value for selenium.

Beans, peas, and lentils

Beans, peas, and lentils are good sources of protein and are high in fiber. They're an excellent replacement for red and processed meats, providing muscle-building protein without the saturated fat. They also contain folate, which can keep the DNA in your cells healthy, and they may offer additional cancer protection via their phytochemicals. It's still unclear exactly how these compounds may protect against cancer, but a variety of effects are likely at work, including hormone regulation, antioxidant activity, and increased *apoptosis* (programmed cell death, as mentioned earlier in this chapter).

Try to replace at least one meat-based meal with a bean-based meal weekly. Just be sure to introduce the beans slowly to reduce gas. Start with a small portion of ⅓ to ½ cup per week. As your tolerance grows, you can increase the frequency with which you use beans in place of meat.

If gas deters you from eating beans, use Beano to help you digest the carbohydrate. Beano contains a natural enzyme that may prevent or minimize unpleasant gas when taken with your beans.

Cruciferous vegetables

Cruciferous vegetables, or *flowering vegetables,* as they're sometimes called, get their name from their appearance. The four-petal flowers from these vegetables resembles a cross or "crucifer," which aptly lead them to be named *cruciferous.* Some of these vegetables form a head, like broccoli, Brussels sprouts, rapini, cabbage, cauliflower, and turnips. Others, like kale and collard greens, don't form a head and are sometimes less recognized as a member of this family of vegetables.

Some studies suggest that women with breast cancer who eat higher amounts of cruciferous vegetables may have a reduced risk of disease recurrence. But even if breast cancer is not your main concern, these vegetable are highly nutritious. To reap their many benefits, try to eat ½ cup to 3 cups daily.

It's unclear whether eating them raw or cooked is best. Some people suggest that raw is better because some of the enzyme activity needed for benefit is lost with cooking, whereas others suggest that cooking them enables your gut to release more of the beneficial compounds they contain. Because the jury is still out, perhaps eating a little of both at a meal may be best to maximize benefit. These vegetables may also introduce gas into your digestive tract. Just as with beans, Beano may help minimize gas production.

Leafy greens

Leafy greens are an excellent source of fiber, folate, carotenoids like lutein and zeaxanthin, and flavonoids. Most of these compounds have antioxidant activity that can protect your cells from damage. Lutein and zeaxanthin are also protective for your eyes and may reduce the risk of developing macular degeneration, which can cause blindness.

Leafy greens include spinach, kale, romaine lettuce, leaf lettuce, mustard and collard greens, chicory, and Swiss chard.

One of the easiest ways to add leafy greens to your diet is to replace iceberg lettuce with romaine or leaf lettuce on your sandwiches or in your salads. You can also make green smoothies by adding some leafy greens to the mix.

Wild salmon

Wild salmon is an excellent source of protein and omega-3 fatty acids. A 3-ounce portion provides about 2,500 mg of omega-3 fatty acids and 500 mg of eicosapentaenoic acid (EPA). The American Heart Association recommends eating fish twice a week as part of a healthy diet. Wild salmon usually has more omega-3 fatty acids than farm-raised salmon. Wild salmon is also preferred over farm-raised salmon because of chemicals that may be present in farm-raised fish. For more on wild salmon versus farm-raised, see Chapter 11.

Berries

Berries are a good source of fiber, vitamin C, ellagic acid, and the phyochemical anthocyanidins, which give many berries their distinctive color. They also contain catechins and the bioflavonoid quercetin.

Berries have garnered considerable media attention regarding their numerous health benefits for a variety of ailments. For example, blueberries have been reported to help reduce memory loss as we age, whereas cranberries are often touted to help with urinary tract infections. They've also shown some potentially positive results in the cancer arena in animal and laboratory studies.

We don't really know yet whether berries can help fight cancer, but we do know that all berries are high in antioxidants and phytochemicals, both of which may help promote the health of all the cells in your body. If you can, try to incorporate 1 cup of berries into your diet on a daily basis. They work great in smoothies, mixed into yogurt, tossed in a salad, or eaten directly out of hand.

Yogurt or kefir

Both yogurt and kefir are good sources of protein from whey, which may help with muscle maintenance and immunity. The good bacteria called *probiotics* in these foods also help to keep your digestive tract and immune system healthy. In addition, they contain bone-building calcium, which also keeps your cells healthy and may help lower blood pressure. Last but not least, these foods contain butyric acid and conjugated linoleic acid (CLA), which, in addition to supporting the immune system, may help to reduce the risk of cancer.

When buying yogurt or kefir, look for low-fat, plain versions and add your own flavors to reduce sugar content. You can mix in some berries and honey, granola (like our Homemade Granola recipe in Chapter 14), low-sugar jam, nuts, or even a bit of dark chocolate.

Dark chocolate

We saved the best superfood for last! Dark chocolate is a good source of antioxidants, which may help lower blood pressure and protect your heart, and an ounce a day is all it takes to reap the benefits of this superfood without getting too many calories.

In addition, dark chocolate appears to contain compounds that have antidepressant qualities. Because cancer can lead to depression, dark chocolate may be a natural way to get a bit of a boost in the mood department.

When buying dark chocolate, go for the highest percentage of cocoa that is still palatable to you. Commercial dark chocolate bars may contain anywhere from 30 percent to 90 percent cocoa, so 60 percent cocoa may be a good place to start. Just keep in mind that the higher the cocoa content, the lower the sugar content, and the better for you. Of course, the more bitter it will also taste.

Cancer-Fighting Culinary Spices and Herbs

Spices and herbs have long been used for medicinal purposes, such as fighting indigestion and other digestive problems. Although we have a long way to go to understand the direct benefits of consuming certain spices and herbs including with regard to protecting against and fighting cancer and its side effects, their indirect beneficial effects may be more easily recognized.

One such effect is their unique flavor profile, which ranges from strong to mild, with only small amounts needed to create a whole new taste sensation. When cancer-related loss of appetite and taste changes occur, which can lead to undesirable weight loss, adding herbs and spices to your cooking may help stimulate your taste buds and reinvigorate your appetite.

In this section, we look at some culinary herbs and spices that have shown promise with regard to cancer, whether by preventing it, fighting it, or reducing its side effects. Not all effects discussed will be direct, but that doesn't make them any less potent.

Ginger

Ginger is the root of the plant *Zingiber officinale*. It has long been used in folk medicine to treat everything from colds to constipation. Ginger can be used fresh, in powdered form (ginger spice), or candied. Although the flavor between fresh and ground ginger is significantly different, they can be substituted for one another in many recipes. In general, you can replace ⅛ teaspoon of ground ginger with 1 tablespoon of fresh grated ginger, and vice versa.

With regard to cancer, there is some evidence that when ginger dietary supplements are taken with standard anti-nausea medications, ginger can be helpful in reducing chemotherapy-induced nausea and vomiting in some people. Other studies suggest that ginger may help with nausea after surgery, and may also help with indigestion or an otherwise upset stomach. Then there are the studies that lead these results to be questioned by showing no such correlations. Consuming ginger and ginger products, in addition to taking any anti-nausea medications as prescribed, may provide some comfort for a queasy stomach during cancer treatment.

Although the Food and Drug Administration (FDA) considers ginger to be a safe food, you shouldn't load up on over-the-counter ginger supplements or start eating a significant amount of ginger. It's also important to speak to your oncologist or another physician about using ginger. This is particularly essential if you're taking blood-thinning medications like warfarin (Coumadin), because excessive amounts of ginger may increase the risk of bleeding.

Rosemary

Rosemary is a hearty, woody Mediterranean herb that has needlelike leaves and is a good source of antioxidants. Its name means "dew of the sea" in Latin because it can survive with no to very little water, often extracting enough moisture from the sea breeze to live. Because of its origin, rosemary is commonly used in Mediterranean cooking and you'll often see it included as a primary ingredient in Italian seasonings. You can use it to add flavor to soups, tomato-based sauces, bread, and high-protein foods like poultry, beef, and lamb.

Rosemary may help with detoxification; taste changes; indigestion, flatulence, and other digestive problems; and loss of appetite. Try drinking up to 3 cups of rosemary leaf tea daily for help with these problems.

Turmeric (curry)

Turmeric is an herb in the ginger family and is what makes curry yellow and gives it its distinctive flavor. Curcumin appears to be the active compound in turmeric. This compound has demonstrated antioxidant and anti-inflammatory properties, potentially protecting against cancer development. Turmeric extract supplements are currently being studied to see if they have a role in preventing and treating some cancers, including colon, prostate, breast, and skin cancers. Although results appear promising, they have largely been observed in laboratory and animal studies, so it's unclear whether these results will ultimately translate to humans.

Used in curry and other foods, turmeric is considered safe; however, use of turmeric supplements may lead to high concentrations in the blood, increasing the risk of various drug–herb interactions. Taking turmeric supplements is not advised unless under medical supervision, because you may be more prone to experiencing bleeding complications if you're taking blood-thinning medications like warfarin (Coumadin), developing low blood glucose levels if you're taking medications to manage diabetes, or experiencing heartburn despite taking acid-reducing drugs.

Chile peppers

Chile peppers contain capsaicin, a compound that can relieve pain. When capsaicin is applied topically to the skin, it causes the release of a chemical called *substance P.* Upon continued use, the amount of substance P eventually produced in that area decreases, reducing pain in the area. But this doesn't mean you should go rubbing chile peppers where you have pain. Chile peppers need to be handled very carefully, because they can cause burns if they come in contact with the skin. Therefore, if you have pain and want to harness the power of chile peppers, ask your oncologist or physician about prescribing a capsaicin cream. It has shown pretty good results with regard to treating *neuropathic pain* (sharp, shocking pain that follows the path of a nerve) after surgery for cancer.

Another benefit of chile peppers is that they may help with indigestion. Seems counterintuitive, right? But some studies have shown that ingesting small amounts of cayenne may reduce indigestion.

Finally, when you have taste changes, adding some chile peppers or a little cayenne to your cooking can help reawaken your taste buds. You can also try sprinkling on some Tabasco sauce. So, even if you never liked chile peppers, you may enjoy them when facing taste changes.

Garlic

Garlic belongs to the *Allium* class of bulb-shaped plants, which also includes chives, leeks, onions, shallots, and scallions. Garlic has a high sulfur content and is also a good source of arginine, oligosaccharides, flavonoids, and selenium, all of which may be beneficial to health. Garlic's active compound, called *allicin,* gives it its characteristic odor and is produced when garlic bulbs are chopped, crushed, or otherwise damaged.

Several studies suggest that increased garlic intake reduces the risk of cancers of the stomach, colon, esophagus, pancreas, and breast. It appears that garlic may protect against cancer through numerous mechanisms, including by inhibiting bacterial infections and the formation of cancer-causing substances, promoting DNA repair, and inducing cell death. Garlic supports detoxification and may also support the immune system and help reduce blood pressure.

According to the World Health Organization, safe daily doses of garlic for health promotion among adults is approximately one garlic clove, up to 1,200 mg of dried garlic powder, and up to 5 mg of garlic oil. Exceeding these doses can cause garlic to interfere with any medications you're on, as well as blood clotting. This is also a reason garlic supplements should be avoided unless specifically prescribed by your doctor.

We recommend getting garlic by using fresh crushed garlic in salad dressings or in cooking, because allicin starts to degrade immediately after it's produced. Garlic goes well with most protein foods, including fish.

Peppermint

Peppermint is a natural hybrid cross between water mint and spearmint. It has been used for thousands of years as a digestive aid to relieve gas, indigestion, cramps, and diarrhea. It may also help with symptoms of irritable bowel syndrome and food poisoning. Peppermint appears to calm the muscles of the stomach and improve the flow of bile, enabling food to pass through the stomach more quickly.

If your cancer or treatment is causing an upset stomach, try drinking a cup of peppermint tea. Many commercial varieties are on the market, or you can make your own by boiling dried peppermint leaves in water or adding fresh leaves to boiled water and letting them steep for a few minutes until the tea reaches the desired strength.

Peppermint can also soothe a sore throat. For this reason, it is also sometimes used to relieve the painful mouth sores that can occur from chemotherapy and radiation, or is a key ingredient in treatments for this condition. However, you should not use peppermint oil before discussing with your oncologist.

Like other herbs, peppermint can interfere with certain medications. For example, combining peppermint oil with cyclosporine (Neoral, Sandimmune), a drug that suppresses the immune system after hematopoietic stem cell transplant, can lead to higher concentrations of this agent in the blood. That's why getting peppermint from food sources is better than using dietary supplements.

Chamomile

Chamomile is a daisy-like plant native to Europe, Asia, and Northern Africa. There are two distinct varieties of chamomile: German and Roman. Both are thought to have similar medicinal benefits and have been used throughout history to treat a variety of conditions. The Egyptians used chamomile to treat fevers, whereas the ancient Greeks and Romans used it for headaches and a variety of intestinal problems.

Chamomile may help with sleep issues; if sleep is a problem for you, try drinking a strong chamomile tea shortly before bedtime.

Chamomile mouthwash has also been studied for preventing and treating mouth sores from chemotherapy and radiation therapy. Although the results are mixed, there is no harm in giving it a try, provided your oncologist is not opposed. If given the green light, simply make the tea, let it cool, and rinse and gargle as often as desired.

Chamomile tea may be another way to manage digestive problems, including stomach cramps. Chamomile appears to help relax muscle contractions, particularly the smooth muscles of the intestines.

Don't consume more than 3 cups of chamomile tea per day to avoid interactions with medications, such as blood-thinning medications. Again, talk with your healthcare team about anything you're consuming, including chamomile.

Protecting Against Food–Drug and Herb–Drug Interactions

You may have heard that certain drugs shouldn't be taken with grapefruit juice. But grapefruit juice isn't the only food that can cause a drug interaction. A vast variety of foods and herbs can decrease a drug's effectiveness or may make the drug's effects more potent. And as you age, your ability to metabolize drugs also changes, so if you're older, this is another factor to keep in mind.

Now, it would be impossible for us to list every possible food–drug and herb–drug interaction, even if we had the space to do so. In some cases, we may not even know yet whether a particular food or herb can pose a problem. New cases describing such events are always popping up in the literature. But here are some steps you can take to minimize risk:

✔ **Consume foods in normal amounts, and use herbs and spices moderately, particularly if you're taking any medications.** Herbs and spices are concentrated foods, so they should be used moderately. This means you shouldn't eat an excessive amount of these foods daily or use them for days on end, unless you're just adding them to your cooking as you normally would. Ideally, rotating the healthy foods that you eat and the herbs and spices that you use is the best way to prevent interactions while ensuring you get the broadest range of cancer-fighting nutrients.

✔ **Unless specifically prescribed by or discussed with your doctor, don't use dietary supplements, which may include capsules, pills, or even oils (if ingested).** Supplements are poorly controlled and can easily lead to interactions, because they generally contain a high concentration of active compounds.

✔ **If you're cleared to take a dietary supplement, only take it according to the package instructions or as prescribed.** Don't take large doses without discussing this with your physician or healthcare team.

✔ **Always talk with your physician or healthcare team if you're on any medications and plan on changing your diet.** This is important because your doctor knows which medications you're on and whether there are any foods you should avoid.

✔ **Do some research to educate yourself.** Several online resources are available by subscription for a minimal cost. A couple examples are ConsumerLab.com (`www.consumerlab.com`) and the Natural Medicines Comprehensive Database (`http://naturaldatabase.therapeuticresearch.com`). Also, some cancer centers, universities, or medical organizations, have information that is accurate and vetted on their websites free of charge. If you're unsure about the information you find, talk to your healthcare team.

Chapter 9

Cooking with the Proper Tools and Techniques

In This Chapter

▶ Identifying which tools are safest for food preparation and storage

▶ Discovering tools that simplify food preparation

▶ Getting a handle on clean cooking methods

*A*fter you've stocked your kitchen with wholesome, cancer-fighting foods, it's time to get cooking! Although this task may seem daunting, particularly if you've spent more time at restaurants than in your kitchen, cooking at home is one of the best things you can do for your and your family's health. When you're involved in selecting and preparing your foods, even if it's from the sidelines (maybe your partner wears the chef's hat), you'll know exactly what's in each bite. And in addition to avoiding unwholesome eats, you won't have to worry about what may be going on behind closed doors at some restaurant kitchen.

Are you now thinking, "That's great, but I just don't know if I have the time or energy to do this"? Guess what? No matter who does the cooking in your household, there's no need for that person to be tethered to the stove. Although there are no cooking robots to be had just yet, there are many tools and gadgets that can make it significantly easier and less time-consuming for you to prepare wholesome meals and to keep those foods fresh and safe.

In this chapter, we show you some must-have kitchen equipment, from items that keep foods safe from pathogens and environmental toxins to gadgets that ease food preparation. After you get a handle on the equipment, we look at some clean food preparation methods. Before you know it, you'll be a clean-eating, cancer-fighting chef.

The Importance of Gearing Up

When you're exhausted from treatment or even the daily grind, you may be too tired to chop a bunch of vegetables, constantly check on the meat baking in the oven, or deal with cleaning multiple pots and dishes. And if you have containers or cookware that are damaged, you may be inadvertently exposing your wholesome eats to cancer-causing substances. To avoid such issues, it's important to have all the right gear at your disposal and to know how to use and evaluate it on a regular basis for safety issues.

In this section, we examine safety issues surrounding some popular kitchen gear. We also look at healthy cookware and gear and gadgets that can make your life in the kitchen easier. With a well-equipped kitchen, your foray into clean eating will go down as smoothly as a milkshake.

Being aware of potential safety issues

These days it seems a new paranoia-inducing report comes out every other day announcing some new *carcinogen* (cancer-causing agent) we need to be aware of. Fortunately, our bodies generally do a really good job keeping us safe from all the potential toxins we're exposed to on a daily basis. If it didn't, we'd have very short life expectancies. Although numerous factors can impact whether a toxin actually causes harm — including the extent of your exposure; how you're exposed; and your age, sex, diet, genes, lifestyle, and general health — you don't want to be oblivious to potential risks or ignore them either, particularly if you can be proactive in taking steps to avoid them.

What follows are some popular kitchen items for which safety concerns have been reported, but if these items are used appropriately and properly maintained, they should pose minimal, if any, risks. So, in the following sections, we examine their potential risks and how you can avoid or minimize them to keep your kitchen safe.

Although it's important to consider and evaluate all health risks to the fullest extent possible, you can't become paralyzed by them. If your cooking tools and vessels are not damaged, discolored, or old (manufactured at a time when lead was commonly used in ceramic glazes), any potential risks should be minimal.

Aluminum cookware

Plain aluminum cookware is inexpensive, lightweight, and thermally responsive, so it's no wonder that a considerable amount of cookware sold today uses this metal. Its potential safety hazard lies in its reactivity. As foods cook, particularly acidic foods like tomato sauce, they can pick up aluminum particles that are then ingested. Some studies have indicated that aluminum exposure can lead to Alzheimer's disease or even cancer, but the findings have been tenuous.

Still, if you want to reduce your risk, consider using stainless steel instead, or avoid cooking acidic foods in aluminum pots. You can also look for anodized aluminum cookware, which treats the cookware to produce a nonstick, scratch-resistant cooking surface that prevents the aluminum from getting into food. But as with all nonstick coatings, you need to make sure it doesn't get scratched up, compromising safety. One way to protect your cookware is to use utensils that are less likely to damage it, such as those made of wood or plastic, rather than metal.

Ceramic and enamel cookware and dishes

Some ceramic and enamel cookware and dishes can be very safe, but it depends on when and where they were produced, as well as which compounds were used to produce their glazing. Older ceramic and enamel cookware may contain lead in their glaze, which can leach out into food and slowly cause lead poisoning. So, if you inherited a colorful ceramic teapot from your grandmother, it's best displayed decoratively. The same is true for ceramic and enamel cookware and dishes made in foreign countries that don't have strict safety regulations, such as China, India, Mexico, India, and Hong Kong.

To enhance safety, look for American- or Canadian-made ceramic and enamel cookware from larger companies; make sure the product is labeled as being safe for food or for cooking; avoid using the product with acidic foods; and prevent the glaze from wearing down by handling the product carefully, such as by hand washing it, not using steel wool on it, and not using metal or other abrasive utensils to scoop food out of it.

Cookware and bakeware with nonstick coatings

Nonstick cookware is convenient, because it's easier to clean and also helps cut down on the amount of fat needed in cooking, but if nonstick coatings become damaged or scratched, they may release little bits of inert plastic and other toxins into the food as it's being cooked. When heated over high heat, the coatings may also release toxic gases that contain carcinogens. Upon inhalation, these gases may cause lung injury. Breathing gases produced by Teflon, for instance, has been associated with a condition called *polymer fume fever,* in which a fever and flu-like symptoms occur four to eight hours after exposure.

To maximize safety, when using nonstick cookware and bakeware, look for nonstick coatings that don't use perfluorooctanoic acid (PFOA) or polytetra-fluoroethylene (PTFE). There are an abundance of nonstick coatings, so do your research. Currently, some nonstick coatings that may be safer include Thermolon (Green Pan), SandFlow (Farberware), and anodized aluminum. Regardless of which coatings your cookware or bakeware features, don't heat them over high heat; use low or medium heat for cooking. When any damage becomes noticeable, such as scratches or gouges, toss them. Because such cookware can scratch easily, handle it with care. Don't use abrasive cleaners on them, like steel wool.

Copper cookware

Cookware made from 100 percent copper is very expensive and can leach copper onto foods. Although copper is an essential mineral that is currently deficient in many U.S. diets, routine use of copper cookware can lead to copper toxicity over time (but no increased cancer risk).

To reduce the likelihood of copper toxicity, use copper cookware sparingly or buy copper cookware that is buffered by stainless steel. Also, avoid cooking acidic foods in copper vessels, because they're more likely to react with the copper.

Plastic containers

Most people have at least one cabinet full of reusable plastic containers to store food in. These containers are lightweight, don't break when dropped, and are inexpensive, making them an ideal choice. But there have been concerns about these containers releasing carcinogenic- and hormone-disrupting compounds such as bisphenol A (BPA) onto the foods stored in them.

Not all plastics are created equal. Plastics are classified by the type of resin they use. The resins that appear to pose the least risk are #1PET, #2HDPE, #4LDPE, and #5PP. To reduce risks, look for containers with these markings on the bottom or inside of the container. If you don't see these markings, check if the container is recyclable. If it is, then it's likely made with a lower-risk resin. Other strategies you can use to further minimize risk include discarding any containers that are damaged, stained, or cloudy; avoiding heating foods in plastic containers; and avoiding single-use plastic containers, which are generally made from less safe resins.

Silicone bakeware

Silicone is a synthetic rubber made of bonded *silicon* (a natural element abundant in sand and rock) and oxygen. It has become popular for bakeware because it's flexible, strong, and comes in lots of colors and shapes. But although the Food and Drug Administration (FDA) has approved silicone as a food-safe substance, there have been anecdotal reports of dyes and of silicone oil oozing out of overheated silicone cookware and of odors being emitted from them. The FDA also hasn't conducted any comprehensive studies to determine whether silicone can leach out of cookware and potentially contaminate food.

If you decide to give this bakeware a try, be sure to buy from a reputable brand, and not an inexpensive unknown manufacturer, and carefully follow the manufacturer's care and use instructions.

Stocking your kitchen with healthy gear

When you're making clean foods, you want those foods to stay as clean and free from toxins as possible. And just as with clean foods, the healthiest kitchen gear is constructed from materials as close to nature as possible. Now, this doesn't mean these items don't pose any risks. After all, just because something is natural doesn't mean it's healthy or risk-free, but the risks are generally lower.

What follows are some kitchen items that are considered safer, along with any risks they may pose and how to minimize these risks.

Bamboo and wooden utensils

You can't get more natural than bamboo and wood. These items won't transfer any carcinogenic or toxic substances to your foods, and they're naturally resistant to bacteria, but they can still pick up pathogens and contaminate foods if not used properly.

To prevent this from happening, never let a utensil that has been in contact with raw meat come in contact with a cooked or ready-to-eat food. Also, look for bamboo or hardwoods when buying such utensils, rather than soft woods, because these are more resilient and not as prone to splitting or deterioration from moisture. Many bamboo and wooden utensils are coated with a food-safe mineral oil, which provides another layer of protection against bacteria. Care is simple — some mild dish detergent and hot water are all that's needed.

Cast-iron cookware

Unlike the metals released by other cookware, iron is considered a healthy food additive by the FDA. Therefore, having iron from this cookware leach into food is generally considered beneficial, particularly because many people are iron deficient. And when you have certain types of cancer or are receiving chemotherapy or other treatments, you may be particularly vulnerable to iron-deficiency anemia. On the other hand, if you have *hemochromatosis* (your body stores too much iron), cast iron use is contraindicated.

If you're experiencing taste changes from your cancer treatment, you may want to avoid cooking any acidic foods using cast-iron cookware, because these foods may pick up a metallic taste, making them particularly unpalatable. More iron is also picked up the longer a food cooks, and newer cookware is more likely to release iron than well-seasoned cookware.

A drawback of cast iron is that it's higher maintenance. The cookware needs to be seasoned before it's first used. This process creates a nonstick coating by infusing the cookware with oil or grease, which can be done by coating it with cooking oil and baking in a 350-degree oven for an hour, repeating this process as needed to maintain the nonstick coating. The cookware is best cleaned by being rinsed with hot water immediately after cooking. Burned-on food can be removed with a mild abrasive, like coarse salt, and a nonmetal brush. If rust appears, you can use steel wool to remove it and then re-season the pan.

Glass bakeware and food storage solutions

Glass bakeware and food storage containers won't release any toxins, nor will they react with any foods. They're also easy to maintain and dishwasher safe. The main safety hazards posed by glassware include breakage from an impact or a sudden temperature change.

Pyrex offers a wide variety of glass bakeware and food storage solutions, including food storage containers with glass lids that feature a silicone rim, which is a good solution if you want to eliminate the plastic lids featured by most glass food storage containers. The benefit of using glass storage solutions is that you can bake, store, reheat, and serve food all by using the same dish. You can also easily grab a dish for a transportable lunch.

Wooden cutting boards

Although the jury is still out regarding which type of cutting board is best, wood appears to be favorable due to its naturally antibacterial properties. Studies indicate that wood pulls bacteria deep below its surface, keeping them well away from foods. In contrast, bacteria on plastic cutting boards sometimes linger on the surface even after properly cleaned, particularly as these boards become scarred from all the knife action.

Regardless of which cutting boards you choose, you should always have at least two of them to optimize food safety: one for fruits, vegetables, bread, and anything that can be safely eaten raw, and the other just for cutting raw meats, poultry, and fish.

Stainless-steel cookware

Stainless steel mixes steel with chromium and nickel to produce a corrosion-resistant metal that is durable and easy to clean. Stainless steel is a great choice for healthy cooking because it's one of the most inert metals, although some reports indicate that it may leach a small amount of nickel or chromium. The chromium leaching may provide some benefits because it's needed in trace amounts and many people are deficient in this mineral. As for the nickel, because the stainless steel is more stable than many other cookware metals, the likelihood of it leaching nickel is low. One drawback of stainless steel is that it doesn't conduct heat evenly, but you can find some stainless steel cookware with an inner core of aluminum or copper or a copper-clad bottom to address this. Because these metals don't come in contact with the food, they're a safe option as well.

Go-go-gadget!: Making your life easier with some simple kitchen tools

If you've ever gone into a kitchen store, you may have found the number of available culinary gadgets and tools overwhelming — there's a gadget or tool for almost every purpose. Some tools are designed to fill very specific needs that likely won't arise very frequently, like the strawberry stem remover. But if you're going to eat clean and optimize your intake of cancer-fighting nutrients, there are gadgets and tools that you may turn to time and time again to help with the prep in the kitchen.

What follows are some gadgets you should consider adding to your cancer-fighting kitchen if you don't already have them.

Blender

Blenders are great for whipping up smoothies, sauces, spreads, and even soups. Numerous different types of blenders are on the market, including

- ✔ **Individual-sized blenders:** Individual-sized blenders with transportable cups are worth the investment if you make a lot of smoothies, have difficulty eating solid foods, or need to get extra calories in your diet due to cancer-related weight loss.

- ✔ **Immersion blenders:** Immersion blenders enable you to blend items in the container they're being prepared in. They're especially handy for making creamy soups, sauces, and batters.

✓ **Traditional blenders:** If you want an all-purpose blender, then a traditional blender is the way to go. When shopping for a traditional blender, look for these features:

- A heavy base to stabilize the blender

- A motor of at least 60 Hz for sufficient ability to blend

- A large-capacity glass beaker to prevent toxin issues with plastic resins

- A two-piece lid to ensure you can add ingredients during the blending process

- The ability to select a variety of speeds or to *pulse* (blend in bursts) ingredients

Coffee grinder

Coffee grinders are great for grinding more than coffee beans and can be used to grind spices, flaxseeds, nuts, and small grains (like rice) to produce a flour. This can be a good way to ensure quality control and for you to get the freshest ingredients. After all, spices you grind fresh will have a lot more aroma and flavor than already-ground versions at the supermarket. And if you have a gluten allergy, for instance, grinding your own rice flour can help to reduce cross-contamination issues.

Digital cooking thermometer

A digital cooking thermometer is a great way to ensure your meat doesn't overcook, making it dry and unpalatable, but also isn't undercooked, posing a health risk. These thermometers generally feature a stainless-steel probe that goes into the meat and that's connected to a digital display via a cable. An alarm sounds when the meat reaches the perfect temperature.

Food processor

Many healthy recipes, including in this book, call for a variety of fresh vegetables and other ingredients chopped, ground, minced, sliced, or shredded. Instead of doing all this work by hand, which can be tiring, toss the ingredients directly into a food processor, and you'll be done dicing and slicing in the blink of an eye.

Although you can process some foods in a blender, blenders really puree ingredients and often require the addition of liquid, so they're not a suitable substitute for a food processor.

Look for units with a heavy base, large capacity, wide feed tube, simple controls with a variety of speeds, and safety features (such as a lid that must lock with the base before the unit turns on).

Slow cooker

Cooking can't get much simpler than a slow cooker. Just toss your ingredients in the slow cooker in the morning, set the timer, and when you come home in the evening, a nice hot meal is waiting for you. Slow cookers are particularly great for making chili, soups, and stews. When buying a slow cooker, look for one with a removable stoneware insert to ease cleaning and with a clear lid to enable monitoring during the cooking process.

Do not use abrasive utensils, such as those made of metal, to remove or shift contents in a slow cooker. You don't want to damage the stoneware glaze. In addition, when you use your slow cooker, avoid extended heat-up and cool-down periods to prevent foodborne illnesses. You can achieve this by setting the cooker on high for at least the first hour of cooking and making sure that cooking temperatures reach the safety zone for the food being cooked.

Steamer basket

A steamer basket is a specially designed basket that fits right inside a pot and keeps food above the water's surface, enabling steam from the boiling water below to cook the food. Not only is this cooking method a speedy and simple way to cook, but it enables foods to retain their nutrients because they don't leach out into any cooking liquid. Look for a steamer basket made of stainless steel.

You can also buy steamer baskets specifically made for the microwave. These are constructed of plastic, so look for versions that are BPA-free.

Oil sprayer/spritzer

To keep your food from sticking and to get a healthy dose of monounsaturated and polyunsaturated fats, you'll want to use plant-based oils in some of your cooking. But instead of pouring large amounts of oil into the pan, you can use an oil sprayer or spritzer to evenly disperse a much smaller amount. Although you can buy a variety of nonstick sprays in the grocery store, a refillable sprayer enables you to know exactly what you're getting (no propellants or chemicals), there won't be any gummy film accumulating on your cookware, and the taste is far superior. Look for one made of stainless steel.

Clean Cooking Methods

Now that you have your cancer-fighting foods on hand and the right equipment to prepare them, you want to get to cooking them. But if you're new to cooking or even to healthy cooking, suddenly immersing yourself in new techniques can be intimidating. Don't worry! In this section, we break down some of the most common healthy cooking techniques and how they work so you'll be cooking like a clean eating guru before you know it!

Baking

This technique cooks food by surrounding it with dry heat in an oven. Everything from lean proteins, to starches, to produce can be cooked by baking. To get started, preheat your oven by turning it on and allowing it to warm to the desired temperature. After your dish is prepared and placed in an oven-safe vessel, place it in the fully preheated oven for the amount of time the recipe calls for.

Ovens can run hotter or cooler than their temperature gauge indicates, which can impact your recipe. To ensure a proper cooking temperature, use an oven thermometer placed inside the oven to check the temperature. These thermometers are typically hung on an oven rack.

Boiling

Boiling cooks foods immersed in a liquid. Two methods are generally used to boil foods. They can be placed into already rapidly boiling liquid (usually water) and then have the heat turned down so the food simmers, such as often occurs with pastas. Alternatively, the food can be placed into the pot with a cold liquid, brought to a boil, and cooked until the food is done, as is often done with produce and eggs. Although nutrients do leach out of foods that are boiled, they still retain a lot of their nutrients. This is also a low-fat way to prepare a variety of whole foods when water or a low-fat liquid (like low-fat milk or broth) is used.

When boiling produce, consider reserving the cooking liquid for use as a base for soups and sauces.

Broiling

Broiling cooks foods by placing them very close to the heating element in the oven. Because broiling uses a direct, high heat, it usually only takes a few minutes to cook lean, non-thick cuts of proteins, like fish fillets and chicken breasts.

Start by preheating the broiler for five to seven minutes. Season your meat and place it on a broiler pan or in a shallow baking pan. Then place the pan in the oven about 5 inches from the heat source, or further if the cut is thicker; very thick cuts of meat should not be broiled. Depending on the thickness of the meat, you can turn it over between the five and ten minute mark. Cook the meat on the other side until it reaches the appropriate internal temperature.

Microwaving

Microwaving produces *microwaves,* a form of electromagnetic radiation that causes water molecules in food to vibrate and produce heat, which cooks the food. In the United States, the FDA has strict safety standards that microwave manufacturers must meet, including that radiation emissions not pose a hazard to public health. Some nutrients break down when foods are microwaved (such as vitamin C) because of their exposure to heat, but because cooking times are shorter with microwaves, microwaves may do a better job of preserving nutrients than other cooking methods.

To ensure safety, always follow the manufacturer's instruction manual for recommended operating procedures and safety precautions, and never operate a microwave if the door doesn't close or is damaged or warped.

Stir-frying

This method enables you to quickly cook food (mainly meats, vegetables, and rice or noodles), in a small amount of oil in either a sauté pan or a skillet. To get started, place your pan over a medium-high heat and allow it to warm before adding oil. When the pan is hot, add in just enough healthy oil to lightly cover the bottom of the pan. Once the oil heats, add your ingredients. Keep a close eye on the food, stirring often, to ensure even cooking and to prevent burning.

Steaming

Steaming enables you to cook vegetables to a crisp texture. Wash and cut your vegetables into equal-sized pieces to promote even cooking. Then place a large pot filled with 1 to 2 inches of water over high heat and bring to a boil. Place your steaming basket into the pot, add your vegetables, and cover the pot. Let the vegetables sit in the steam for a few minutes until they achieve the desired tenderness. Remove the lid carefully to prevent the steam from burning your hands, and serve the vegetables immediately.

Making grilling a healthier option

Grilling can occasionally be a healthy cooking method, but you need to be careful. This is because cooking foods — particularly meat, chicken, and fish — at a high temperature over an open flame can lead to the production of several carcinogens, which form in the foods themselves or get deposited on the food from the smoke produced during the cooking process. Although there is little evidence to connect grilled foods to cancer risk in humans, they have been shown to cause cancer in animals. Because it's better to be safe than sorry, here are a few ways you can make grilled, broiled, and even baked foods safer:

✔ **Give preferential treatment to grilled veggies and fruits.** Kebobs that contain small cuts of meat also tend to be safer, because they cook faster and have a lower chance of charring or being exposed to smoke.

✔ **Always use the lowest temperature possible when grilling, baking, or broiling foods, and avoid eating burned or charred meats, poultry, and fish.** In a pinch, you can eat around the charred parts.

✔ **Choose foods prepared with acidic marinades that use lemon juice or vinegar.** These marinades reduce the amount of smoke that sticks to the food's surface, cutting down on the carcinogens. If the marinade contains spicy peppers and other herbs and spices, you'll also benefit from an antioxidant boost.

✔ **Choose leaner cuts of meats, trim all visible fats, and remove the skin from poultry before cooking, because fats char more easily.**

✔ **Prevent meat juices from dripping down onto the heat source.** Strategies include thawing meats before cooking them; precooking meats on high in the microwave for 60 to 90 seconds to reduce their juices; avoiding flattening burgers during cooking and instead flipping them more frequently; and cooking meats on top of aluminum foil or in a foil packet.

Part III
Wholesome Recipes

The Best Sources of Vitamins

	Vegetarian	Nonvegetarian
Vitamin A	Carrots, leafy greens, sweet potatoes	Eggs, cheddar cheese, fortified milk, liver
B-complex*	Beans, leafy greens, nutritional yeast, whole grains	Chicken, eggs, salmon
Vitamin C	Bell peppers, broccoli, papaya, pineapple, strawberries	Liver, oysters
Vitamin D	Shitake mushrooms	Eggs, fortified milk, salmon, sardines
Vitamin E	Almonds, leafy greens, papaya, sunflower seeds	None
Vitamin K	Broccoli, Brussels sprouts, leafy greens, parsley	Eggs, liver

* All the known essential water-soluble vitamins except for vitamin C. These include vitamin B1 (thiamine), vitamin B2 (riboflavin), vitamin B3 (niacin), vitamin B5 (pantothenic acid), vitamin B6 (pyridoxine), vitamin B7 (biotin), vitamin B9 (folic acid), and vitamin B12 (the cobalamins). No single food has all the B-complex vitamins, but the foods listed here contain many members of the B-complex.

Find out how to build your own smoothies in a free article at www.dummies.com/extras/cancernutritionrecipes.

In this part . . .

- Discover why breakfast may be the most important meal of the day.

- See what constitutes a complete meal, whether you're preparing an entrée with sides or a one-dish meal.

- Improve your nutrition and beat treatment-related side effects with snacks, whether you whip up a snack to go or a spread to please a crowd.

- Nourish your body while satisfying even the most ravenous sweet tooth.

Chapter 10

Invigorating Breakfasts

*P*eople generally belong to one of two camps: breakfast lovers and breakfast skippers. If you're a breakfast lover, you probably don't need any convincing that breakfast is a very important meal. But if you're used to plowing through your morning without eating until lunch, this is a habit you may want to reconsider, and this chapter gives you some food for thought (pun intended) on that front. After we convince you of the many benefits that a wholesome breakfast provides, we offer more than a dozen recipes to get you started.

Now, we recognize there are times when eating may be difficult due to cancer or its treatments, making it tempting to skip breakfast — even if breakfast is a meal you typically enjoy. But it's important to make every effort to nourish yourself to the fullest extent possible during such times, including when it comes to breakfast. In addition, making sure you have food in your stomach first thing in the morning can help ease some side effects. One way to get nutrients during such times is via smoothies, which are easier to consume and digest and require very little effort to prepare. We include two smoothie recipes in this chapter to get you started.

And even if eating isn't an issue, we realize you may have very little energy to prepare meals. Most of the recipes we include in this chapter are easy to prepare. If you find a recipe to be too involved, you can reserve it for times when you have more energy, or ask a loved one to prepare it for you. You can also consider preparing some of the recipes in advance and freezing or refrigerating them for later consumption. Just remember to wrap them well and label them so that they stay fresh and you don't end up eating something that has long since expired. The last thing you need to contend with is a food-borne illness.

Why Breakfast Matters

Cancer and its treatments can suck all the energy right out of you, leaving you wondering how to get your energy back. Although a good night's sleep and relaxation can be important in giving you energy while enabling your body to recover, another important source of energy is food. And if you're fortunate enough to get a good night's sleep, you've gone a long stretch of time without eating. So, it's important to "break" the "fast" (get it?) and fuel up with breakfast to help bolster the energy that sleep has granted you.

In addition to providing energy, studies have shown that eating breakfast promotes the ability to perform tasks better and provides a sense of well-being. Cancer and its treatments can impede your ability to perform the activities of daily life and rob you of a sense of well-being, but eating breakfast may help offset some of these effects. Also, putting the right food in your stomach when you get up in the morning may help combat some side effects, like an upset stomach from treatment.

Another benefit of breakfast is that it reduces the risk of becoming overweight or obese, both of which are risk factors for cancer, including cancer recurrence and secondary cancers.

It's unclear how eating breakfast prevents obesity, but a variety of interrelated factors are probably at work. For example, some studies have shown that people who skip breakfast eat more calories throughout the rest of the day, whereas other studies have found that eating fewer, larger meals can lead to more fat accumulation, even if the same amount of calories are eaten throughout the day via smaller, more frequent meals.

Breakfast is also a good way to consume fiber, which can help you feel full longer, causing you to eat less throughout the day. Because most people only eat half the fiber they should, breakfast is a good way to try to fill that gap (provided you aren't on a low-fiber diet for diarrhea or other gastrointestinal issues).

Finally, when you first wake up, because you've gone many hours without eating, you're in a catabolic state. This means your valuable muscle tissue may be broken down for nutrients. Breakfast stops this process. There's also some research to suggest that eating first thing in the morning may help lower your liver's production of harmful low density lipoprotein (LDL) cholesterol and improve your insulin response.

So, as you can see, breakfast is a very important meal for a variety of reasons and shouldn't be skipped. Even if you don't feel like preparing any recipes in this book, we encourage you to eat a little something in the morning. A bowl of whole-grain cereal, some yogurt, and a piece of fruit, or a whole-grain piece of bread with some nut butter and/or fruit spread can make for a good breakfast.

If you don't care for traditional breakfast fare, that's fine, too. Take a look at some of the other recipe chapters in this book to see if anything inspires you. Chapters 14 and 15, which offer recipes for snacks and desserts, may be good places to start.

Filling Up on Whole Grains

Breakfast foods often feature grains. After all, most of us have eaten cereal, bread, pancakes, or other baked goods in the morning, all of which contain a variety of grains. When these foods contain all components of a grain, including the germ, endosperm, and bran, they're considered *whole grains.* Compared with refined grains, which strip away the germ and bran, whole grains provide more nutrients and fiber, so those are the grains you should give preferential treatment to when you can.

Because whole grains digest slowly, they can keep you feeling satisfied until lunch. Now, just because whole grains are nutrient dense doesn't mean they create foods that are dense. So, if you think eating whole grains means you'll be eating a bunch of gritty and dense foods, we think you'll be pleasantly surprised when you try the whole-grain recipes in this chapter. Many of these whole-grain recipes also contain some fruits and healthy sources of fats, including some omega-3s from walnuts, wheat germ, and even flax.

Some people have an intolerance or sensitivity to *gluten,* the protein portion of some grains, such as wheat, rye, barley, and even oats if they've been contaminated with gluten during preparation. If you're on a gluten-free diet, you should be able to use the Warm Blueberry and Pumpkin Spice Quinoa recipe, as well as the following oat recipes (provided you buy gluten-free oats): Soothing Apple Cinnamon Oatmeal, Breakfast Cookies, Unchunky Monkey Baked Oatmeal, and Overnight Raspberry Icebox Oatmeal. Also, most of the recipes in the "Finding Satisfaction with Fruits and Vegetables" section in this chapter will be okay for you.

Whole-Wheat Blender Batter Waffles or Pancakes

Prep time: 5 min • **Cook time:** 12–15 min • **Yield:** 4 servings

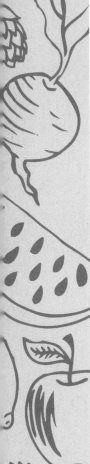

Ingredients	Directions
¾ **cup whole-wheat flour**	**1** Add all ingredients to a blender, and blend until well combined.
1½ **teaspoons baking powder**	
1 teaspoon cinnamon	**2** Set aside.
3 tablespoons liquid egg whites (or 1 whole egg)	**3** *For pancakes:* Spray a griddle with cooking spray, and heat until hot. (Drops of water will quickly and noisily evaporate if dropped on the griddle.) Pour the desired amount onto the griddle. When bubbles start to form on the pancake, flip it with a spatula, and cook the other side until browned. Cook the remaining batter the same way.
1 teaspoon honey	
1 tablespoon olive oil	
1 cup milk	
	For waffles: Spray a nonstick waffle iron with cooking spray. Then pour approximately one-quarter of the mixture into the waffle iron and cook for approximately 2 to 3 minutes, or until the waffle iron indicates that the waffle is done. Remove and keep warm. Cook the remaining batter the same way.

Per serving: Calories 156 (From Fat 53); Fat 6g (Saturated 2g); Cholesterol 8mg; Sodium 192mg; Carbohydrate 21g (Dietary Fiber 3g); Protein 6g.

Vary It! If you don't like cinnamon, feel free to omit it. You can also add 1 teaspoon of vanilla to the batter if you like.

Tip: Get an additional nutrient boost by topping these pancakes or waffles with warmed applesauce, fruit puree, berries, yogurt, or a nut butter.

Breakfast Cookies (Chapter 10), Pomegranate Antioxidant Smoothie (Chapter 10), and Simple Vegetable Omelet (Chapter 10)

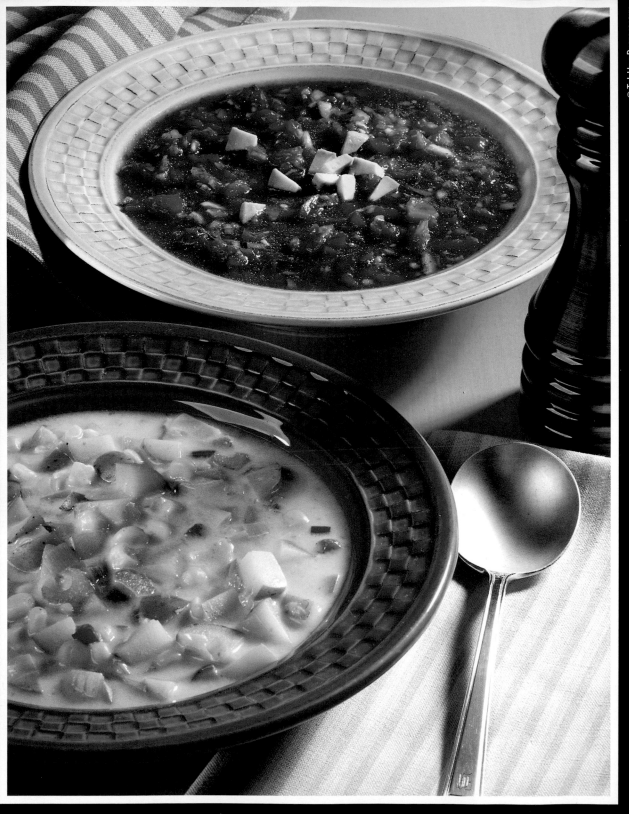

Refreshing Gazpacho (Chapter 11) and Potato, Leek, and Corn Soup (Chapter 11)

Pasta Salad with Pecans and Grapes (Chapter 13), Crispy Kicked-Up Multi-Grain Chicken (Chapter 12), and Gingered Honey-Glazed Carrots (Chapter 13)

Orange-Glazed Asparagus (Chapter 13) and Easy Baked Salmon (Chapter 12)

Balsamic Green Beans (Chapter 13), Moroccan Shrimp (Chapter 12), and Confetti Couscous (Chapter 13)

Onion and Garlic Roasted Chickpeas (Chapter 14), Homemade Granola (Chapter 14), and Fruit and Nut Trail Mix (Chapter 14)

Vibrant Fruit Salsa with Cinnamon Chips (Chapter 14) and Garden Guacamole (Chapter 14)

Super Antioxidant Peach Raspberry Crisp (Chapter 15), Gingered Fruit Salad (Chapter 15), and Chilled Minty Strawberry Soup (Chapter 15)

Whole-Wheat Pumpkin Pie Muffins

Prep time: 10 min • **Cook time:** 18 min • **Yield:** 12 muffins

Ingredients	*Directions*
1½ **cups whole-wheat flour**	*1* Preheat the oven to 350 degrees.
½ **cup packed brown sugar**	*2* Grease a 12-cup muffin pan or line with paper liners.
½ **teaspoon cinnamon**	
¼ **teaspoon ground cloves**	*3* In a large bowl, stir together the whole-wheat flour, brown sugar, cinnamon, cloves, ginger, baking powder, baking soda, and salt.
¼ **teaspoon ground ginger**	
¼ **teaspoon baking powder**	
½ **teaspoon baking soda**	*4* Make a well in the center, and add the eggs, pumpkin, oil, and honey.
½ **teaspoon salt**	
2 **eggs**	*5* Mix just until the dry ingredients are absorbed.
1 **cup canned pumpkin**	*6* Divide dough evenly between the muffin cups.
½ **cup canola oil**	
½ **cup honey**	*7* Bake for 18 minutes, or until the tops spring back when lightly touched.
	8 Cool in the pan before removing the muffins.

Per serving: Calories 230 (From Fat 95); Fat 11g (Saturated 1g); Cholesterol 31mg; Sodium 174mg; Carbohydrate 33g (Dietary Fiber 3g); Protein 4g.

Storing whole-wheat flour

Properly storing whole-wheat flour is important, because it can become rancid very quickly. You can tell your flour has gone rancid if it has a strong oily or moldy odor. Whole-wheat flour should have very little, if any, smell. You're unlikely to get sick if you eat whole-wheat flour that has turned, but it won't taste good.

The best place to store your whole-wheat flour is in the freezer. For ultimate freshness, place the flour in an airtight container or bag. Stored this way, the flour should last for at least six months. When you need the flour for a recipe, let it sit at room temperature for approximately 15 minutes before use.

Warm Blueberry and Pumpkin Spice Quinoa

Prep time: 5 min • **Cook time:** 25 min • **Yield:** 4 servings

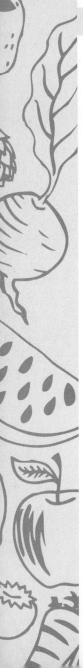

Ingredients	Directions
1 cup skim milk or soymilk	**1** In a medium saucepan, combine the milk, water, and quinoa. Bring to a boil over high heat.
1 cup water	
1 cup quinoa	
2 cups blueberries	**2** Reduce the heat to medium and cover, simmering for 15 minutes or until most of the liquid is absorbed.
½ teaspoon ground pumpkin spice	**3** Turn off the heat and let stand covered for an additional 5 minutes.
4 teaspoons agave nectar	
⅓ cup chopped almonds	**4** Stir in the blueberries and pumpkin spice. Divide into 4 bowls, and garnish each bowl with 1 teaspoon of the agave nectar and 4 teaspoons of the chopped almonds.

Per serving: Calories 287 (From Fat 62); Fat 7g (Saturated 1g); Cholesterol 1mg; Sodium 45mg; Carbohydrate 50g (Dietary Fiber 6g); Protein 10g.

Vary It! If you don't care for blueberries, try another berry or fruit. And if you're not a fan of pumpkin spice, try cinnamon instead.

Soothing Apple Cinnamon Oatmeal

Prep time: 5 min • **Cook time:** 15 min • **Yield:** 2 servings

Ingredients	*Directions*
1 cup milk	*1* In a medium saucepan over medium-high heat, bring the milk and water to a boil.
½ cup water	
¾ cup uncooked rolled oats	*2* Mix in the oats, and then add the applesauce, wheat germ, cinnamon, and maple syrup. Mix well.
½ cup unsweetened applesauce	
2 tablespoons wheat germ	*3* Return to a boil. Then reduce the heat and simmer for 8 to 10 minutes or until the oatmeal reaches the desired consistency. For thinner oatmeal, add more water.
½ teaspoon cinnamon	
1 teaspoon pure maple syrup	

Per serving: Calories 243 (From Fat 56); Fat 6g (Saturated 3g); Cholesterol 17mg; Sodium 63mg; Carbohydrate 39g (Dietary Fiber 5g); Protein 10g.

Vary It! If you don't care for apples, mix in another fruit instead, like blueberries, raspberries, or bananas.

Tip: Add an additional nutrient boost by sprinkling with some chopped nuts or mixing in a little flaxseed oil, ground flaxseed, or whey protein.

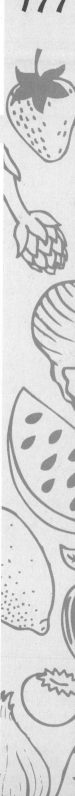

Breakfast Cookies

Prep time: 10 min • **Cook time:** 15–20 min • **Yield:** 4 servings

Ingredients

¾ cup whole-wheat flour

¼ teaspoon salt

¼ teaspoon baking soda

½ teaspoon cinnamon

¼ teaspoon ground allspice

1 cup uncooked quick-cooking oats

⅓ cup dried cranberries

¼ cup chopped walnuts

1 large egg white

3 tablespoons unsweetened applesauce

½ cup dark brown sugar

1 small banana, peeled and cut into 1-inch pieces

1 teaspoon vanilla extract

Directions

1 Preheat oven to 400 degrees, and line baking sheets with parchment paper.

2 In a mixing bowl, whisk together the whole-wheat flour, salt, baking soda, cinnamon, and allspice. Mix in the oats, cranberries, and walnuts. Set aside.

3 In a blender on medium speed, mix the egg white, applesauce, and brown sugar until smooth. Then blend in the banana and vanilla until smooth.

4 Pour the banana mixture into the bowl with the dry ingredients, mixing with a spatula until well combined. The batter will be fairly stiff.

5 Drop the batter by spoonfuls onto the baking sheets, spacing each drop about 2 inches apart, for a total of 12 cookies. Flatten them slightly with the back of a wet spoon, wetting the spoon frequently between cookies.

6 Bake for 10 minutes in a preheated oven.

7 Turn the pans 180 degrees to enable even baking and bake an additional 5 to 8 minutes or until the cookies are golden brown and almost firm in the center when pressed with a finger.

Per serving: Calories 375 (From Fat 61); Fat 7g (Saturated 1g); Cholesterol 0mg; Sodium 251mg; Carbohydrate 74g (Dietary Fiber 7g); Protein 9g.

Unchunky Monkey Baked Oatmeal

Prep time: 10 min • **Cook time:** 40 min • **Yield:** 9 servings

Ingredients	*Directions*
1 ripe banana, peeled	**1** Preheat the oven to 350 degrees and spray an 8-x-8-inch pan with nonstick cooking spray.
⅓ cup honey	
2 cups milk	**2** Mash the banana in a bowl. Then add the honey, milk, vanilla, and flaxseed oil to it and mix until well combined.
2 teaspoons vanilla paste or extract	
1 tablespoon flax seed oil (optional)	**3** Add the oats, nuts, and dark chocolate and mix well.
2 cups uncooked quick oats	
¼ cup toasted almond slices (or chopped nut of choice)	**4** Pour into the baking pan and bake for approximately 40 minutes, until the middle is set. Remove from oven and cut into bars.
1 ounce dark chocolate chips	

Per serving: Calories 185 (From Fat 47); Fat 5g (Saturated 2g); Cholesterol 7mg; Sodium 35mg; Carbohydrate 30g (Dietary Fiber 3g); Protein 6g.

Vary It! This recipe is very versatile. Feel free to omit the nuts and/or chocolate or add different fruits.

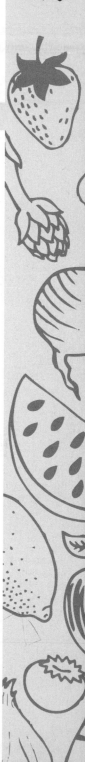

Overnight Raspberry Icebox Oatmeal

Prep time: 5 min • **Yield:** 1 serving

Ingredients	Directions
¼ cup uncooked old-fashioned rolled oats	**1** In a half-pint (1-cup) jar or bowl, combine the oats, milk, yogurt, chia seeds, and honey. If in a jar, put the lid on the jar and shake until well combined; if in a bowl, stir until well combined.
⅓ cup skim milk	
¼ cup low-fat Greek yogurt	
1½ teaspoons chia seeds	**2** Add the raspberries and stir until mixed.
2 teaspoons honey (more or less to taste)	**3** Return the lid to the jar or cover the bowl and refrigerate overnight or up to 2 days. Eat chilled.
¼ to ½ cup fresh or frozen raspberries	

Per serving: Calories 315 (From Fat 39); Fat 4g (Saturated 2g); Cholesterol 5mg; Sodium 63mg; Carbohydrate 61g (Dietary Fiber 6g); Protein 12g.

Vary It! This recipe can be modified to incorporate any fruits you like. You can also consider adding nut butter or flaxseed oil to get more nutrients.

Finding Satisfaction with Fruits and Vegetables

Breakfast is a great time to get in one or more servings of fruits and vegetables. Fruits are the stars of smoothies and can be paired with dairy like yogurt or cottage cheese to create a wholesome and delicious breakfast. Vegetables, particularly greens such as spinach and kale, can also work great in smoothies.

Don't worry if you don't like these veggies — their flavors almost disappear when combined with the other ingredients. Just start with a few leaves and try increasing the amount the next time. If you end up adding too much, you can always add more liquid or more of another ingredient to balance the texture and flavors. That's the great thing with smoothies — you can tinker with them until you get them just right.

For even more great smoothie recipes, check out *Juicing & Smoothies For Dummies,* by Pat Crocker (Wiley).

Another great vehicle for getting vegetables in the morning is eggs. Whether added to an omelet, incorporated into a scramble, or baked into a frittata, vegetables and eggs make a delicious pairing. For a while, eating eggs was considered unhealthy because the yolk contains a considerable amount of cholesterol (approximately 186 mg per egg). As a result, they were thought to increase artery-clogging cholesterol levels. But more recent studies have found no increased risk in heart disease among people who ate one egg a week compared with those who ate more than one egg. Based on such findings, the American Heart Association has deemed consumption of one egg per day acceptable, but if you're concerned about your cholesterol levels, you can substitute whole eggs with egg whites, which have no cholesterol. You can also extend the amount of egg you consume by adding additional whites to a whole egg. You'll see this done in both of the egg-based recipes we include in this chapter.

If you want to use organic ingredients for these recipes, that's great but not necessary. However, you *should* avoid any dairy products that contain recombinant bovine growth hormone (rBGH), which some farmers use to increase their cows' milk production. To avoid rBGH, look for labeling that says "produced without rBGH." You should also look for dairy products from grass-fed cows, so if this means buying organic, this is an area where the investment is worth it. Also, keep in mind that pesticides are more concentrated in the fat of animal products, including dairy products, so choosing low-fat products will help minimize pesticide exposure if you don't buy organic.

Pomegranate Antioxidant Smoothie

Prep time: 5 min • **Yield:** 2 servings

Ingredients	Directions
8 ounces pomegranate juice	**1** In a blender, add the pomegranate juice, strawberries, blackberries, and blood orange. Cover and blend on high until the fruits are well mixed.
¼ cup strawberries	
¼ cup blackberries	
¼ blood orange, peeled	**2** Add the yogurt and crushed ice, and blend on high until the mixture is smooth.
½ cup blueberry yogurt	
1 cup crushed ice	**3** Taste and add agave nectar, maple syrup, or honey, if needed. Start with a tablespoon. If adding the nectar, maple syrup, or honey, blend again. Pour into two glasses and serve immediately.
Agave nectar, pure maple syrup, or honey (optional, to taste)	

Per serving: Calories 172 (From Fat 8); Fat 1g (Saturated 0g); Cholesterol 4mg; Sodium 38mg; Carbohydrate 39g (Dietary Fiber 3g); Protein 3g.

Tropical Tummy-Taming Smoothie

Prep time: 5 min • **Yield:** 4 servings

Ingredients	Directions
One 20-ounce can diced pineapple in juice, chilled	**1** In a blender, add the pineapple, crystallized ginger, and protein powder, and blend on high speed until smooth (approximately 45 seconds).
¼ cup crystallized ginger	
½ cup whey protein powder	**2** Add the Greek yogurt, banana, and agave nectar and blend until smooth, another 30 to 40 seconds. Pour into glasses and enjoy.
½ cup plain fat-free Greek yogurt	
1 cup sliced bananas, frozen	
1 tablespoon agave nectar	

Per serving: Calories 262 (From Fat 11); Fat 1g (Saturated 0g); Cholesterol 0mg; Sodium 41mg; Carbohydrate 41g (Dietary Fiber 2g); Protein 24g.

Simple Vegetable Omelet

Prep time: 5 min • **Cook time:** 15 min • **Yield:** 1 serving

Ingredients	Directions
1 tomato, diced	**1** Preheat a large skillet over medium heat and spray the pan with cooking spray.
1 green onion, sliced	
1 cup baby spinach	**2** Add the tomato (with juices), green onion, and spinach to the pan. Stir and cook the vegetables until soft and the spinach is wilted. Remove the vegetables from the pan.
1 egg	
2 egg whites	
1 tablespoon milk	**3** Rinse out the pan, return the pan to the stove, reduce the temperature to medium-low heat, and spray the pan again with cooking spray.
¼ cup shredded low-fat cheddar cheese	
	4 In a small bowl, whisk the egg, egg whites, and milk, and pour into the pan. While the omelet cooks, lift the edges and allow the uncooked egg to flow underneath. When the egg is mostly cooked, flip it.
	5 Place the vegetables on top of the egg and sprinkle with cheese. Turn off the heat.
	6 When the cheese is melted, fold the egg in half. Serve warm.

Per serving: Calories 206 (From Fat 68); Fat 8g (Saturated 3g); Cholesterol 192mg; Sodium 391mg; Carbohydrate 12g (Dietary Fiber 3g); Protein 22g.

Baby spinach

Baby spinach is not a particular variety of spinach — it's just spinach that has been harvested at an early stage of plant growth, usually between 15 and 35 days after planting. Baby spinach leaves are small, have a tender texture, and taste sweet. Their nutrient profile is similar to that of mature spinach.

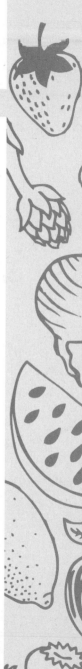

Cheesy Spinach Breakfast Squares

Prep time: 15 min • **Cook time:** 25 min • **Yield:** 8 servings

Ingredients	Directions
1 egg	**1** Preheat the oven to 350 degrees.
⅓ cup liquid egg whites (or the egg whites from 2 large eggs)	**2** In a large mixing bowl, beat the egg, egg whites, both flours, baking powder, butter, and milk. Set aside.
½ cup all-purpose flour	
½ cup whole-wheat flour	**3** In a large pot or Dutch oven, heat the olive oil and add the onions and garlic. Sauté the onions a few minutes, until glassy.
1 teaspoon baking powder	
2 tablespoons butter, melted	
1 cup milk	**4** Add the spinach and salt, toss with the onions, and cover for 2 minutes.
1 tablespoon olive oil	
1 onion, chopped	**5** Uncover the pot and toss the spinach. Continue cooking until the spinach is wilted, approximately another minute.
2 tablespoons garlic, chopped	
1½ pounds fresh baby spinach	
½ teaspoon salt	**6** Add the spinach mixture to the moist flour mixture and mix until well combined.
16 ounces low-fat sharp cheddar cheese, grated	
	7 Add the cheese, and mix until well combined.
	8 Spray a 9-x-9-inch baking dish with cooking spray, and then pour the mixture into the baking dish.
	9 Bake 25 minutes or until the center is set.
	10 Cool slightly before cutting.

Per serving: Calories 271 (From Fat 94); Fat 10g (Saturated 5g); Cholesterol 47mg; Sodium 716mg; Carbohydrate 26g (Dietary Fiber 6g); Protein 21g.

Tip: If you like a bit of heat and can tolerate some spice, consider adding a few shots of hot pepper sauce to the batter.

Southwestern Egg Scramble

Prep time: 10 min • **Cook time:** 5 min • **Yield:** 4 servings

Ingredients	*Directions*
10 egg whites (about 1½ cups liquid egg whites)	*1* In a bowl, combine the egg whites, egg, and cayenne pepper and whip together.
1 whole egg	
⅛ teaspoon cayenne pepper	*2* In a separate bowl, mix the bell pepper, chilies, onion, and tomato together and season with salt and pepper.
¼ cup bell pepper, diced	
2 tablespoons mild green chilies, diced	
¼ cup green onion, diced	*3* Spray a medium skillet with cooking spray, add the vegetable mixture, and stir for about 1 minute.
¼ cup tomato, diced	
Salt and pepper (to taste)	*4* Pour the egg mixture into a pan and stir when the eggs begin to cook. Serve when the eggs are cooked through.

Per serving: Calories 72 (From Fat 13); Fat 1g (Saturated 0g); Cholesterol 56mg; Sodium 306mg; Carbohydrate 3g (Dietary Fiber 1g); Protein 11g.

Vary 1t! If you don't like Southwestern flavors, omit the spices and use vegetables you do like. Mushrooms, onions, broccoli, spinach, and zucchini are just a few that are great mixed with eggs in a scramble.

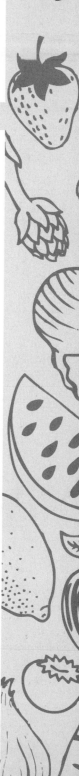

Fresh Fruit Porridge

Prep time: 5 min • **Yield:** 2 servings

Ingredients	Directions
2 bananas	*1* In a food processor or blender, add the bananas, strawberries, peach, and plum and puree until smooth.
10 strawberries	
1 peach	
1 plum	*2* Pour into bowls and add ½ cup of the blueberries and 1 tablespoon of the hemp or flaxseeds to each bowl.
1 cup blueberries	
2 tablespoons ground hemp or flaxseeds	

Per serving: Calories 247 (From Fat 37); Fat 4g (Saturated 1g); Cholesterol 0mg; Sodium 9mg; Carbohydrate 55g (Dietary Fiber 10g); Protein 4g.

Tip: If any of the fruits in this recipe are not in season, feel free to use frozen. You can also use dried plums, but may have to add a little fruit juice to help them puree.

American Parfait

Prep time: 15 min • **Yield:** 4 servings

Ingredients	Directions
½ cup blueberries	*1* In a large bowl, mix the blueberries, raspberries, strawberries, and juice, and allow to marinate in the refrigerator for at least 15 minutes.
½ cup raspberries	
1 cup strawberries	
¼ cup 100 percent pineapple or orange juice	*2* In each of four small cups or bowls, layer ¼ cup of the yogurt, ½ cup of the fruit mixture, and 2 tablespoons of the granola. Serve cold.
1 cup low-fat vanilla yogurt	
½ cup low-fat granola	

Per serving: Calories 117 (From Fat 13); Fat 2g (Saturated 1g); Cholesterol 2mg; Sodium 34mg; Carbohydrate 24g (Dietary Fiber 3g); Protein 3g.

Tip: Granola can often be fattening. Read labels carefully to find brands low in fat and sugar. The Bear Naked brand makes a few versions that have pretty decent stats. Alternatively, you can make your own (see the Homemade Granola recipe in Chapter 14).

Chapter 11

Soothing and Nourishing Soups

In This Chapter

▶ Uncovering the nourishing power of soups

▶ Getting a primer on soup making

▶ Starting a meal with soup

▶ Making soup your main course

*W*e've all been told that chicken soup can help us feel better when we have a cold or the flu. In fact, some studies have suggested that chicken soup and other hot liquids can help with a runny nose. But chicken soup is just the tip of the iceberg when it comes to the health benefits of incorporating soups into your diet when you're undergoing treatment for cancer. Soups are a great way to get whole grains, vegetables, fruits, and beans into one dish, particularly if you're short on time or energy. You can't get more wholesome than that!

In this chapter, we offer some insight into why soups are a great way to nourish yourself and look at a few things to keep in mind as you prepare soups. We also provide you with some recipes to get you started, whether you're looking for a soup that serves as a meal or one that whets the appetite.

Why Soups Are So Nourishing

How do we love soups? Let us count the ways. First, they can be one of the most easily prepared, nutrient-dense dishes. You cook all the ingredients in one pot using a healthy base that you consume, so you benefit from any nutrients that leach out into the cooking liquid instead of discarding them.

We also love soups because they don't require much effort to prepare. Because everything goes into one pot, there are also considerably fewer dirty dishes you have to tackle at the end of the cooking process. In addition, soups freeze well and can be easily reheated for those times when you don't have the time or strength to prepare a meal from scratch.

To safely store your leftover soup, pour it into smaller containers so it will cool faster. Plan to use leftover soup within three to four days or freeze in small containers for use within three to four months after frozen. Just be sure to use it within three to four days after thawing.

In addition, soups are often well tolerated and can be a comfort food during cancer treatment, warming the body and soul. Many of the soups in this chapter will go down a little easier than solid foods if you have a sore mouth or throat. In addition, some of the soups may tempt your taste buds if you're experiencing taste changes.

Another tremendous benefit of soups is that they're exceedingly versatile — ingredients can be easily swapped and the nutrient density enhanced. For example, you can try adding a cup or two of whole or pureed beans to your favorite soup to add protein and give the soup a creamy texture without adding extra saturated fat. Protein powders or nonfat dry milk also can be added to a milk-based soup to boost protein content without changing flavor. If a soup recipe contains a vegetable you don't like or can't tolerate, you can simply replace it with another. You can also hide vegetables you normally wouldn't eat in soups. You can puree them so they disappear or even try adding whole pieces for pops of color. Even if you don't like eating certain vegetables, the other flavors of the soup will transform how they taste.

Getting Started with Soups

A unifying trait of soups is that they all have a base, but you have a lot of flexibility in terms of what you use as a base. You can use a low-sodium homemade or store-bought stock, broth, or bouillon (including cubes) in vegetable, chicken, beef, or another flavor. Other healthy base options include any variety of non-paste canned tomatoes (such as diced, crushed, or stewed), nonfat milk, or even a dairy substitute like rice milk or soy milk.

If you have the time and energy, you can try making your own stock or base (see the vegetable stock recipe later in this section). If making a homemade base sounds too involved for you, look for premade, low-sodium, low-fat broth that comes in a soft-pack quart container. Don't feel bad about splurging on the base — it's important to find one that suits your palate, because it'll add flavor and nutrients to your soup.

Vegetable Stock

Prep time: 5 min • **Cook time:** 45 min • **Yield:** 8 cups

Ingredients	*Directions*
1 tablespoon olive oil	*1* Heat the oil in a soup pot over medium heat, and add the onions, leek, celery, carrots, garlic, parsley, and thyme. Cook for 5 to 10 minutes, stirring frequently so the vegetables don't brown.
2 large onions, quartered	
1 medium leek (white and green parts), chopped	
2 celery stalks with leaves intact, chopped	*2* Add the water, sea salt, and bay leaves, and bring to a boil. Then lower the heat and simmer for at least 35 minutes.
2 large carrots, quartered	
8 cloves garlic, crushed	*3* Remove the broth from the heat, strain the liquid, and discard the vegetables.
8 sprigs fresh parsley or 4 teaspoons dried parsley	
6 sprigs fresh thyme or 3 teaspoons dried thyme	
2 quarts water	
1 teaspoon sea salt	
2 bay leaves	

Per cup: Calories 18 (From Fat 15); Fat 2g (Saturated 0g); Cholesterol 0mg; Sodium 290mg; Carbohydrate 1g (Dietary Fiber 0g); Protein 0g.

Tip: If you prefer, instead of following this recipe, you can make vegetable stock by saving all the trimmings from the vegetables you eat during the week and adding them to a pot of water with some garlic, onion, parsley, bay leaves, and other desired herbs and simmering them for 35 minutes to a few hours. Then strain them out and toss them. Use the stock within a week or freeze it for up to six months for later use.

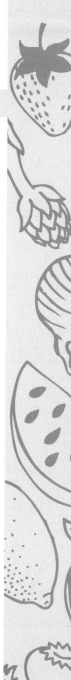

Enjoying Soups as Starters

Soups make fantastic starters. They can be nice and light, leaving plenty of room for the main meal, while also getting the appetite going. At the same time, they can help you increase your vegetable consumption and keep you feeling full longer.

Keep in mind that any of our starter soups can also serve as a great meal — simply add a little protein to the soup itself (for example, by incorporating some beans, tofu, chicken, or other lean meat, or by having a small piece of baked fish or chicken on the side), and enjoy the soup with some whole-grain bread. This is a particularly good idea if you don't have much of an appetite and don't feel like eating much. Soup makes a great mini meal.

The starter soup recipes in this section focus heavily on vegetables. You can make these recipes any time, but to extract the best flavors, consider preparing them when the produce they contain is in season, or feel free to add additional seasonal produce to the recipes. You can find a handy reference guide at www.fruitsandveggiesmorematters.org/what-fruits-and-vegetables-are-in-season.

If you can afford to buy organic ingredients for the recipes in this book or any other soup recipes you'd like to make, go for it. However, using organic ingredients isn't necessary. Just be sure to wash and trim your produce well to minimize pesticide exposure. If you don't have the energy to chop and prepare produce, you can buy frozen vegetables instead or see if your grocery store sells packs with washed and trimmed vegetables in the produce section. Just look for versions that aren't packed in any sauces and don't have added seasonings or sodium.

The recipes in this chapter are just a guideline to get you started with soups. Feel free to modify the ingredients to suit your taste or to use what you have on hand. Don't be afraid to experiment. Soups are very forgiving!

Apple Carrot Ginger Soup

Prep time: 10 min • **Cook time:** 40 min • **Yield:** 4 servings

Ingredients	*Directions*
1½ teaspoons olive oil	*1* Heat the oil in a large pot, and then add the celery, carrot, onion, garlic, ginger, thyme, and curry. Sauté lightly for 2 to 3 minutes.
¼ cup diced celery	
1 cup shredded carrot	
¼ cup onion, peeled and chopped	*2* Stir in the flour and cook while stirring for about two minutes.
1½ teaspoons minced garlic	
1 tablespoon minced fresh ginger root or 1 teaspoon ground ginger	*3* Add the milk, broth, and applesauce. Cook for 30 minutes, stirring occasionally.
1 teaspoon fresh thyme or ¼ teaspoon dried thyme	*4* Remove the soup from the heat, place in a blender, and puree until smooth.
¼ teaspoon curry powder	
2 teaspoon whole-wheat flour	*5* Return the soup to the stove and simmer for 10 more minutes.
2 cups skim milk	
2 cups vegetable broth	
½ cup unsweetened applesauce	

Per serving: Calories 128 (From Fat 47); Fat 5g (Saturated 1g); Cholesterol 2mg; Sodium 546mg; Carbohydrate 16g (Dietary Fiber 2g); Protein 5g.

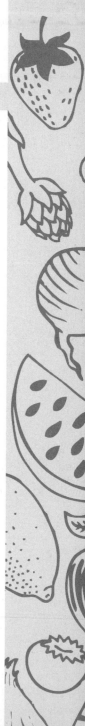

Potato, Leek, and Corn Soup

Prep time: 15 min • **Cook time:** 40 min • **Yield:** 8 servings

Ingredients	*Directions*
1 tablespoon olive oil	*1* Heat the oil in a large Dutch oven over medium heat, and add the leek, celery, and bell pepper. Cook for 4 minutes or until the vegetables are tender, stirring frequently.
1½ cups coarsely chopped leek (about 1 large)	
½ cup finely chopped celery	
½ cup finely chopped bell pepper	*2* In a small microwavable bowl, heat the milk slightly and then add the flour to it, stirring with a whisk.
2 cups milk	
3 tablespoons all-purpose flour	*3* Slowly add the milk-and-flour mixture to the Dutch oven, stirring constantly. Stir in the broth, corn, potatoes, salt, and freshly ground black pepper; bring to a boil.
3 cups chicken broth	
2 cups fresh corn kernels (about 4 ears)	
2 pounds cubed Yukon gold or red potato (with skin)	*4* Reduce the heat, and simmer for 20 minutes or until the potatoes are tender. Top with shredded cheddar cheese, if desired.
¼ teaspoon freshly ground black pepper	
⅛ teaspoon salt	
Cheddar cheese, shredded (optional)	

Per serving: *Calories 217 (From Fat 41); Fat 4g (Saturated 1g); Cholesterol 6mg; Sodium 432mg; Carbohydrate 37g (Dietary Fiber 3g); Protein 7g.*

Butternut Squash and Apple Soup

Prep time: 15 min • **Cook time:** 40 min • **Yield:** 4 servings

Ingredients	*Directions*
2 teaspoons olive oil	*1* Preheat the oven to 350 degrees.
¼ cup diced carrot	
2 tablespoons onion, peeled and diced small	*2* In a soup pot, heat the oil and sauté the carrots, onions, and celery until tender.
2 tablespoons celery, diced small	
⅛ teaspoon fresh ginger root or ⅛ teaspoon ground ginger	*3* Add the ginger, thyme, butternut squash, broth, apple juice, and milk. Bring to a boil, stirring frequently.
⅛ teaspoon fresh thyme or ⅛ teaspoon dried thyme	
One 10-ounce package frozen butternut squash cubes, thawed and mashed	*4* Reduce the heat to low and simmer for 40 minutes. If the soup is too thick, add hot broth to thin it out. Add the salt and pepper to taste.
1 cup vegetable or chicken broth	
1 cup unsweetened 100 percent apple juice	
3 cups milk	
Salt and pepper to taste	

Per serving: *Calories 174 (From Fat 79); Fat 9g (Saturated 4g); Cholesterol 26mg; Sodium 314mg; Carbohydrate 18g (Dietary Fiber 1g); Protein 6g.*

Vary It! Instead of butternut squash, try acorn squash or yams for a whole new taste sensation.

Creamy Potato Soup

Prep time: 15 min • **Cook time:** 30 min • **Yield:** 6 servings

Ingredients	*Directions*
4 medium potatoes, peeled and cubed	*1* In a large saucepan, combine the potatoes, onions, carrots, celery, and chicken broth and bring to a boil. Reduce the heat; cover and simmer for 12 to 15 minutes or until the vegetables are tender.
¾ cup onion, peeled and chopped	
1 medium carrot, peeled and chopped	*2* Using a potato masher, lightly mash the vegetables. Alternatively, for a smoother consistency, place the vegetable mixture in a blender and blend until smooth; then return to the saucepan.
2 stalks celery, chopped	
1½ cups chicken broth	
3 tablespoons canola oil	*3* In a small saucepan, heat the canola oil. Stir in the flour until smooth. Gradually stir in the milk. Heat milk without boiling and cook, stirring for about 2 minutes or until thickened.
3 tablespoons all-purpose flour	
2½ cups milk	
1 tablespoon minced fresh parsley or 1 teaspoon dried parsley	*4* Stir the milk-and-flour mixture into the vegetable mixture. Cook and stir until thickened and bubbly.
¾ teaspoon salt	*5* Add the parsley, salt, and pepper.
½ teaspoon pepper	
1 cup shredded low-fat Swiss cheese	*6* Remove from the heat and stir in the cheese until melted.

Per serving: Calories 282 (From Fat 113); Fat 13g (Saturated 4g); Cholesterol 22mg; Sodium 889mg; Carbohydrate 32g (Dietary Fiber 3g); Protein 11g.

Roasted Cauliflower and Sage Soup

Prep time: 10 min • **Cook time:** 1 hr 30 min • **Yield:** 4 servings

Ingredients	*Directions*
1½ large cauliflower heads, broken into small florets	*1* Preheat the oven to 350 degrees.
2 tablespoons olive oil, divided	*2* Place all the cauliflower in a bowl with 1 tablespoon of the olive oil and pepper; toss to coat.
Dash of pepper	
¼ cup onion, peeled and diced small	*3* Place the cauliflower in a roasting pan and roast in the oven for 45 minutes or until lightly brown.
¼ cup celery, diced small	
½ teaspoon fresh chopped sage or ¼ teaspoon dried sage	*4* In a medium pot, add the remaining olive oil and sauté the onions, celery, sage, thyme, and garlic until the onions are translucent.
⅛ teaspoon fresh thyme or ⅛ teaspoon dried thyme	
1 teaspoon garlic, peeled and minced	*5* Add the flour, and cook for two minutes, stirring often.
3 tablespoons unbleached all-purpose flour	*6* Whisk in the milk and broth.
3 cups milk	*7* Add the roasted cauliflower and bring to a boil. Reduce the heat to low and simmer for 30 minutes.
3 cups chicken or vegetable broth	
	8 Remove the soup from the heat, place in a blender, and puree. Return the soup to the pot and heat on the stove for another 15 minutes.
	9 Place the soup in bowls and serve.

Per serving: *Calories 169 (From Fat 74); Fat 8g (Saturated 1g); Cholesterol 1mg; Sodium 771mg; Carbohydrate 19g (Dietary Fiber 5g); Protein 6g.*

Vary It! Not sure about the sage? Feel free to try other herbs, like oregano and rosemary.

Creamy Asparagus Soup

Prep time: 15 min • **Cook time:** 30 min • **Yield:** 6 servings

Ingredients	*Directions*
1 tablespoon canola oil	*1* In a large saucepan, heat the oil, and add the asparagus, onions, celery, leek, and potatoes. Cook for 5 minutes covered, stirring occasionally.
24 asparagus spears, cut into 1-inch lengths	
1 small white onion, peeled and diced small	*2* Add the vegetable broth. Simmer for 20 minutes or until the vegetables are softened.
1 celery stalk, diced small	
1 leek (white part only), split, washed, and diced small	*3* Carefully transfer the soup to a blender in small batches. Puree until smooth, add the fresh spinach, and puree again.
2 small to medium Yukon gold potatoes, peeled and diced small	*4* Return the pureed mixture to the saucepan. Add the sour cream and stir on low heat until blended.
5 cups vegetable broth	
4 ounces (about 2½ cups) fresh spinach, washed	*5* Season with salt and pepper.
1 cup low-fat sour cream	
Salt and pepper to taste	

Per serving: Calories 212 (From Fat 84); Fat 9g (Saturated 3g); Cholesterol 13mg; Sodium 444mg; Carbohydrate 26g (Dietary Fiber 3g); Protein 7g.

What's with that smell?

Some people find that their urine smells like sulfur after consuming asparagus. If your urine smells reminiscent of cooked cabbage after eating asparagus, don't be alarmed and don't let this deter you from eating asparagus. The odor doesn't signify anything harmful. Studies indicate that asparagus contains various sulfuric compounds that, when acted upon by certain enzymes in the digestive system, produce the smell. Not everyone has those digestive enzymes, so your urine may not smell any different than usual.

Why eat up asparagus? Prized since ancient times, this vegetable is a great source of numerous vitamins, including vitamins A, C, E, and K, as well as folate and the trace mineral chromium. It's also a good source of fiber.

Root Vegetable and Mushroom Soup

Prep time: 20 min • **Cook time:** 40 min • **Yield:** 6 servings

Ingredients	*Directions*
2 low-sodium chicken or vegetable bouillon cubes	*1* In a 4-quart saucepan, bring 3 cups of water to a boil and add the bouillon cubes, stirring until they're dissolved. Add the soy sauce and ginger, and stir to mix. Then add the potato, yam, carrot, and apple. Reduce the heat to low and simmer.
½ teaspoon ground ginger powder	
1 large potato, peeled and cubed small	
1 medium sweet potato, peeled and cubed small	*2* In a skillet, heat the olive oil over medium heat. Add the mushrooms, onion, and garlic, and sauté 5 to 10 minutes, until the mushrooms are tender and the onions start to soften.
1 large carrot, peeled and chopped	
1 apple, peeled and chopped	*3* Add the mushroom and onions to the 4-quart saucepan containing the soup. Add more water, if needed. Stir, cover, and cook for 20 to 30 minutes.
3 tablespoons olive oil	
¾ pound button mushrooms, chopped	
1 large onion, peeled and chopped	
6 small garlic cloves, peeled and pressed	
1 tablespoon dried parsley	
3 cups water, plus more as needed during cooking	

Per serving: *Calories 191 (From Fat 63); Fat 7g (Saturated 1g); Cholesterol 0mg; Sodium 189mg; Carbohydrate 30g (Dietary Fiber 3g); Protein 3g.*

Vary It! The root vegetables in this soup are available year-round, but in the winter, when other root vegetables are in season, consider adding or substituting parsnips, turnips, rutabagas, and kohlrabi.

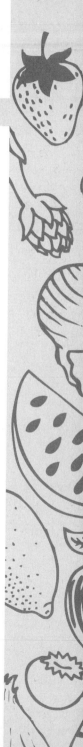

Escarole and Rice Soup

Prep time: 10 min • **Cook time:** 30 min • **Yield:** 6 servings

Ingredients	Directions
1 tablespoon olive oil	*1* Heat the olive oil in a large pot. Add the onion and garlic, and sauté for about 3 minutes.
1 small onion, peeled and chopped	
2 teaspoons garlic, peeled and minced	*2* Turn the heat to low, add the escarole, sprinkle with salt, and cook another 3 minutes.
1 escarole, washed, separated, and roughly chopped	*3* Add 1 cup of the broth and cook 10 to 15 minutes, until the escarole is wilted and tender.
¾ teaspoon coarse salt	
5 cups chicken broth	*4* Add the remaining broth and bring to a boil.
3 cups Arborio rice (or any short-grain rice), cooked	*5* Add the rice, cover, and simmer over low heat for another 10 minutes.
Pepper to taste	
Freshly grated Parmesan cheese, to taste	*6* Season as desired with pepper.
	7 Ladle into bowls and sprinkle with Parmesan cheese before serving.

Per serving: Calories 333 (From Fat 55); Fat 6g (Saturated 1g); Cholesterol 4mg; Sodium 1,092mg; Carbohydrate 62g (Dietary Fiber 4g); Protein 7g.

Refreshing Gazpacho

Prep time: 10 min • **Yield:** 6 servings

Ingredients	Directions
1 cucumber, seeded, peeled, and diced	*1* Puree the cucumber, bell peppers, tomatoes, onion, and garlic in a blender or food processor for about 30 seconds.
2 red bell peppers, seeded and diced	
4 plum tomatoes, seeded and chopped	*2* Add the tomato juice, vinegar, olive oil, oregano, basil, and salt and pepper (as desired), and pulse a few times to mix.
½ small red onion, peeled and chopped	
2 garlic cloves, peeled and minced	*3* Chill for at least 1 hour before serving.
3 cups low-sodium tomato juice	
¼ cup red wine vinegar	
¼ cup olive oil	
1 teaspoon fresh oregano or ¼ teaspoon dried oregano	
1 teaspoon fresh basil or ¼ teaspoon dried basil	
Salt and black pepper to taste	

Per serving: Calories 135 (From Fat 83); Fat 9g (Saturated 1g); Cholesterol 0mg; Sodium 172mg; Carbohydrate 12g (Dietary Fiber 2g); Protein 2g.

Tip: To get some additional healthy fat or to add creaminess, consider serving with half a diced avocado. To dice an avocado, cut it in half, remove the pit, and slice the flesh inside the skin in parallel slices. Then cut across the slices you already made to form squares. Scoop the avocado out of the flesh with a spoon.

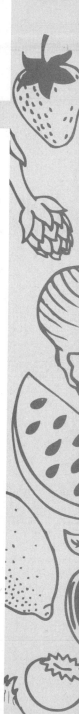

Digging Into Meal-Based Soups

Almost no meal is more comforting to dig into when it's cold outside or after a long and tiring day than soup, which quickly warms and soothes the body and soul. Although soups are often used as starters, they can also serve as fantastic meals when they incorporate heartier ingredients, including whole grains and lean proteins. Meal based soups are a particularly good idea when you're feeling tired, because they're so easy to eat.

Some whole grains that are great for meal-based soups include quinoa, barley, farro, and bulgar wheat. These grains are high in fiber, digesting more slowly than refined grains like white rice and pasta, which means you'll be full longer and reduce the impact on your blood glucose levels.

You have many options for adding lean protein to your soups. Tofu and beans are a great vegetarian option. (If you're concerned about eating soy, see the nearby sidebar.) Dried beans are preferable to canned varieties to reduce sodium content, but you can certainly use canned beans for convenience. When buying canned beans, look for brands that use BPA-free cans. Also, compare labels to find the brand that contains the least amount of sodium.

Although eating a largely plant-based diet has been associated with numerous health benefits, including reduced cancer risk, some nutrients that are best obtained from animal sources (such as conjugated linoleic acid [CLA], a fatty acid that has also been associated with cancer prevention), improve immunity and provide a host of other beneficial effects. You have many options for animal sources of lean protein, including grass-fed beef, free-range chicken, bison, ostrich, turkey, and pork. If you don't like to eat meat or poultry, you can consider marine sources of lean protein, including tuna, wild Alaskan salmon, and even shellfish like oysters, clams, crab, lobster, scallops, and shrimp.

The soy debate

Although there is controversy regarding soy intake when it comes to breast cancer for people with estrogen-receptor-positive disease, it isn't a concern for people with estrogen-receptor-negative disease. Soy intake is also encouraged for certain types of cancer, such as prostate cancer. Most experts agree that moderate intake (two to three servings per day) of whole soy foods is safe, even for those with estrogen-receptor-positive breast cancer. These experts also recommend getting soy from more natural sources as opposed to the many processed soy foods that are on the market. Recommended sources are whole soybeans, edamame, tofu, or even fermented soy like tempeh and miso. Sources that are *not* recommended are soy supplements, bars, powders, and soymilks with added soy isoflavones or soy isolates. Soy burgers and hot dogs or protein bars containing these ingredients should also be consumed very sparingly, if at all. If you're actively being treated for breast cancer, as a precaution, be sure to discuss your soy intake with your healthcare provider or dietitian.

Quick Black Bean Soup

Prep time: 10 min • **Cook time:** 30 min • **Yield:** 8 servings

Ingredients	*Directions*
2 teaspoons peeled and minced garlic	*1* In a heated medium saucepan, add a small amount of water, and sauté the garlic, onions, and bell pepper until soft.
½ cup onion, peeled and diced	
½ cup red or green bell pepper, diced	*2* Add the beans with liquid, salsa, cumin, chili powder, corn, and broth to the saucepan, and mix well. Bring to a boil.
Two 15-ounce cans no-salt-added black beans, undrained	
½ cup salsa	*3* Reduce the heat and bring to a low simmer for 10 minutes.
2 teaspoons cumin	
1 tablespoons chili powder	*4* Ladle the soup into bowls and top with shredded cheese and cilantro.
1 cup frozen corn, thawed	
One 15-ounce can chicken broth	
½ cup shredded low-fat sharp cheddar cheese	
2½ tablespoons chopped, fresh cilantro or 1 teaspoon dried cilantro (optional)	

Per serving: Calories 202 (From Fat 21; Fat 2g (Saturated 1g); Cholesterol 3mg; Sodium 394mg; Carbohydrate 35g (Dietary Fiber 7g); Protein 12g.

Tip: You can also garnish this soup with a tablespoon of low-fat sour cream and chopped green onion.

Wild Salmon Soup

Prep time: 15 min • **Cook time:** 40 min • **Yield:** 5 servings

Ingredients	*Directions*
2 cups water	*1* Add the water to a large pot, and bring to a boil.
4 ounces carrots, peeled and diced small	*2* Add the carrots, onion, bay leaf, and peppercorns. Reduce the heat to low, and cook for 15 minutes.
1 small onion, peeled and diced small	
1 bay leaf	*3* Add the potatoes, salmon, and dill, and cook for 15 to 20 minutes.
14 ounces (about 4 medium) Yukon gold potatoes, peeled and cubed small	
4 ounces raw wild salmon, cubed and fine pin bones and skin removed	*4* Check the potatoes for doneness. When soft, add the milk, butter, salt, and parsley. Cook for an additional 5 minutes. Remove bay leaf and peppercorns before serving.
1 tablespoon fresh dill weed or 1 teaspoon dried dill	
5 whole peppercorns	
2 cups milk	
1 tablespoon butter	
1 teaspoon sea salt	
1 tablespoon fresh parsley or 1 teaspoon dried parsley	

Per serving: Calories 194 (From Fat 64); Fat 7g (Saturated 4g); Cholesterol 30mg; Sodium 540mg; Carbohydrate 22g (Dietary Fiber 2g); Protein 11g.

Wild versus farmed salmon: Does it matter?

Most of the salmon on the market is farm raised. Farm-raised salmon is considerably less expensive than wild salmon, but farmed salmon is fattier, has less protein, contains less of the desirable omega-3 fatty acids and more of the undesirable omega-6 fatty acids, and contains more toxins than wild salmon, making it a far inferior choice.

When buying wild salmon, look for Alaskan salmon. All Alaskan salmon is guaranteed wild — it's illegal to farm salmon in Alaska. In addition, most canned salmon is wild because farm-raised salmon doesn't can well. Buying canned salmon is a good way to get wild salmon at a good price.

Asian Chicken Soup with Rice

Prep time: 10 min • **Cook time:** 30 min • **Yield:** 8 servings

Ingredients	*Directions*
1 tablespoon olive oil	*1* In a large pot, heat the olive oil and then add the onions and garlic. Sautee until the onions are translucent, stirring frequently.
1 small onion, peeled and chopped	
2 garlic cloves, peeled and minced	
2 quarts chicken broth	*2* Add the broth to the pot and bring to a simmer.
1 pound boneless, skinless chicken breast, cubed	*3* Add the chicken and continue to simmer on low heat for 15 minutes.
4 ounces fresh shiitake mushrooms, chopped	*4* Add both types of mushrooms, rice, ginger, soy sauce, and parsley. Season with salt and pepper to taste, and simmer an additional 10 minutes.
4 ounces fresh button mushrooms, chopped	
2 cups brown jasmine rice, cooked	
1 tablespoon fresh ginger, peeled and minced or 1 teaspoon dried ginger	
1 tablespoon low-sodium soy sauce	
3 tablespoons fresh parsley or 3 teaspoons dried parsley (optional)	
Salt and pepper to taste	

Per serving: Calories 157 (From Fat 40); Fat 4g (Saturated 1g); Cholesterol 31mg; Sodium 1,109mg; Carbohydrate 13g (Dietary Fiber 1g); Protein 15g.

Vary It! Don't have brown jasmine rice? Try white rice, regular brown rice, quinoa, or another whole grain — or omit the rice altogether.

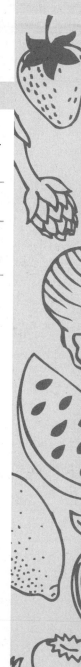

Curried Lentil Soup

Prep time: 10 min • **Cook time:** 45 min • **Yield:** 6 servings

Ingredients	Directions
3¾ cups vegetable broth	**1** In a large pot, add the vegetable broth, lentils, carrot, celery, onion, and garlic and bring to a boil.
¾ cup red lentils	
1 carrot, peeled and chopped	**2** Turn the heat to low, add the curry powder and tumeric, and cover the pot.
1 celery stick, chopped	
1 onion, peeled and chopped	**3** Let simmer for 45 minutes, stirring occasionally.
1 clove garlic, peeled and minced	
1 teaspoon curry powder	**4** Add the salt and pepper to taste.
1 teaspoon turmeric	
Salt and pepper, to taste	

Per serving: Calories 158 (From Fat 14); Fat 2g (Saturated 1g); Cholesterol 0mg; Sodium 452mg; Carbohydrate 28g (Dietary Fiber 7g); Protein 9g.

Looking at lentils

Lentils are a type of dried bean that comes in brown, green, and red varieties. Red lentils tend to taste sweeter and nuttier than their brown and green counterparts. Regardless of the lentil, they pack a powerful nutritional punch, serving as a good source of cholesterol-lowering fiber.

Because of their high fiber content, they also help you maintain steady blood sugar levels. In addition, they serve as a good source of protein, many minerals, vitamin B1 (thiamin), and folate, while containing virtually no fat.

Hearty Vegetarian Minestrone

Prep time: 15 min • **Cook time:** 50 min • **Yield:** 6 servings

Ingredients	*Directions*
2 tablespoons olive oil	*1* In a large pot, heat the olive oil and add the onion, garlic, and celery, and cook and stir over medium heat until the onion is translucent and the celery is tender.
1 small onion, peeled and chopped	
2 cloves garlic, peeled and minced	
1 stalk celery, chopped	*2* Add the broth, tomatoes (with juice), carrot, cabbage, zucchini, chickpeas, parsley, basil, and oregano. Bring to a boil, and then reduce the heat.
3 cups low-sodium vegetable broth	
One 28-ounce can low-sodium diced tomatoes, undrained	*3* Cover and simmer for 20 to 30 minutes on low heat, or until the vegetables are tender.
1 carrot, peeled and chopped	
½ cup green cabbage, finely shredded	*4* Add your pasta of choice. Return to a boil, and then reduce the heat and cover and simmer until the pasta is al dente (about 10 minutes).
1 small zucchini, chopped	
1 cup canned chickpeas, drained	*5* Season with salt and pepper, as desired.
2 tablespoons minced fresh parsley or 2 teaspoons dried parsley	
1½ tablespoons fresh basil or ½ teaspoon dried basil	
1½ tablespoons fresh oregano or ½ teaspoon dried oregano	
½ cup uncooked pasta of choice	
Salt and pepper, to taste	

Per serving: Calories 161 (From Fat 47); Fat 5g (Saturated 1g); Cholesterol 0mg; Sodium 201mg; Carbohydrate 23g (Dietary Fiber 7g); Protein 5g.

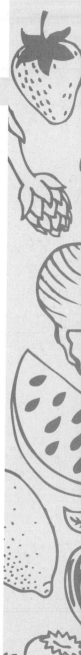

Chapter 12

Enticing Main Dishes

In This Chapter

▶ Getting to the point of main dishes

▶ Coming up with entrees that are meals unto themselves

▶ Making main dishes you can build a meal around

An entrée is usually the main dish or focus of a meal. If you're like many people, when you think of a main dish or an entrée to plan your meal around, you think of a big piece of meat, chicken, or fish. You may add a starch and a few vegetables to your plate, but in much smaller portions.

However, as we've learned more about optimal eating and health, the recommendations of what foods and food ratios make up a healthy plate have changed, leading to new objectives for eating.

In this chapter, we discuss how to meet the new recommendations for eating to meet your nutritional needs. We also get you started with some recipes to help you meet these objectives. Some of the entrées in this chapter are *complete entrées* (meaning they don't need much added to them to make them nutritionally balanced). Others are protein-based dishes that require sides to become a complete meal. (For vegetable- and whole-grain-based side dishes, turn to Chapter 13.)

Entrée Objectives

Much of what we know about what to eat before, during, and after a cancer diagnosis comes from epidemiologic studies. In these studies, the diets of different populations of people with cancer are compared to see if there are potential associations between foods they've eaten and their cancer. Although these types of studies don't prove cause and effect, they do suggest that some diets may be more or less associated with cancer development or recurrence.

Generally speaking, epidemiologic studies have indicated that people who eat a typical Western diet — which is high in animal fat, sugar, and excess calories — have a higher incidence of many cancers than do people who eat a diet focused on plant-based foods. For this reason, many organizations that make healthy diet recommendations encourage meal planning that focuses less on meat and more on whole grains, vegetables, beans, fruits, and dairy products.

For example, the New American Plate from the American Institute for Cancer Research (AICR) recommends meals that are two-thirds grains, vegetables, and beans, and only one-third meat or another animal protein. The United States Department of Agriculture (USDA) also recently replaced the Food Pyramid with MyPlate, which recommends about three-fourths of your plate be grains, colorful vegetables, and fruits, and one-fourth of your plate be protein. For more on these recommendations, see Chapter 4.

Based on the AICR and USDA recommendations, the more colorful your plate the better. Whole grains, vegetables, fruits, and beans should dominate, with just a small portion of animal protein. Keep in mind that a serving size of meat is just 3 ounces, which is roughly the size of a bar of soap. This is in stark contrast to a restaurant plate, which may consist of a 12-ounce steak and a few string beans.

An ideal entrée would include whole grains, vegetables or fruits, and protein all in one recipe, and we include a few such recipes in this chapter. But it would be pretty boring to eat one-pot meals all the time, so we also include many entrées that require side dishes to make them a complete meal. After all, as they say, "Variety is the spice of life." And, nutritionally speaking, variety is also one of the best ways to make sure you're getting optimal nutrition.

Complete Entrées

Some entrées or main dishes contain just about everything you need to make a healthy, balanced meal. The recipes in this section all include grains, vegetables, and a protein source as ingredients. Serve these with some fresh fruit or a fruit salad for dessert and maybe low-fat milk or a milk alternative and you have everything you need to meet your nutritional requirements for a meal. *Bon appétit!*

Mexican Lasagna

Prep time: 25 min • **Cook time:** 35 min • **Yield:** 6 servings

Ingredients:	Instructions
2 onions, peeled and chopped	*1* In a large frying pan, sauté the onions and garlic for a few minutes in the olive oil. Add the beans, chilies, tomatoes, chili powder, and cumin. Simmer for 20 minutes, stirring occasionally.
3 cloves garlic, peeled and minced	
1 tablespoon olive oil	
Two 15-ounce cans pinto beans, drained and rinsed	*2* Preheat the oven to 350 degrees.
One 4-ounce can green chilies	*3* Spread one-third of the bean mixture in a 9-x-13-inch baking dish. Top with 4 of the tortillas and 1 cup of the cheese. Top with half of the remaining bean mixture, the remaining 4 tortillas, and the remaining 1 cup of cheese. Top with the remaining bean mixture.
Two 15-ounce cans chili-style or fire-roasted tomatoes	
1 to 2 tablespoons chili powder (or to taste)	
1 tablespoon cumin (or to taste)	*4* Cover with foil and bake about 35 minutes.
8 corn tortillas	
2 cups low-fat shredded Mexican-style cheese	

Per serving: Calories 374 (From Fat 113); Fat 13g (Saturated 4g); Cholesterol 27mg; Sodium 1,261mg; Carbohydrate 51g (Dietary Fiber 11g); Protein 21g.

Tip: If you're on a sodium-restricted diet, this recipe can be modified to use no-salt-added tomatoes or fresh tomatoes.

Note: If you're making this recipe for dinner, leftovers are great warmed up for lunch the next day.

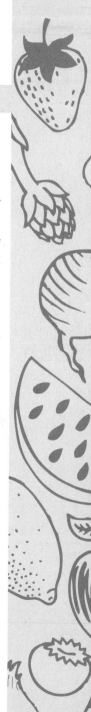

Moroccan Shrimp

Prep time: 5–10 min • **Cook time:** 25 min • **Yield:** 4 servings

Ingredients	*Instructions*
One 28-ounce can unsalted whole plum tomatoes, drained and with ¼ cup of the liquid reserved	**1** Individually remove the tomatoes from the can. Holding each tomato over a deep skillet, crush each tomato by hand, letting the flesh squeeze through your fingers into the pan.
1 medium onion, peeled, halved, and cut lengthwise into ½-inch crescents	**2** Add the onion, garlic, cumin, paprika, and ginger to the pan.
2 garlic cloves, peeled and chopped	**3** Over medium-high heat, bring the tomatoes to a simmer, stirring to combine all the ingredients.
1 teaspoon ground cumin	
1 teaspoon ground sweet paprika	**4** Mix in the cilantro, parsley, salt, and a generous pinch of pepper.
½ teaspoon ground ginger	
½ cup chopped cilantro	**5** Cover and simmer the sauce over medium-low heat until the tomatoes are soft, about 15 minutes.
¼ cup chopped flat-leaf parsley	
¼ teaspoon salt	**6** Add the shrimp and chickpeas, pushing them into the sauce. If the sauce seems dry, pour ¼ cup of the reserved canned tomato juice into the pan.
Ground black pepper, to taste	
20 large shrimp, peeled, deveined, and tails removed (see Figure 12-1)	**7** Cover and simmer gently until the shrimp are an opaque white and the chickpeas are heated through, about 8 to 10 minutes.
One 15-ounce can chickpeas, rinsed and drained	
2 cups cooked couscous	**8** Serve immediately over the couscous.

Per serving: *Calories 229 (From Fat 16); Fat 2g (Saturated 0g); Cholesterol 54mg; Sodium 365mg; Carbohydrate 40g (Dietary Fiber 7g); Protein 15g.*

Tip: For additional flavor, you can use fire-roasted tomatoes in place of the unsalted whole plum tomatoes.

Vary It! This recipe is also great using cod in place of the shrimp. Both shrimp and cod contain some omega-3 fatty acids to help support your immune system.

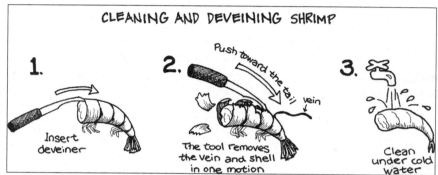

Figure 12-1: Cleaning and deveining shrimp.

CLEANING AND DEVEINING SHRIMP

1. Insert deveiner

2. Push toward the tail — vein — The tool removes the vein and shell in one motion

3. Clean under cold water

Illustration by Elizabeth Kurtzman

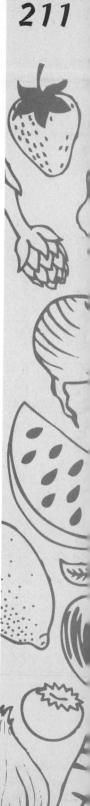

Chicken Teriyaki Stir Fry

Prep time: 10 min • **Cook time:** 35 min • **Yield:** 2 servings

Ingredients	*Directions*
½ **pound boneless, skinless chicken breast, sliced**	*1* Add the teriyaki to the chicken and let it sit in the refrigerator for 15 to 30 minutes.
1½ **teaspoons teriyaki sauce**	
⅛ **cup chicken broth**	*2* In a small bowl, combine the chicken broth, soy sauce, rice wine vinegar, and sesame oil. Set aside.
⅛ **cup soy sauce**	
1 **teaspoon rice wine vinegar**	*3* Heat a skillet or wok and add 1 tablespoon of the canola oil. Then stir-fry the chicken until cooked through, remove from the heat, and set aside.
1 **teaspoon sesame oil**	
2 **tablespoons canola oil**	
½ **medium onion, peeled and chopped**	*4* Add the remaining tablespoon of canola oil to the pan and stir-fry the onion for 1 to 2 minutes, followed by the garlic and ginger. Then add the carrots, broccoli, mushrooms, and water chestnuts, one type of vegetable at a time. Continue stir-frying for 4 to 5 minutes.
2 **cloves garlic, peeled and minced**	
½ **tablespoon peeled and minced fresh ginger**	
1 to 2 **carrots, peeled and sliced fine**	*5* Return the cooked chicken to the pan, and add the reserved sauce.
1 to 2 **cups broccoli florets**	*6* In a small cup, mix the cornstarch with a tablespoon of water and then add this mixture to the pan to thicken the sauce.
½ to 1 **cup mushrooms, sliced**	
1 **small can water chestnuts, drained**	
½ **teaspoon cornstarch**	*7* Serve over the cooked brown rice.
2 **cups cooked brown rice**	

Per serving: Calories 567 (From Fat 192); Fat 21g (Saturated 3g); Cholesterol 63mg; Sodium 1,256mg; Carbohydrate 61g (Dietary Fiber 8g); Protein 33g.

Vary It! Try this recipe with different protein sources (shrimp, tofu, and even a lean red meat can be used once in a while). Vary the vegetables based on what's in season. Add some pineapple, and mix up the sauce by adding fruit juices. If brown rice isn't your thing, try serving over another whole grain like quinoa.

Italian Eggplant and Rice Casserole

Prep time: 10 min • **Cook time:** 45 min • **Yield:** 4 servings

Ingredients	Directions
1 cup uncooked brown rice	*1* Cook the rice according to the package instructions and set aside.
2 tablespoons olive oil	
½ cup onions, peeled and chopped	*2* Heat 1 tablespoon of the olive oil in a large skillet over medium heat, and sauté the onions and garlic until the onions are tender. Then add the turkey and brown, approximately 5 minutes.
2 cloves garlic, peeled and minced	
12 ounces lean ground turkey	
3 cups chopped fresh tomatoes	*3* Stir in the tomatoes, agave nectar, basil, allspice, and thyme. Cover, reduce the heat, and simmer for 20 minutes.
1 tablespoon agave nectar	
2 teaspoons dried basil	
½ teaspoon ground allspice	*4* Preheat the oven to 350 degrees.
¼ teaspoon dried thyme	*5* In another large skillet, heat the remaining tablespoon of olive oil and lightly fry the eggplant in batches, just until slightly tender.
One 12-ounce eggplant, peeled and cut into thin slices	
1⅓ cups low-fat mozzarella cheese, grated	*6* Spoon enough of the tomato mixture into the bottom of an 8-x-8-inch baking pan to thinly cover the bottom. Then layer as follows: eggplant, tomato/turkey mixture, rice, and a sprinkling of both cheeses. Repeat until all the ingredients are used up, making sure to end with a cheese layer. Bake for 30 minutes or until bubbly.
½ cup grated Parmesan cheese	

Per serving: Calories 485 (From Fat 157); Fat 17g (Saturated 5g); Cholesterol 62mg; Sodium 316mg; Carbohydrate 60g (Dietary Fiber 5g); Protein 24g.

Note: If you're dealing with cancer-related weight loss, you can add calories to this dish by adding a little Béchamel sauce to each layer. You'll need the following: ¼ cup butter; ¼ cup flour; 1½ to 2 cups milk; and ¾ cup grated Parmesan cheese, Gruyere, or another salty cheese. Melt the butter in a pan and add all the flour to it, stirring to get rid of any lumps. Cook this for about 5 minutes, stirring occasionally, and then add a little milk at a time, stirring as you do; the more milk you add, the thinner the sauce. Finally, add the cheese.

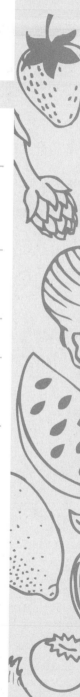

Chicken Tomato Curry

Prep time: 10 min • **Cook time:** 45 min • **Yield:** 4 servings

Ingredients

2 tablespoons extra-virgin olive or canola oil

1 onion, peeled and chopped

1 small red pepper, seeded and diced

1 small yellow pepper, seeded and diced

⅔ cup vegetable stock

One 10.75-ounce can fire-roasted tomatoes

1 teaspoon curry powder

1 teaspoon dried or fresh basil

½ teaspoon ground black pepper

3 boneless, skinless chicken breast halves, cut into bite-size pieces

¼ cup grated Parmesan cheese (optional)

2 cups uncooked brown rice

Directions

1 Cook the rice according to the package instructions.

2 While the rice is cooking, preheat the oven to 350 degrees. Place the chicken in a 9-x-13-inch baking dish.

3 In a medium skillet, heat the oil over medium heat, and then sauté the onion and peppers for about 5 minutes, just to soften slightly. Stir in the vegetable stock, tomatoes, curry powder, basil, and black pepper. Reduce the heat to low and simmer about 10 minutes.

4 Pour the mixture over the chicken. Bake for 1 hour, sprinkling with Parmesan cheese, if desired, for the last 10 minutes of baking.

5 Serve the chicken tomato curry over the rice.

Per serving: Calories 583 (From Fat 92); Fat 10g (Saturated 2g); Cholesterol 55mg; Sodium 317mg; Carbohydrate 91g (Dietary Fiber 4g); Protein 30g.

Vary It! Curry is an easy food to experiment with. Some spices you can consider incorporating include cumin, garam masala, coriander, turmeric, and paprika. Spicy peppers like serrano and chili peppers can add additional kick, but if you give them a try, you may want to consider balancing the heat with a cooling ingredient like yogurt or coconut milk. For a vegetarian curry, try using chickpeas, butternut squash, or any starchy veggies you have on hand.

Rainbow Paella

Prep time: 15 min • **Cook time:** 30 min • **Yield:** 6 servings

Ingredients	*Directions*
2 tablespoons olive oil	*1* In a large skillet, heat 1 tablespoon of the olive oil over medium heat. Then add the onion, garlic, pepper, carrots, and zucchini. Cook for 5 minutes, stirring frequently. Add the turkey sausage. Cook for an additional 2 to 3 minutes.
1 onion, peeled and chopped	
2 cloves garlic, peeled and chopped	
1 red bell pepper, seeded and chopped	
1 cup peeled and sliced carrots	*2* Stir in the vegetable broth, thyme, and saffron. Bring the mixture to a boil and simmer for 10 minutes, stirring occasionally.
1 zucchini, quartered and sliced	
4 ounces lean turkey sausage (plain or mild Italian), sliced	*3* In a separate large skillet, heat the remaining tablespoon of olive oil over medium heat. Add the shrimp and cook until pink. Remove from the pan and set aside.
¾ cup vegetable broth	
½ teaspoon dried thyme	
¼ teaspoon dried saffron	*4* Add the tomatoes, peas, and rice to the vegetable/sausage mixture and continue to stir and cook for another 5 minutes or until heated through.
24 large shrimp, peeled, deveined, and tails removed (refer to Figure 12-1)	
3 tomatoes, seeded and chopped	*5* Remove from the heat. Stir in the lemon juice, parsley, and cooked shrimp. Season with salt and pepper to taste.
½ cup frozen green peas, thawed	
3 cups cooked brown or white rice	
2 tablespoons lemon juice	
¼ cup flat-leaf parsley, chopped	
Salt and pepper, to taste	

Per serving: Calories 264 (From Fat 61); Fat 7g (Saturated 1g); Cholesterol 48mg; Sodium 481mg; Carbohydrate 39g (Dietary Fiber 6g); Protein 13g.

Tip: Add more broth if you prefer to have a more soupy paella.

Vary It! If you don't want to spend the money on saffron or don't have it on hand, feel free to substitute turmeric.

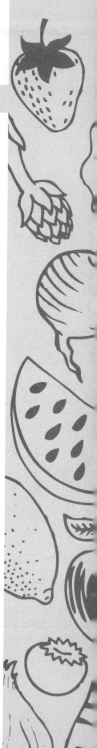

Scandinavian Salmon and Potato Casserole

Prep time: 15 min • **Cook time:** 1 hr 30 min • **Yield:** 8 servings

Ingredients

2 eggs

2 cups milk

3 tablespoons Parmesan cheese

1 teaspoon salt

⅛ teaspoon white pepper

1 tablespoon fresh dill, chopped

1 tablespoon dried parsley

5 medium russet potatoes, peeled and cut into ¼-inch slices

1 small onion, peeled and chopped

½ pound fresh carrots, peeled and sliced

½ pound frozen peas, thawed

One 14.75-ounce can boneless, skinless pink salmon, drained

½ cup whole-wheat seasoned bread crumbs

1 tablespoon butter, cut into small pieces

Directions

1 In a medium bowl, mix the eggs, milk, Parmesan cheese, salt, white pepper, dill, and parsley. Set aside.

2 Spray an 11-x-17-inch baking dish with cooking spray. Then layer the sliced potatoes, onion, carrots, peas, and salmon. Repeat until all ingredients are used up, making sure the layer ends with potato.

3 Pour the milk/egg mixture on top to cover the potatoes. Then sprinkle on the bread crumbs and randomly place some pats of butter on them.

4 Cover the casserole dish with aluminum foil and bake at 375 degrees for 30 minutes. Lower the heat to 350 degrees and let bake for 1 hour, removing the foil 20 minutes before the end of baking time to enable the bread crumbs to brown. Check the potatoes for doneness, adding time, if needed.

Per serving: Calories 269 (From Fat 62); Fat 7g (Saturated 3g); Cholesterol 88mg; Sodium 531mg; Carbohydrate 35g (Dietary Fiber 4g); Protein 17g.

Vary It! You can substitute canned tuna for the salmon. If you don't like carrots and peas, feel free to use other vegetables instead.

Slow-Cooker Stew

Prep time: 5–10 min • **Cook time:** 8 hr • **Yield:** 4 servings

Ingredients	Instructions
5 to 6 small potatoes, washed thoroughly and cut into quarters	**1** Combine all ingredients in a 5- to 6-quart slow cooker, add water to cover the ingredients, cover the slow cooker, and cook on low for about 8 hours.
¾ small bag of carrots, washed and sliced	
One 10-ounce bag frozen, mixed vegetables	**2** Season with pepper, paprika, and other herbs as desired. Add a packet of low-sodium beef stew seasoning mix.
12 ounces beef broth	
½ small bag frozen peeled pearl onions	
1 small onion, peeled and chopped	
2 cloves garlic, peeled and minced	
5 to 6 stalks celery, chopped	
1½ pounds beef stew meat	
Pepper, to taste	
Paprika, to taste	
1 packet low-sodium beef stew seasoning mix	

Per serving: Calories 536 (From Fat 85); Fat 10g (Saturated 4g); Cholesterol 126mg; Sodium 952mg; Carbohydrate 60g (Dietary Fiber 10g); Protein 53g.

Vary It! This is a very basic stew recipe. Experiment by substituting chicken or other protein sources, using chicken or vegetable broth instead of beef broth, or thickening with cornstarch, if a thicker consistency is desired. Also, vary the vegetables in the stew based on season, availability, and your taste preferences.

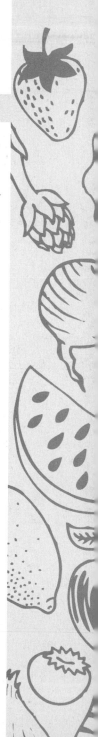

Entrées Requiring Side Dishes

The entrées in this section require more side dishes of whole grains, and colorful vegetables and fruits to make complete meals. These entrées are more traditional protein-based entrées, where a meal is planned around a protein food, such as chicken, lean beef, fish, or even tofu.

In this section, you find two fish dishes. Cooking fish is intimidating to many people, but as you can see from these recipes, it's very easy to prepare. Even if you're not a fan of fish, give it a try. Your palate may have changed during your cancer treatment, and the health benefits of fish are worth it. Most people get only half the amount of omega-3 fatty acids that they should be getting for optimal health.

Fish consumption has been consistently linked to health in numerous studies. The American Heart Association recommends two servings of fish a week for a healthy diet. And it doesn't sit heavy in the stomach either, which may be beneficial when you're dealing with the gastrointestinal effects of cancer treatment. If you find you enjoy the fish recipes we provide, feel free to change up the fish you use in them to get some variety. Just avoid using shark, swordfish, king mackerel, or tilefish, because these species contain the highest levels of mercury.

Finally, quite a few dishes in this chapter, such as the Vegetarian Chili, can be turned into a complete meal simply by adding a few whole grains to the pot. In addition, all the recipes are incredibly versatile and can be easily modified to suit your tastes and needs. For example, you can remove the heat-conferring spices from the Crispy Kicked-Up Multi-Grain Chicken, such as the crushed red pepper flakes and the hot sauce, if you have a sensitive stomach, or you can add more of these and other spices if you want to kick it up a few more notches.

Vegetarian Chili

Prep time: 5 min • **Cook time:** 1 hr • **Yield:** 10 servings

Ingredients	Instructions
1 onion, peeled and chopped	**1** Sauté the onion and garlic in the olive oil until tender.
4 cloves garlic, peeled and minced	
1 tablespoon olive oil	**2** Add the beans, corn, tomatoes, chili powder, cayenne pepper, cumin, black pepper, oregano, basil, and bay leaf.
One 15-ounce can red beans, drained and rinsed	
One 15-ounce can garbanzo beans, drained and rinsed	**3** Simmer for 1 hour, and then remove the bay leaf.
One 15-ounce can pinto beans, drained and rinsed	**4** Season to taste with salt and pepper.
1 cup frozen corn kernels, thawed	
4 cups canned chopped tomatoes	
⅓ cup chili powder	
1 teaspoon cayenne pepper (optional)	
2 teaspoons cumin	
1 tablespoon ground black pepper	
2 tablespoons dried oregano	
1 teaspoon dried basil	
1 bay leaf	
Salt and pepper, to taste	

Per serving: Calories 176 (From Fat 32); Fat 4g (Saturated 1g); Cholesterol 0mg; Sodium 510mg; Carbohydrate 30g (Dietary Fiber 6g); Protein 9g.

Note: You could easily turn this recipe into a complete meal by adding some brown rice or other grain during cooking. If you do so, you'll probably need to add a little more tomatoes or other liquid so it doesn't get too thick.

Tip: If you're dealing with unwanted cancer-related weight loss, you can boost the nutrient density by topping your chili with some diced avocado. You can also consider sprinkling on some cheese, sour cream, or plain yogurt.

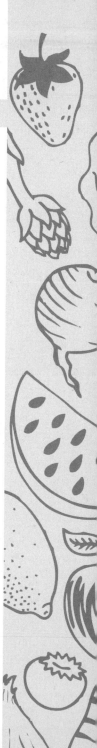

Tofu Loaf

Prep time: 5–10 min • **Cook time:** 1 hr • **Yield:** 6 servings

Ingredients	Directions
1½ pounds firm tofu	**1** Preheat the oven to 350 degrees.
1 egg	
⅓ cup ketchup	**2** Drain the tofu and remove as much moisture as possible. Then mash it in a large bowl.
⅓ cup soy sauce	
2 tablespoons Dijon mustard	**3** Add all the other ingredients to the bowl.
½ cup fresh parsley, chopped	
1 medium onion, peeled and finely chopped	**4** Spray a meatloaf pan with cooking spray or coat the bottom of the pan with a little oil to keep the loaf from sticking during cooking.
1 carrot, peeled and finely grated	
¼ teaspoon garlic powder	**5** Press the mixture into the pan and bake for 1 hour.
1 cup whole-wheat bread crumbs	**6** Let cool 10 to 15 minutes before trying to remove the loaf from the pan.

Per serving: Calories 129 (From Fat 52); Fat 6g (Saturated 1g); Cholesterol 10mg; Sodium 1,144mg; Carbohydrate 10g (Dietary Fiber 1g); Protein 11g.

Note: Tofu is a great alternative to meat in this loaf. It's a great source of protein without the saturated fat and cholesterol found in meat. Leftover loaf makes great lunch sandwiches.

Pasta with Bolognese Sauce

Prep time: 10 min • **Cook time:** 40 min • **Yield:** 6 servings

Ingredients	*Directions*
2 tablespoons olive oil	***1*** In a large skillet, heat the oil over medium heat. Add the onion, garlic, and celery, and cook until soft, about 5 minutes, stirring frequently. Add the beef to the pan and brown, about 5 minutes.
½ onion, peeled and chopped fine	
2 cloves garlic, peeled and chopped fine	
2 stalks celery, chopped fine	***2*** Pour in the wine. Cook, stirring until the wine is cooked off (about 5 minutes). Then pour the crushed tomatoes into the skillet. Add the oregano, nutmeg, and red pepper to the skillet. Simmer, stirring occasionally, until thick, about 25 minutes. Stir in the mascarpone cheese just before serving.
½ pound lean grass-fed ground beef	
½ cup dry red wine	
Two 28-ounce cans crushed tomatoes	
1 teaspoon dried oregano	***3*** While the sauce is simmering, cook the pasta as directed. Drain and toss with the sauce.
½ teaspoon nutmeg	
½ teaspoon dried red pepper flakes	***4*** Sprinkle with Parmesan cheese, as desired.
4 tablespoons mascarpone cheese	
One 1-pound box whole-grain pasta of choice	
Parmesan cheese, grated	

Per serving: Calories 528 (From Fat 168); Fat 19 (Saturated 7g); Cholesterol 41mg; Sodium 402mg; Carbohydrate 77g (Dietary Fiber 12g); Protein 23g.

Note: You don't need to use the wine in this recipe if you don't want to. You can add broth or water instead or forgo the additional liquid altogether.

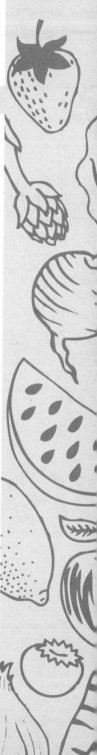

Crispy Kicked-Up Multi-Grain Chicken

Prep time: 10 min • **Cook time:** 35–40 min • **Yield:** 8 servings

Ingredients	*Directions*
1 cup plain Greek yogurt	*1* Line a baking sheet with parchment paper.
1 tablespoon hot sauce (optional)	*2* In a large bowl, combine the yogurt and hot sauce. Then add the chicken pieces to coat.
8 chicken drumsticks, skinless	
8 boneless, skinless chicken breasts (4 ounces each)	*3* Add the cereal, onion powder, garlic powder, black pepper, paprika, and hot pepper flakes to a 1-gallon zip-top plastic bag. Shake the bag to mix and slightly crush some of the flakes. Then add the chicken one or two pieces at a time to the bag, seal, and shake to coat until all the chicken is coated.
1½ cups multi-grain cereal flakes, crushed	
1½ teaspoons onion powder	
1½ teaspoons garlic powder	
2 teaspoons ground black pepper	*4* Place the chicken on the baking sheet and refrigerate for 30 minutes. Do not cover the chicken.
1 teaspoon paprika	*5* Preheat the oven to 400 degrees. Then transfer the chicken to the oven and bake for 35 to 40 minutes.
2 teaspoons crushed hot pepper flakes (optional)	

Per serving: Calories 250 (From Fat 55); Fat 6g (Saturated 2g); Cholesterol 105mg; Sodium 149mg; Carbohydrate 8g (Dietary Fiber 1g); Protein 39g.

Note: If you don't have multi-grain cereal, you can use whole-wheat bread crumbs along with the seasonings, unless you're using seasoned bread crumbs.

Easy Baked Salmon

Prep time: 2 min • **Cook time:** 15–20 min • **Yield:** 4 servings

Ingredients	Directions
1 to 2 tablespoons butter or margarine, melted	*1* Preheat the oven to 375 degrees.
2 teaspoons lemon juice	*2* In a small bowl, combine the butter or margarine, lemon juice, tarragon, and garlic powder.
1 teaspoon dried tarragon leaves	
¼ teaspoon garlic powder	*3* Slightly grease a baking dish or spray with cooking spray. Then place the salmon filets in the dish.
4 salmon filets (about 4 ounces each)	*4* Pour the butter or margarine mixture over the salmon.
	5 Bake for 15 to 20 minutes or until the fish flakes with a fork.

Per serving: Calories 171 (From Fat 64); Fat 7g (Saturated 2g); Cholesterol 72mg; Sodium 84mg; Carbohydrate 1g (Dietary Fiber 0g); Protein 25g.

Tip: For a moister salmon, you can wrap the filets in aluminum foil or parchment paper, or cover the baking dish with foil prior to baking.

Vary It! This recipe can also be made with fresh tarragon. Mix butter, lemon juice, and garlic powder and pour over the fish. Top each filet with a small, fresh sprig of tarragon and bake.

Note: Cooking temperatures and times can vary based on the thickness of the fish filets. Generally, 10 minutes of cooking per inch is required.

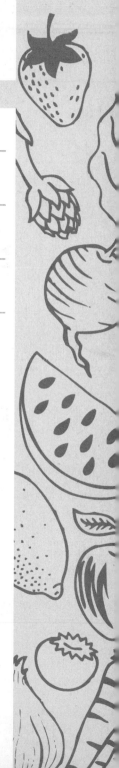

Baked Lemon Cod

Prep time: 5 min • **Cook time:** 20 min • **Yield:** 3 servings

Ingredients	Instructions
12 ounces fresh cod	*1* Preheat the oven to 350 degrees.
2 teaspoons olive oil	
4 teaspoons lemon juice	*2* Spray an 8-x-8-inch pan with cooking spray and place fish in the pan in a single layer.
1 teaspoon grated lemon rind	
⅛ teaspoon lemon pepper	*3* In a bowl, mix the olive oil, lemon juice, lemon rind, and lemon pepper.
2 teaspoons dried parsley	
	4 Pour over the fish.
	5 Sprinkle with the dried parsley, cover the baking dish with aluminum foil, and bake for 20 minutes or until the fish flakes easily with a fork.

Per serving: Calories 112 (From Fat 33); Fat 4g (Saturated 1g); Cholesterol 43mg; Sodium 76mg; Carbohydrate 1g (Dietary Fiber 0g); Protein 18g.

Vary It! You can substitute any number of fish in this recipe, including orange roughy, tilapia, or whitefish.

Chapter 13

Light Yet Satisfying Sides

In This Chapter

▶ Recognizing the power of a simple side dish

▶ Going for grains and starchy vegetables

▶ Making fruits and vegetables the focus of your side dish

Most Americans don't eat enough fruits, vegetables, and grains to optimize their health. When you consider that french fries remain the dominant side dish from sea to shining sea, this probably doesn't come as a big surprise. Now, there is nothing wrong with enjoying french fries and other decadent fare on occasion. Life should be about enjoying experiences, including food. But if you have these experiences every day, they're no longer special, and they become unhealthy, increasing your risk of cancer and a host of other health problems, such as obesity, high blood pressure, high cholesterol, and diabetes.

In this chapter, we look at how side dishes can be a great way to create a plate that's both appetizing and nutritious. The recipes in this chapter are all very versatile and can be paired with the protein-based entrees outlined in Chapter 12 or with entrees of your own creation. If you give these recipes a try, you'll see that grains, fruits, and vegetables can get your taste buds soaring without requiring an overdose of sodium and fat.

Creating an Appetizing and Nutritious Plate with Sides

According to recommendations by the American Institute for Cancer Research, two-thirds of your plate should be filled with vegetables, fruits, whole grains, or beans, and only one-third of the plate should be an animal protein (see Chapter 4). Now, don't feel like each and every plate of food you eat has to meet that ratio. You may have some meals where you just have a protein source with a grain *or* a vegetable, and other meals where maybe you just have vegetables (such as a salad). That's okay. The ultimate goal is to pack as many nutritious foods into your day as you can, with the majority of those nutrients coming from plant-based foods. The good news is, there are numerous ways for you to achieve this goal.

For example, instead of compartmentalizing your plate (two-thirds this, one-third that), you may want to work toward creating color-dominated plates. If you're eating a turkey sandwich on whole-grain bread, for instance, instead of reaching for potato chips, you might consider having some carrot sticks and broccoli on the side and adding some romaine lettuce and tomato slices to your sandwich. With these veggies added to your plate, it has suddenly become much more colorful and nutritious.

Many cancer-fighting nutrients are in the compounds that give fruits and vegetables their color, so "eating the rainbow" — getting as many different colored foods into your diet as possible — can be a good strategy for optimizing nutrition.

Every day, strive to eat at least 1½ to 2 cups of fruit, 2 to 3 cups of vegetables, and 6 or 7 servings of grains (at least half from whole grains). For more information on what counts as a cup or an ounce, visit `www.choosemyplate.gov/food-groups`.

Gobbling Up Grains and Starchy Vegetables

Despite the United States being a major wheat-producing country, many Americans eat only half the recommended amount of whole grains daily. Some people may be afraid to eat grains, thinking they're nothing but fattening carbs; others just don't know how to incorporate grains into their diet. But no matter where you fall on the issue, the fact is, grains are a tremendous source of energy. And when you're battling cancer, you need to harness whatever energy you can to get through your treatment and move toward recovery.

Whole grains are generally preferable to refined grains (like white pasta, white bread, and white rice) because whole grains contain more nutrients and fiber, but if you're having bowel problems (like diarrhea or a bowel obstruction), eating refined grains that are lower in fiber is best until your gastrointestinal issues resolve. Don't worry — you'll still get lots of nutrients and energy from grains, but you'll give your innards a break. On the other hand, if you're not having bowel problems or you're constipated, focusing on high-fiber whole grains is ideal.

The recipes in this section feature a variety of grains, as well as a variety of starchy vegetables. If a recipe is based around a particular type of grain you can't eat, feel free to replace it with one that you can.

Confetti Couscous

Prep time: 10 min • **Cook time:** 20 min • **Yield:** 6 servings

Ingredients	*Directions*
5 cups low-fat, low-sodium chicken stock	*1* In a large pot, bring the chicken stock to a boil.
4 cups uncooked couscous	*2* In a casserole dish, place the couscous and spread it so that it evenly covers the bottom of the dish. Carefully pour the hot chicken stock into the casserole dish; there should be just enough stock to cover the couscous. Tightly cover the dish with plastic wrap and steam until all the stock is absorbed (approximately 15 minutes). Remove the plastic wrap and fluff with a fork.
2 tablespoons olive oil	
½ teaspoon cumin	
½ teaspoon cinnamon	
½ cup flat-leaf parsley, chopped fine	
Kosher salt and white pepper to taste (optional)	*3* In a small bowl, mix 1 tablespoon of the oil, cumin, cinnamon, parsley, salt, and white pepper until well combined; set aside.
¼ cup red onion, peeled and diced fine	
¼ cup red bell pepper, peeled and diced fine	*4* In a large nonstick skillet, sauté the onion, bell pepper, squash, and zucchini in the remaining table-spoon of oil for 5 minutes or until tender. Then fold these vegetables into the couscous in the casserole dish and pour the dressing on top.
¼ cup yellow squash, diced fine	
¼ cup zucchini, diced fine	
Fresh lemon juice (optional)	*5* Sprinkle with lemon juice, if desired.

Per serving: Calories 495 (From Fat 47); Fat 5g (Saturated 1g); Cholesterol 0mg; Sodium 73mg; Carbohydrate 91g (Dietary Fiber 6g); Protein 17g.

Tip: If you don't have the energy to sauté vegetables, buy the kind that come in steamer bags and then just mix those into the couscous. You can even use veggies that already have a sauce, if you don't feel like mixing up your own.

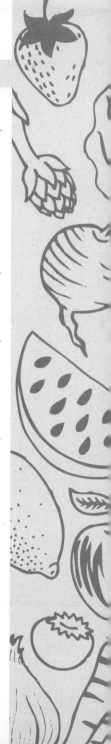

Harvest Pilaf

Prep time: 10 min • **Cook time:** 1 hr • **Yield:** 6 servings

Ingredients	*Directions*
2¾ cups vegetable broth ½ cup wild rice, uncooked	*1* In a large saucepan, bring the vegetable broth to a boil; then add the wild rice. Cook for 30 minutes.
¾ cup brown rice, uncooked 2 tablespoons olive oil 1 onion, peeled and diced 4 cloves garlic, peeled and minced	*2* Add the brown rice to the saucepan, cover, and cook for another 50 minutes, or until the rice is done cooking. Be sure to keep an eye on the rice during the cooking process. You may need to add additional broth (up to ½ cup) and cooking time (the entire process can take up to 80 minutes) to get both the wild and brown rice to be cooked properly.
3 cups fresh button mushrooms, sliced 2 celery stalks, sliced ½ teaspoon thyme ½ teaspoon marjoram	*3* In a large skillet, heat the oil and sauté the onions and garlic until the onions start to caramelize, approximately 8 to 10 minutes. Add the mushrooms, celery, thyme, and marjoram, and cook for another 5 minutes. If more moisture is needed, add some broth to the pan.
⅓ cup chopped fresh parsley ⅓ cup toasted sliced almonds Salt and pepper (to taste)	*4* Add the cooked rice, parsley, and almonds, and stir well to combine. Cook for a few more minutes until the pilaf is heated through.

Per serving: Calories 243 (From Fat 75); Fat 8g (Saturated 1g); Cholesterol 0mg; Sodium 418mg; Carbohydrate 37g (Dietary Fiber 4g); Protein 7g.

Note: If you don't want to spend time cooking rice, you can use Uncle Ben's Ready Rice, which heats in the microwave in 90 seconds. The Whole Grain Brown version doesn't have any added sodium, but the Long Grain & Wild version has a considerable amount, so if you use it, avoid adding any additional salt to this recipe. If you go the Ready Rice route, you can use one pack of each and start with Step 3 in this recipe. Then break apart the rice in the pack before adding to the skillet (you don't need to heat it in the microwave first), and then add broth as needed for moisture.

Tip: For instructions on how to toast almonds see the Balsamic Green Beans recipe, later in this chapter.

Pasta Salad with Pecans and Grapes

Prep time: 5 min • **Cook time:** 10 min • **Yield:** 8 servings

Ingredients	Directions
12 ounces uncooked bow-tie (farfalle) pasta	**1** Cook the pasta according to package directions. Drain and set aside.
5 tablespoons pecans, chopped	**2** Preheat the oven to 350 degrees. Lightly spray a baking sheet with cooking spray or line with nonstick aluminum foil. Evenly distribute the pecans on the baking sheet, and place them in the oven until they toast and just become aromatic, about 5 minutes. Shake the pan while toasting if needed, to prevent burning. Remove from baking pan and set aside.
1 cup low-fat sour cream	
2 tablespoons low-fat mayonnaise	
1 tablespoon sherry vinegar	
Salt and ground black pepper to taste	
1 cup seedless green grapes, halved	**3** In a large bowl, add the sour cream, mayonnaise, vinegar, and salt and pepper (if desired), and mix until well combined.
1 cup seedless red grapes halved	**4** Add the pasta and toss to coat the noodles.
1 stalk celery, chopped	**5** Add the green and red grapes, celery, pecans, and mint, and gently fold the ingredients together. Refrigerate a few hours before serving.
1 tablespoon chopped fresh mint or 1 teaspoon dried mint	

Per serving: Calories 289 (From Fat 96); Fat 11g (Saturated 3g); Cholesterol 18mg; Sodium 200mg; Carbohydrate 42g (Dietary Fiber 2g); Protein 8g.

Vary It! You can use virtually any type of pasta to make this recipe. Other good shapes include rotini (spiral-shaped), penne, rigatoni, ziti, and elbow macaroni. It all depends on what type of texture you prefer. For instance, rotini tends to hold onto more ingredients than a flatter noodle like farfalle.

Tip: For additional nutrients, you can make this recipe with whole-grain pasta or boost your vegetable intake by looking for pastas that incorporate veggies, like Barilla's Veggie Farfalle.

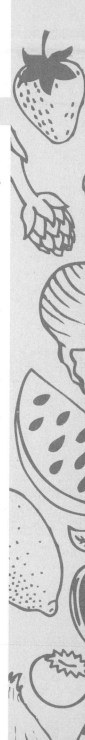

Mediterranean Mixed Grains Salad

Prep time: 10 min • **Cook time:** 1 hr • **Yield:** 5 servings

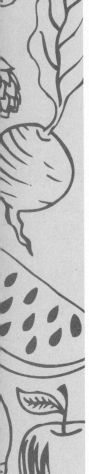

Ingredients

½ **pound quick-cooking barley**

¼ **pound rye berries**

¼ **pound wheat berries**

½ **cup Kalamata olives, pitted and sliced**

½ **cup feta cheese**

½ **cup cucumber, diced small**

½ **cup tomatoes, diced small**

¼ **cup red onion, diced small**

½ **cup roasted red bell peppers, peeled, seeded, and chopped**

¼ **cup flat-leaf parsley, chopped**

¼ **cup apple cider vinegar**

1 **teaspoon garlic, minced**

¼ **cup plus 1 tablespoon olive oil**

Salt and white pepper to taste (optional)

Directions

1 Bring 14 cups of water to a boil in a large pot, add the wheat berries, reduce the heat to simmer, and cook for 15 minutes. Then add the rye berries and cook for 30 minutes. Finally, add the quick-cooking barley and cook for an additional 15 minutes. Drain, and set grains aside to cool.

2 After all the grains have cooled, mix them together in a large bowl with the olives, feta, cucumber, tomatoes, red onion, roasted red peppers, and parsley.

3 In a separate bowl, whisk together the vinegar, garlic, and olive oil until well blended. Pour over the salad, mix well, and season with salt and pepper to taste.

Per serving: Calories 471 (From Fat 196); Fat 22g (Saturated 5g); Cholesterol 13mg; Sodium 575mg; Carbohydrate 60g (Dietary Fiber 12g); Protein 13g.

Note: Your barley is done cooking when 20 percent of the grains have burst open. You can also make the rye berries softer by soaking them in water the night before cooking them.

Tip: If serving immediately, the flavors meld together a little quicker when you mix the warm grains with the dressing and other veggies. Otherwise, make this the night before to maximize flavor. Enjoy as a side or as a meal over a bed or arugula or baby spinach.

Spaghetti Squash with Marinara Sauce

Prep time: 10 min • **Cook time:** 40 min • **Yield:** 6 servings

Ingredients	*Directions*
2 whole spaghetti squash	*1* Preheat the oven to 400 degrees, and line a baking sheet with nonstick aluminum foil.
¼ cup extra-virgin olive oil	
⅛ teaspoon salt	*2* Split the squashes in half, and scrape out the seeds. Season the squash with olive oil, salt, and pepper. Place on baking sheet flesh side down, and roast for approximately 40 minutes, or until fully cooked. Then remove from the oven and let rest until cool enough to handle, approximately 10 minutes.
Pepper (to taste)	
Marinara Sauce (see the following recipe)	
	3 Use a large kitchen spoon to scrape the strands of squash from the inside of the skin. Add the spaghetti squash to the pan with the hot Marinara Sauce just long enough to heat.

Marinara Sauce

¼ cup extra-virgin olive oil	*1* In a large pot, heat the oil over medium-high heat. Add the onions and garlic, and sauté until the onions start to brown, a little after 5 minutes.
1 small onion, peeled and finely chopped	
1 garlic clove, peeled and finely chopped	*2* Add to the pot the celery, carrot, salt, and pepper, and continue sautéing until all vegetables are soft, about 5 minutes.
1 stalk celery, finely chopped	
1 carrot, peeled and finely chopped	*3* Add the tomatoes and bay leaf, and simmer uncovered over low heat until the sauce thickens, about 30 to 40 minutes.
¼ teaspoon salt	
¼ teaspoon freshly ground black pepper	
One 32-ounce can crushed tomatoes	
1 dried bay leaf	

Per serving: *Calories 256 (From Fat 165); Fat 19g (Saturated 3g); Cholesterol 0mg; Sodium 651mg; Carbohydrate 20g (Dietary Fiber 3g); Protein 3g.*

Twice-Baked Potatoes

Prep time: 5 min • **Cook time:** 1 hr • **Yield:** 6 servings

Ingredients	*Directions*
4 medium russet potatoes	**1** Preheat the oven to 400 degrees.
1½ cups low-fat cottage cheese	**2** Thoroughly wash the potatoes, scrubbing the skins, and then prick each potato in several places with a fork.
¼ cup plain low-fat yogurt	
1 cup low-fat sharp cheddar cheese, grated	**3** Bake potatoes directly on the center rack until tender, 45 to 60 minutes. Let cool slightly, and then carefully cut each potato in half lengthwise and scoop out the pulp into a bowl, taking care not to break the skins.
2 tablespoons fresh flat-leaf parsley or 2 teaspoons dried parsley	
¼ teaspoon salt	**4** Reduce the oven temperature to 350 degrees.
¼ teaspoon black pepper	**5** In a food processor or blender, process the cottage cheese, yogurt, cheddar, parsley, salt, and pepper. Then add this mixture to the bowl with the potato pulp and stir by hand until well combined.
Paprika for sprinkling (optional)	
	6 Divide the mixture among the potato shells, and place the shells on a cookie sheet. Bake for 10 to 15 minutes until slightly browned on top. Sprinkle with paprika, if desired.

Per serving: Calories 187 (From Fat 20); Fat 2g (Saturated 1g); Cholesterol 7mg; Sodium 461mg; Carbohydrate 27g (Dietary Fiber 3g); Protein 15g.

Note: The best baking and mashing potatoes are also called starchy potatoes, and they tend to be long and have a coarse skin. You may see these sold in the supermarket as Russets (Arcadia, Burbank, Norkotah, among others), Goldrush, Long White, White Rose, California Long White, or Idaho.

Creamy Cashew Rutabaga Gratin

Prep time: 20 min • **Cook time:** 1 hr 15 min • **Yield:** 6 servings

Ingredients	Directions
2 small rutabagas	*1* Preheat oven to 375 degrees.
1 cup raw cashews	
1 tablespoon nutritional yeast	*2* Peel and cut the rutabaga, and slice or use a mandolin to get rounds that are about ⅛ inch in thickness. Set aside.
Salt to taste (optional)	
4 teaspoons fresh thyme, chopped	*3* Boil enough water to make 1½ cups, and then pour this over the cashews in a blender (but don't blend). Let sit for 15 to 30 minutes until the nuts soften. Then add the yeast, and blend on the highest setting until smooth and creamy, about 3 minutes. Scrape down the sides if needed. Season with a little salt, if desired.
4 teaspoons fresh marjoram, chopped	
¼ teaspoon ground nutmeg	
Salt and pepper to taste (optional)	
2 slices hearty whole-grain bread	*4* Cover the bottom of an 8-inch round baking dish with a single layer of rutabaga slices, overlapping the edges and working in a circle. Sprinkle on a little of the chopped thyme, marjoram, and salt and pepper (if desired). Then do the same with a second layer of rutabaga, but add enough of the cashew sauce to cover both layers (about one-third of the sauce). Continue in this pattern until all the rutabaga is used up, making sure the top layer is covered in cashew sauce. Sprinkle the top with nutmeg.
1 tablespoon olive oil	
	5 Tear the bread into small pieces, and toss with olive oil in a small bowl. Then spread on top of the gratin.
	6 Bake for approximately 1 hour and 15 minutes, or until the rutabagas are tender when pierced and the breadcrumbs are golden brown.

Per serving: Calories 204 (From Fat 125); Fat 14g (Saturated 2g); Cholesterol 0mg; Sodium 59mg; Carbohydrate 16g (Dietary Fiber 3g); Protein 7g.

Note: Rutabagas can generally be bought year-round, but they're in season during the fall and winter. When buying, look for unwaxed roots. (Wax is used to improve storage, but it seals in rot and mold.) Rutabagas should be firm and have a yellow flesh.

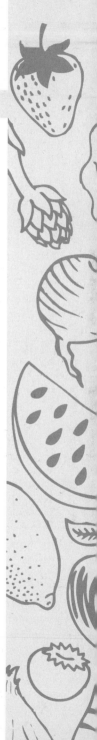

Fueling Up with Fruits and Vegetables

On the New American Plate (see Chapter 4), fruits and vegetables are given preferential treatment over grains and protein. This isn't surprising, considering they're among the most nutrient-dense foods on the planet. But although we all know that fruits and vegetables are good for us, many of us still aren't making enough of an effort to get them. According to a 2006 study that examined data from the National Health and Nutrition Examination Survey, only 40 percent of Americans ate an average of five or more servings of fruits and vegetables daily.

There are likely many reasons for this. Some people may think that produce costs more than convenience foods, others may not like vegetables or know how to prepare them, and others may simply not think to eat them. If you're among the majority not getting your daily dose of fruits and vegetables, we recommend you make the effort. They truly do a body good and may help provide your body with the resources it needs to beat your cancer and protect you from a recurrence, a secondary cancer, or other potential treatment-related health issues.

You can get your fruits and vegetables through juices, as well as fresh, frozen, dried, or canned produce, giving you lots of options. Ideally, you should eat as many different types of fruits and vegetables as you can in any given day to get the greatest variety of cancer-fighting nutrients, but that isn't absolutely necessary.

It's not about perfection. Just try to add as much in the way of fruits and vegetables as you can.

All the recipes in this chapter provide at least one serving of produce. We include a variety of vegetables for you to try, and there are both cold and warm dishes. As these recipes show, produce doesn't have to be bland or boring. Enjoy!

Cauliflower Italiano

Prep time: 5 min • **Cook time:** 25–40 min • **Yield:** 6 servings

Ingredients	Directions
⅔ cup mayonnaise	*1* Preheat the oven to 425 degrees.
1 tablespoon hot sauce	
6 cups fresh cauliflower florets	*2* In a large bowl with a lid, mix the mayonnaise with the hot sauce until well combined.
1 cup seasoned whole-wheat breadcrumbs	*3* Add the cauliflower florets to the bowl, cover with the lid, and shake until the florets are well coated. Then add the breadcrumbs to the bowl, cover, and shake again.
	4 Pour the cauliflower florets onto an ungreased baking sheet and arrange in a single layer, avoiding having the pieces touch.
	5 Bake 25 to 40 minutes, or until golden brown.

Per serving: Calories 210 (From Fat 182); Fat 20g (Saturated 3g); Cholesterol 15mg; Sodium 239mg; Carbohydrate 7g (Dietary Fiber 3g); Protein 2g.

Vary It! Try this recipe with a variety of other vegetables, including broccoli, bell peppers, and zucchini. Broccoli works especially well, because the branches on the broccoli heads work like a sponge to absorb the flavors.

Tip: If you don't have seasoned whole-wheat breadcrumbs, try mixing ⅓ cup Parmesan cheese with 1 cup plain breadcrumbs and any seasonings you like.

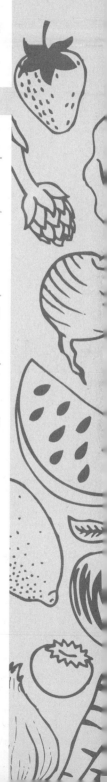

Gingered Honey-Glazed Carrots

Prep time: 5 min • **Cook time:** 12–20 min • **Yield:** 4 servings

Ingredients	Directions
2 tablespoons extra-virgin olive oil 1½ tablespoons honey 1 tablespoon lemon juice ½ teaspoon ground ginger 1 pound baby carrots ¼ cup chopped flat-leaf parsley	**1** In a small bowl, mix the oil, honey, lemon juice, and ginger until well combined. **2** In a medium saucepan, bring the carrots and enough cold water to cover them to a boil. Reduce the heat to medium-high and simmer for 10 to 15 minutes, or until the carrots are tender-crisp. Drain and return to the pan over medium-low heat. **3** Add the honey mixture to the pan, and stir the carrots until well coated. Continue stirring and cooking until a glaze forms, about 2 to 5 minutes. Then mix in the parsley.

Per serving: Calories 137 (From Fat 68); Fat 8g (Saturated 1g); Cholesterol 0mg; Sodium 43mg; Carbohydrate 18g (Dietary Fiber 2g); Protein 1g.

Orange-Glazed Asparagus

Prep time: 5 min • **Cook time:** 7–9 min • **Yield:** 2 servings

Ingredients	Directions
½ pound fresh asparagus, wood ends trimmed ¼ cup orange marmalade 1 tablespoon white wine vinegar ⅛ teaspoon allspice ⅛ teaspoon ground ginger	**1** In a skillet, bring 1 inch of water to a boil. Place the asparagus in a steamer basket over the water for 5 minutes. (You can also use microwave steamer bags or an electric steamer to cook the vegetables.) Drain the asparagus and set aside. **2** In a medium saucepan, mix the remaining ingredients and bring to a boil. Reduce the heat and simmer for 2 to 4 minutes; then remove from the heat and allow the sauce to cool. Pour the sauce over the asparagus and serve.

Per serving: Calories 113 (From Fat 2); Fat 0g (Saturated 0g); Cholesterol 0mg; Sodium 29mg; Carbohydrate 29g (Dietary Fiber 1g); Protein 2g.

Wholesome Cheesy Creamed Spinach

Prep time: 10 min • **Cook time:** 15–20 min • **Yield:** 4 servings

Ingredients	Directions
One 10-ounce package frozen chopped spinach	**1** Cook the spinach per the package directions. Drain and let the spinach sit over a bowl in a colander for continued draining.
¾ cup evaporated skim milk	
2 teaspoons cornstarch	**2** In a small bowl, combine the milk and cornstarch; set aside.
1 tablespoon olive oil	
½ cup onions, peeled and finely chopped	**3** In a nonstick skillet, heat the olive oil over medium heat, and then sauté the onions, basil, oregano, and nutmeg. Cook until tender, about 2 to 5 minutes.
¼ teaspoon dried basil	
¼ teaspoon dried oregano	
⅛ teaspoon nutmeg	**4** Add the milk mixture to the skillet, and cook and stir until thickened and bubbly. Add the cheeses and continue stirring until they're melted and well combined. Then stir in the spinach and heat through.
½ cup reduced-fat Monterey Jack cheese, shredded	
¼ cup Parmesan cheese, shredded	

Per serving: Calories 159 (From Fat 72); Fat 8g (Saturated 3g); Cholesterol 16mg; Sodium 363mg; Carbohydrate 12g (Dietary Fiber 2g); Protein 11g.

Vary It! You can also make this as a baked recipe. Instead of cooking the spinach, let it thaw and then wring it out to remove as much water as possible. Follow steps 2 through 4, and then pour into a baking dish. Sprinkle the top with a little extra cheese, and then bake for 15 to 20 minutes in an oven that has been preheated to 350 degrees, or until the spinach is hot and bubbly and the cheese is slightly browned in spots.

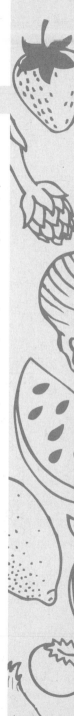

Balsamic Green Beans

Prep time: 5 min • **Cook time:** 10–15 min • **Yield:** 2 servings

Ingredients	*Directions*
2½ **cups fresh green beans**	**1** Rinse the green beans and remove both ends (top and tail).
2 cloves garlic, peeled and minced	
5 teaspoons balsamic vinegar	**2** In a large mixing bowl, combine the garlic, vinegar, agave, and olive oil until well combined; set aside.
1 teaspoon agave nectar	
2½ **teaspoons olive oil**	**3** Steam the beans until tender but firm, approximately 10 to 15 minutes.
¼ **cup toasted sliced almonds**	
	4 Add the beans to the bowl and mix. Then mix in the toasted sliced almonds.
	5 Serve at room temperature or chilled.

Per serving: Calories 189 (From Fat 109); Fat 12g (Saturated 1g); Cholesterol 0mg; Sodium 8mg; Carbohydrate 37g (Dietary Fiber 5g); Protein 10g.

Note: You can always substitute frozen green beans for fresh. Buy the steamer bags and prepare the beans in the microwave per the package directions, or toss the beans into boiling water for approximately 4 minutes or use a basket steamer.

Tip: Some stores sell already toasted almonds, typically in the produce section by the salads, but if you can't find them, you can just buy the plain slices or slivers and toast them yourself. Heat the oven to 350 degrees, spread the almonds on an ungreased baking sheet in a single layer, and place into the oven for 5 to 10 minutes, depending on the quantity you toast. Stir the almonds every 3 minutes to ensure even browning. Remove from the oven when golden brown. You'll need to keep a close eye on them as they're browning because they can burn easily.

Mexican Bean Salad with Lime Dressing

Prep time: 5 min • **Yield:** 4 servings

Ingredients	*Directions*
Two 15-ounce cans black beans, rinsed and drained	*1* In a large bowl, combine the beans, corn, red bell pepper, tomatoes, scallions, and cilantro. Pour the Lime Dressing over them and mix together. Then gently mix in the avocado.
1½ cups frozen corn kernels, thawed	
1 red bell pepper, seeded and diced	*2* Serve at room temperature or cold.
2 tomatoes, seeded and chopped	
4 scallions, ends trimmed and diced	
½ cup fresh cilantro, chopped (optional)	
Lime Dressing (see the following recipe)	
2 avocados, pitted, peeled and diced	

Lime Dressing

¼ cup fresh lime juice (3 or 4 limes)	*1* In a small bowl, mix all ingredients until well blended.
⅓ cup olive oil	
1 tablespoon agave	
2 cloves garlic, minced	
½ teaspoon salt	
⅛ teaspoon chili powder	

Per serving: Calories 249 (From Fat 93); Fat 10g (Saturated 2g); Cholesterol 0mg; Sodium 79mg; Carbohydrate 33g (Dietary Fiber 13g); Protein 10g.

Note: If you make this salad ahead of time, wait until just before serving to mix in the tomato, avocado, and cilantro. This prevents the tomato and avocado from breaking down and causing a mushy texture, and it retains cilantro's fresh flavor.

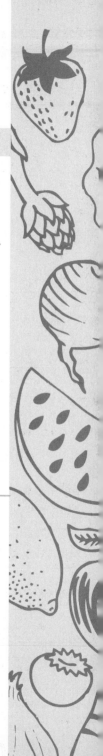

Broccoli Salad

Prep time: 5 min • **Yield:** 6 servings

Ingredients	Directions
½ cup mayonnaise	*1* In a large bowl, mix the mayonnaise, vinegar, and agave. Stir until well combined.
3 tablespoons vinegar (apple cider, red, or white)	
¼ cup agave nectar	*2* Add the broccoli, cranberries, onion, cheese, sunflower seeds, and the salt and pepper (if desired) to the bowl and mix until the ingredients are evenly distributed.
3 cups fresh broccoli florets, broken into small pieces	
1 cup dried cranberries	*3* Refrigerate until ready to serve, preferably at least 1 hour.
1 small red onion, chopped	
1 cup low-fat cheddar cheese, shredded	
1 cup sunflower seeds	
Salt and pepper to taste (optional)	

Per serving: Calories 411 (From Fat 240); Fat 27g (Saturated 4g); Cholesterol 15mg; Sodium 231mg; Carbohydrate 37g (Dietary Fiber 5g); Protein 10g.

Vary It! If you prefer to have your salads more dressed, you can use up to 1 cup of mayonnaise in this recipe. Or, for a less fattening option, try adding ½ cup plain Greek yogurt.

Chapter 14

Energy-Boosting Snacks

In This Chapter

▶ Snacking your way to more energy

▶ Making snacks you can take on the go

▶ Preparing snacks for social situations

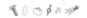

Cancer and its treatments are physically and emotionally draining. Not only is your body fighting the cancer, but you're having to run around to numerous appointments while keeping up with all or most of your usual activities. So, it's not surprising that low energy is one of the most commonly reported side effects of cancer and its treatments. A great way to combat this side effect and keep your energy levels up throughout your cancer journey is snacking. Even if you're constantly running from one appointment to another, many of the recipes we include in this chapter are highly portable, enabling you to nourish yourself even while on the go.

In addition to numerous transportable snacks, you'll find many recipes that are suitable for entertaining. Because family and friends may want to visit you more often, and holidays and other events will continue on, these snacks enable you to reap the benefits of cancer-fighting nutrients on these occasions, when more nutritionally deficient foods may otherwise be the only fare available.

Boosting Nutrition and Combating Side Effects with Snacks

Snacks are a great way to maintain adequate blood glucose levels, preventing you from feeling energy depleted. Certain snacks can also prevent insulin surges. For example, we include a recipe for Onion and Garlic Roasted

Chickpeas (chickpeas are also called *garbanzo beans*) because several studies have shown that eating legumes like chickpeas just before a meal or with a meal can reduce blood glucose surges, thereby reducing the body's insulin response. So, you may even consider having some legumes with a particularly carbohydrate-heavy meal to keep your blood glucose levels steady.

When snacks include wholesome foods, they're also a great way to get in some additional cancer-fighting nutrients. And for those times when you're unable to eat regular meals because of treatment- or cancer-related side effects, snacks can serve as mini meals, ensuring that you don't become malnourished and experience the additional ill effects that accompany it. In addition, they prevent an empty stomach, which may reduce the risk of nausea, particularly when you're going through active treatment.

If your appetite is poor, try having a small snack every three or four hours, or taking little nibbles every hour. For example, you can keep a bag of the Fruit and Nut Trail Mix beside you and eat a little bit at a time, with a goal to finish a portion in three hours and then have a meal or start another snack. If solid foods are difficult for you to eat, consider making yourself a smoothie. (We include a few good smoothie recipes in Chapter 10.) In addition, soft foods, like the Frosty Yogurt Bowls recipe in this chapter, may be good to try and may go down easier.

Snacking on the Run

When you're receiving chemotherapy, eating a little something to prevent a sour stomach is particularly important. Many treatment facilities make snacks available, but they may not be as nutritious or as pleasing to your palate as your own. So, it's generally best to bring your own snacks when you can. Fortunately, there are a vast variety of transportable snacks, and in this section, you find numerous options to try, from wholesome baked goodies to nutritious bites that can be easily bagged.

To enhance the portability of these snacks, parcel them out and package them into individual servings after you prepare them. Be sure to store these snacks appropriately so that they stay fresh. They should be wrapped or placed in an airtight container and then refrigerated.

If you don't have the energy to prepare any snacks, you can ask friends and family to prepare them for you. Of course, there are plenty of options that require no preparation at all. Some of these options include nuts, plain popcorn, whole-wheat crackers with some hard cheese or a nut butter, yogurt, bananas, or carrot sticks.

Homemade Granola

Prep time: 10 min • **Cook time:** 30 min • **Yield:** 8 servings

Ingredients	Directions
2½ cups old-fashioned rolled oats	**1** Preheat the oven to 350 degrees.
¾ cup untoasted sunflower seeds	**2** In a large bowl, combine the oats, sunflower seeds, almonds, coconut, cinnamon, nutmeg, and salt. Toss well to evenly distribute all ingredients.
¾ cup untoasted almonds	
½ cup shredded coconut (unsweetened, if possible)	**3** Add the honey or maple syrup and the vanilla to the dry ingredients, and mix well to combine all ingredients.
1 teaspoon cinnamon	**4** Spread the mixture on a rimmed baking sheet.
¼ teaspoon nutmeg	
¼ teaspoon salt	**5** Bake for 30 minutes, stirring occasionally for even browning.
½ cup honey or pure maple syrup	
½ teaspoon vanilla	**6** Remove from the oven, add the raisins and cranberries, and stir to combine.
½ cup raisins	
½ cup dried cranberries	**7** Let cool, stirring occasionally until the granola reaches room temperature.
	8 Store in an airtight container up to 7 to 10 days in the pantry or up to a month in the refrigerator.

Per serving: Calories 403 (From Fat 167); Fat 19g (Saturated 4g); Cholesterol 0mg; Sodium 81mg; Carbohydrate 55g (Dietary Fiber 7g); Protein 9g.

Vary It! Substitute whatever nuts, seeds, and dried fruits you like. Chopped walnuts, pecans, cashews, and pistachios all work great, as do pumpkin seeds and sesame seeds. Other dried fruits to consider include chopped dried apricots, currents, and cherries.

Tip: If you prefer chunky granola, pat down the mixture into the baking sheet using the back of a spatula, and don't mix the granola as it's baking. When it's done baking, you can remove it from the pan in chunks.

Note: The darker your granola gets without burning, the crunchier it will be.

Note: Avoid buying dried fruits and nuts from bulk bins — particularly if you have a low white blood cell count — to reduce the risk of foodborne illnesses. Instead, look for smaller packages of nuts and dried fruits in the baking section of the grocery store.

Berry and Walnut Granola Bars

Prep time: 15 min • **Cook time:** 20–30 min • **Yield:** 16 servings

Ingredients	*Directions*
2 cups old-fashioned rolled oats	*1* Preheat the oven to 350 degrees. Line a 9-x-13-inch baking pan with parchment, leaving extra parchment to hang over all sides.
½ cup chopped walnuts	
1 large egg	*2* Spread the oats and walnuts on a baking pan and bake for 10 to 12 minutes, stirring occasionally, until lightly browned.
2 large egg whites	
¾ cup Sucanat	
1 teaspoon cinnamon	*3* Reduce the oven temperature to 300 degrees.
2 teaspoons vanilla	
1 tablespoon unbleached flour	*4* In a large bowl, whisk together the egg and egg whites until foamy, and then continue whisking to keep the eggs foamy as you add the Sucanat, cinnamon, and vanilla. Stir in the toasted oats and walnuts, flour, blueberries, and cranberries.
½ cup dried blueberries	
½ cup dried cranberries	
	5 Spread into the prepared pan. Bake 20 minutes for chewy bars or 25 to 30 minutes for crispier bars.
	6 Remove from oven, cool, and cut into bars.

Per serving: Calories 142 (From Fat 31); Fat 3g (Saturated 0g); Cholesterol 13mg; Sodium 15mg; Carbohydrate 25g (Dietary Fiber 2g); Protein 3g.

Tip: If you don't have parchment paper, you can use nonstick foil or regular foil and then grease it with either nonstick spray or butter.

Note: Sucanat is sugarcane juice that's dehydrated. It retains the molasses that gets stripped away when sugar is refined. Because it contains molasses, it has a distinct molasses flavor and provides iron, calcium, vitamin B6, potassium, and chromium. If you don't have Sucanat, you can substitute sugar or another granulated sweetener in this recipe.

Nature's Power Bars

Prep time: 15 min • **Cook time:** 30 min • **Yield:** 24 servings

Ingredients	Directions
One 16-ounce box sprouted whole-grain cereal (Food for Life Ezekiel 4:9)	**1** Preheat the oven to 350 degrees. Line an 11-x-15-inch glass pan with parchment.
3 teaspoons baking powder **2 cups cranberries**	**2** In a food processor or blender, grind the sprouted cereal in batches to a flourlike consistency (it will yield approximately 4 cups) and place into a large bowl.
1 cup sunflower seeds **1 cup pumpkin seeds** **2 cups walnuts or almonds, chopped or slivered**	**3** Add the baking powder to the flour and mix to combine. Then mix in the cranberries, sunflower seeds, pumpkin seeds, nuts, and chocolate chips until well distributed.
1 cup dark chocolate chips (optional) **4 eggs** **1 cup Sucanat**	**4** In another large bowl, beat the eggs, Sucanat, and honey with a hand mixer until light and fluffy. Then beat in the orange juice and olive oil until well combined.
1 cup honey **⅓ cup orange juice**	**5** Add the dry ingredients to the egg mixture, mixing by hand until well combined.
⅓ cup olive oil **Flaxseeds and/or sesame seeds for sprinkling (optional)**	**6** Spread dough evenly on the baking sheet. Sprinkle with flaxseeds and/or sesame seeds, if desired.
	7 Bake approximately 30 minutes, or until lightly browned.

Per serving: Calories 297 (From Fat 134); Fat 15g (Saturated 1g); Cholesterol 0mg; Sodium 130mg; Carbohydrate 39g (Dietary Fiber 4g); Protein 7g.

Vary It! Instead of mixing the chocolate chips into the bars in Step 3, you can sprinkle them on top of the bars once they come out of the oven. The chocolate then melts on the bars, giving them a nice chocolate layer on top.

Note: Food for Life makes the only sprouted whole-grain cereal we've seen on the market. It comes in a variety of flavors. Any type is fine for this recipe. If you can't find this cereal in your supermarket, you can order it online through sites like Amazon.com, or you can opt to use a 16-ounce box of Grape Nuts cereal instead.

Note: For more on Sucanat, see the preceding recipe.

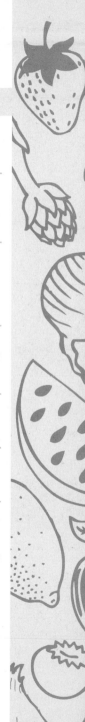

Sour Cream Banana Walnut Muffins

Prep time: 10 min • **Cook time:** 15–20 min • **Yield:** 18 servings

Ingredients	*Directions*
2 cups whole-wheat flour	*1* Preheat the oven to 350 degrees. Prepare the muffin pan with liners or spray with nonstick spray.
1 teaspoon baking soda	
½ teaspoon salt	*2* In a large bowl, combine the flour, baking soda, salt, and Sucanat until well blended.
1 cup Sucanat	
¼ cup olive oil (not extra virgin)	*3* In another large bowl, whisk together the olive oil, egg whites, sour cream, and vanilla until well blended. Then mix in the mashed bananas.
⅓ cup egg whites	
⅓ cup sour cream	
1 teaspoon vanilla extract	*4* Add the dry ingredients to the wet ingredients, mixing by hand until well incorporated. Then mix in the walnuts.
4 very ripe bananas, mashed	
1 cup walnuts, coarsely chopped	*5* Spoon the batter into muffin tins. Bake 15 to 20 minutes until golden brown and a toothpick inserted in the center of a muffin comes out clean.
	6 Cool a few minutes, and then move the muffins to a wire rack to cool completely.

Per serving: Calories 197 (From Fat 76); Fat 8g (Saturated 1g); Cholesterol 2mg; Sodium 150mg; Carbohydrate 29g (Dietary Fiber 3g); Protein 4g.

Vary It! If you don't feel like spooning the batter into individual muffin tins or want to avoid baking these in batches, turn it into banana bread instead. Simply pour the batter into a greased 9-x-5-inch metal or glass loaf pan and bake at 350 degrees for about an hour, or until a toothpick inserted in the center comes out clean.

Tip: If you have diarrhea, it's best to avoid whole grains and nuts, because they can be difficult to digest, making the diarrhea worse. Instead, substitute white flour for the whole-wheat flour in this recipe and use only three mashed bananas and omit the walnuts. You can substitute ¾ cup of whole-wheat flour for every 1 cup of white flour in most recipes, or you can try to increase the moisture content by adding additional milk.

Note: For more on Sucanat, see the Berry and Walnut Granola Bars recipe, earlier in this chapter.

Fresh Strawberry Bread

Prep time: 10 min • **Cook time:** 45–55 min • **Yield:** 14 servings

Ingredients	Directions
1¾ cups whole-wheat flour	**1** Preheat the oven to 350 degrees and grease a 9-x-5-inch metal or glass loaf pan and set aside.
½ cup sugar	
1 teaspoon baking soda	**2** In a large bowl, combine the flour, sugar, baking soda, and nutmeg.
¼ teaspoon nutmeg	
2 eggs	**3** In another large bowl, whisk together the eggs, yogurt, butter, and vanilla.
One 6-ounce container strawberry yogurt	
¼ cup butter, melted and cooled	**4** Add the dry ingredients to the wet ingredients, and mix until well blended. Then fold in the strawberries.
1 teaspoon vanilla extract	
2 cups strawberries, hulled and coarsely chopped	**5** Pour the batter into the prepared loaf pan. Bake for 45 to 55 minutes, or until a toothpick inserted in the center comes out clean.
	6 Cool for 10 minutes and then transfer to a wire rack. Serve warm or cooled.

Per serving: Calories 139 (From Fat 41); Fat 5g (Saturated 2g); Cholesterol 37mg; Sodium 108mg; Carbohydrate 27g (Dietary Fiber 2g); Protein 4g.

Vary It! This recipe is very versatile. Try different yogurt and fruit combinations. For example, you can make blueberry bread by using blueberries and blueberry yogurt instead. Or you can try vanilla yogurt and any fruit or berry of your choice.

Fruit and Nut Trail Mix

Prep time: 5 min • **Yield:** 8 servings

Ingredients	*Directions*
½ **cup dried apricots (preferably unsulphured), diced**	**1** In a large bowl, combine all the ingredients. Gently toss them with clean hands or mix them with a spoon.
½ **cup dried apples, diced**	
½ **cup cranberries**	**2** Place the trail mix in an airtight container or divide it into 8 equal servings and place in snack bags for future enjoyment.
½ **cup golden raisins**	
½ **cup unsalted sunflower seeds (toasted, if desired)**	
½ **cup pumpkin seeds**	
½ **cup chopped unsalted almonds (toasted, if desired)**	
½ **cup chopped unsalted walnuts**	

Per serving: Calories 281 (From Fat 156); Fat 17g (Saturated 2g); Cholesterol 0mg; Sodium 43mg; Carbohydrate 27g (Dietary Fiber 5g); Protein 8g.

Mix it up!

Trail mix is one of the most versatile, easy-to-prepare, and satisfying snack foods out there. If you'd like to develop your own trail mix, consider some of these ingredients:

✔ **Cereal:** If you have a favorite cereal, consider adding it to the mix, particularly if it contains whole grains. The Homemade Granola recipe in this chapter is a great addition to this mix.

✔ **Dried fruit:** Trail mix can accommodate any type of dried fruit (unsulphured, if possible). Some to consider include apples, apricots, banana chips, blueberries, cranberries, currents, figs, ginger, mangos, pears, peaches, plums, raisins, and strawberries.

✔ **Nuts:** Good nut choices include almonds, cashews, peanuts, and walnuts. You can opt to use them raw, roasted, or flavored. Generally, unflavored and unsalted varieties are best.

✔ **Seeds:** You'll want to get shelled seeds or seeds that can be eaten in the shell, such as pumpkin seeds. If you're experiencing digestive issues, shelled seeds are best. Some good seed options include sunflower seeds, pumpkin seeds, and hemp seeds.

✔ **Sweets:** If you're making a sweet trail mix, you can consider adding a few dark chocolate chips, peanut butter chips, M&M's, and yogurt-covered fruits.

✔ **Savory snack foods:** Crackers, pretzels, popcorn, Goldfish-type crackers, mini sesame sticks, dried peas, and carrot chips are some snack foods that can be added to trail mix.

Cookie Dough Energy Balls

Prep time: 5 min • **Yield:** 14 servings

Ingredients	Directions
⅓ cup natural peanut butter	**1** In a large bowl, mix together all ingredients except for the wheat germ. The dough should resemble Play-Doh.
¼ cup honey	
1 scoop chocolate or vanilla whey protein powder	
3 tablespoons ground flaxseeds	**2** Roll into 14 small balls and then roll balls in the wheat germ to coat. Refrigerate overnight for best results.
3 tablespoons mini dark chocolate chips	
3 tablespoons wheat germ	

Per serving: Calories 87 (From Fat 40); Fat 4g (Saturated 1g); Cholesterol 2mg; Sodium 9mg; Carbohydrate 9g (Dietary Fiber 1g); Protein 4g.

Tip: If you don't have any wheat germ, there are plenty of other roll toppings to use. Some options include flaxseeds, chia seeds, cocoa powder, crushed nuts, toasted sunflower seeds, and toasted coconut flakes.

Vary It! Feel free to experiment with other nut butters, including almond and cashew. If you don't want to use dark chocolate chips, consider trying some chopped dried fruit.

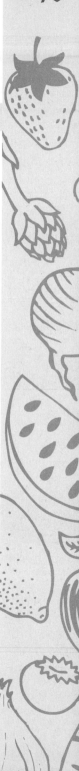

Onion and Garlic Roasted Chickpeas

Prep time: 5 min • **Cook time:** 45–60 min • **Yield:** 8 servings

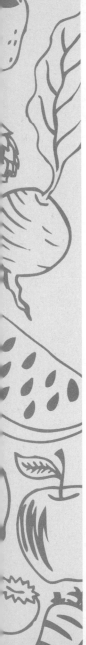

Ingredients	Directions
Two 15-ounce cans chickpeas	***1*** Preheat the oven to 400 degrees.
2 tablespoons olive oil	
Salt to taste	***2*** Pour the chickpeas into a strainer over the sink and rinse them well with cool water. Shake the strainer to remove additional water, and let them drain while proceeding.
1 teaspoon garlic powder	
1 teaspoon onion powder	
	3 Cover a rimmed baking sheet with nonstick foil. If you don't have nonstick foil, you can spray it with cooking spray.
	4 Blot the chickpeas with a paper towel to remove some moisture. Then pour them onto the baking sheet and spread them into a single layer. Blot the chickpeas again, using a few more sheets of paper towel to remove as much moisture as possible.
	5 Place the baking sheet on the lowest rack in the oven. Shake the chickpeas every 15 to 20 minutes to ensure even browning and to prevent burning. Remove when crispy, generally after 45 to 60 minutes.
	6 Add the olive oil, salt, garlic powder, and onion powder to a bowl with a tight-fitting lid. Then carefully pour the chickpeas into the bowl, replace the lid, and toss to distribute the oil and spices.

Per serving: Calories 86 (From Fat 38); Fat 4g (Saturated 0g); Cholesterol 0mg; Sodium 158mg; Carbohydrate 9g (Dietary Fiber 2g); Protein 3g.

Vary It! Try roasting other beans. Red kidney beans and black beans both work well. You'll just have to adjust the roasting times.

Tip: Use whatever spices you like for these beans. Other options to consider include Cajun seasonings, cayenne pepper, cinnamon, coriander, cumin, and paprika.

Entertaining Guests with Homemade Snack Food

Snacks are essential for entertaining, but you don't need to resort to potato chips and fat-laden dips. There are many delicious and nutritious snacks that are just as enjoyable *and* that pack a powerful, nutritional punch. These healthy snacks are what you'll find in this section.

You don't need to reserve these recipes just for entertaining. They can also make great mini meals and many are portable, such as the Original Hummus packed with whole-grain pita wedges or carrot sticks.

You'll find many dips among the recipes that follow. After all, when you're entertaining, dips are often a must-have. Grocery stores carry all kinds of dips, but their nutritional stats generally leave a lot to be desired. So, it's no wonder that dips often get a bad rap. But when made with wholesome ingredients, dips become a great way to obtain additional nutrients with each bite. In addition to getting the nutrients from the item being dipped, you're picking up additional nutrients from the dip itself. And when your dipper is a super food, like carrots, cucumbers, broccoli, and other veggies, you're getting lots of cancer-fighting nutrients.

Did we mention that dipping can be fun? Just be sure no one double dips or take your portion in advance. An episode of *MythBusters* showed that double dipping only adds a few more microbes to the mix, leading them to bust this myth, but when your immune system is suppressed, it's better not to take any chances. It's impossible to protect yourself from *all* bacteria, and you certainly shouldn't make yourself anxious over every potential exposure, but when you can take easy safety precautions, it's definitely worth it.

In addition to the dips, we include a few sweet snacks that can make for fun entertaining, including a Vibrant Fruit Salsa and a treat that simulates the frozen yogurt served at all the self-serve frozen yogurt bars that have popped up in many strip malls across the country. Both of these recipes are highly versatile and enable you to easily customize the fruits you include.

If you decide to make the Frosty Yogurt Bowls when entertaining, consider putting toppings out for your guests to top their own bowls of frosty goodness. You can also easily make the recipe as a single serving, particularly if you have a single-serving blender. For more on this type of blender, see Chapter 9.

Red Lentil Spread

Prep time: 15 min • **Cook time:** 25 min • **Yield:** 8 servings

Ingredients	Directions
3 cups vegetable broth	*1* In a medium saucepan, add the broth, lentils, onion, garlic, and coriander and bring to a boil. Then reduce to a low simmer and cook for 25 minutes, or until the lentils are tender.
2 cups red lentils	
1 medium onion, peeled and chopped (yields ½ cup)	
1 teaspoon chopped garlic	*2* Remove the lentils from the heat, strain, and then chill in the refrigerator.
1 teaspoon ground coriander	
2 tablespoons sour cream	*3* Once the lentils are cooled, place them in a blender and blend. Then add the sour cream, lime juice, cilantro, salt, and pepper, and blend until well combined, scraping down the sides of the blender, as needed.
1 tablespoon lime juice	
2 tablespoons finely chopped fresh cilantro	
⅛ teaspoon salt	
⅛ teaspoon pepper	

Per serving: Calories 170 (From Fat 11); Fat 1g (Saturated 0g); Cholesterol 2mg; Sodium 429mg; Carbohydrate 29g (Dietary Fiber 7g); Protein 12g.

Tip: This spread works great on baked tortilla chips or whole-grain crackers.

Vary It! If you can't find red lentils, try any of the other colors you find. Just follow the package instructions for cooking times, because some lentils require longer cooking times than others.

Original Hummus

Prep time: 5 min • **Yield:** 16 servings

Ingredients	Instructions
Two 19-ounce cans chickpeas, drained but reserving ½ cup of the liquid	**1** In a food processor, combine the chickpeas, reserved liquid, tahini, and garlic and process until smooth.
½ cup liquid from the chickpeas	
¼ cup tahini	**2** Add the remaining ingredients and continue processing to evenly distribute the flavors.
6 garlic cloves, peeled and chopped	
¼ cup lemon juice	
1 tablespoon extra-virgin olive oil	
½ teaspoon salt	
¼ teaspoon pepper	

Per serving: Calories 101 (From Fat 49); Fat 5g (Saturated 1g); Cholesterol 0mg; Sodium 236mg; Carbohydrate 10g (Dietary Fiber 3g); Protein 4g.

Vary It! For a super-spicy variation, do the following: Bump up the amount of pepper to 1 tablespoon and add 1 tablespoon cumin, 1 tablespoon paprika, 1 tablespoon chili powder, and 1 teaspoon crushed red pepper flakes to the recipe.

Tip: If you don't want to make the spicy version of this recipe, but you'd like to add additional flavor, consider adding any of the following to the recipe: 2 tablespoons horseradish, 2 tablespoons roasted red peppers, or 2 tablespoons pesto.

Make your own tahini

Tahini is a paste made from ground sesame seeds. It's commonly used in Middle Eastern cuisine, often as a dip on its own or in hummus and other dishes. If you don't have tahini at home, can't find it at the supermarket, or would rather make your own, it's easy to do. Follow this simple recipe:

1. Preheat the oven to 350 degrees.

2. Place 5 cups of sesame seeds on a baking sheet and toast for 5 to 10 minutes, tossing frequently with a spatula to prevent browning.

3. Cool and then pour the sesame seeds and 1½ cups olive oil into a food processor. Blend for 2 minutes, adding more olive oil if needed to obtain a thick but pourable consistency.

4. Pour into an airtight container and place in the refrigerator. It should keep for up to three months.

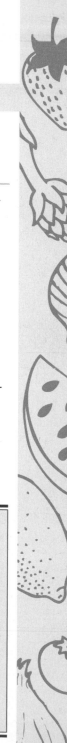

Wholesome Spinach Dip

Prep time: 10 min • **Yield:** 2 servings

Ingredients	Directions
½ **cup low-fat cream cheese, softened**	**1** Place the cream cheese, cottage cheese, and Greek yogurt into a food processor and blend until well combined, scraping down the sides and reprocessing as needed.
½ **cup cottage cheese**	
½ **cup plain low-fat Greek yogurt**	
¼ **cup chopped green onion**	**2** Add the remaining ingredients (except the milk) to the food processor and blend until well combined. If the mixture is too thick, add a little milk and reprocess. Repeat until the desired consistency is achieved.
¼ **teaspoon dill weed**	
½ **teaspoon chopped garlic**	
⅛ **teaspoon salt**	
½ **cup frozen spinach, thawed and water extracted**	**3** Refrigerate for 2 hours before serving to allow flavors to meld.
½ **cup water chestnuts**	
¼ **cup canned artichoke hearts, drained and chopped**	
Milk (only if needed for consistency)	

Per serving: *Calories 284 (From Fat 142); Fat 16g (Saturated 10g); Cholesterol 52mg; Sodium 674mg; Carbohydrate 15g (Dietary Fiber 3g); Protein 22g.*

Note: This dip can be stored in the refrigerator for up to 4 days.

Tip: Getting as much liquid out of the spinach as possible is important. You can do this by grabbing small batches and wringing the water out by hand. This can be uncomfortable if the spinach is still icy, so you may want to run warm water as you do this so that you can warm up your hands between batches. Alternatively, if you have a potato ricer, you can use it to extract the water from the spinach.

Garden Guacamole

Prep time: 5 min • **Yield:** 6 servings

Ingredients	*Directions*
2 ripe avocados	**1** Cut the avocados in half, remove the seeds, and scoop the avocado into a mixing bowl.
1 tablespoon fresh lime juice	
1 tablespoon cilantro, chopped	**2** Mash the avocado, leaving it chunky. Add the remaining ingredients, except for the tomato, and mix until just combined. Don't overmix.
½ red onion, finely minced	
1 clove garlic, passed through a garlic press	**3** Cover the guacamole so that plastic wrap directly skims its surface. (The goal is to prevent oxidation, which causes guacamole to turn an unpalatable brown color. Leaving an avocado pit in the bowl until serving also helps to reduce browning.) Refrigerate until ready to serve.
½ teaspoon coarse salt	
⅛ teaspoon freshly ground black pepper	
1 ripe tomato	
	4 Just before serving, remove and discard the seeds and pulp from the tomato, and then chop the flesh, add it to the guacamole, and mix.

Per serving: Calories 104 (From Fat 76); Fat 8g (Saturated 2g); Cholesterol 0mg; Sodium 162mg; Carbohydrate 8g (Dietary Fiber 5g); Protein 2g.

Vary It! To get an extra protein boost, try mixing in a cup of cottage cheese. Another twist on guacamole that has become popular lately is adding mashed peas to the mix. Peas add a nice vibrant color and provide an additional layer of flavor. If you'd like to give them a try in this recipe, substitute 1 to 2 cups of thawed frozen peas for the tomatoes. Be sure to mash or puree them before mixing them in. Because of their distinctive flavor, if you're not a huge fan of peas, start with 1 cup, but if you love them, then feel free to try 2 cups.

Tip: If you're simply too tired to gather a bunch of ingredients to make guacamole, just slightly mash an avocado with a bit of salsa and enjoy. If you don't have salsa, a little salt will do.

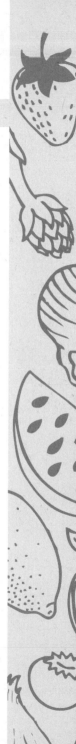

Vibrant Fruit Salsa with Cinnamon Chips

Prep time: 10 min • **Yield:** 10 servings

Ingredients	*Directions*
2 kiwis, peeled and diced	***1*** Preheat the oven to 350 degrees.
1 cup raspberries	
1 cup hulled and diced strawberries	***2*** In a large bowl, mix together the kiwis, raspberries, strawberries, blueberries, apple, honey, lemon juice, and fruit preserves. Cover and place in the refrigerator to chill for at least 15 minutes.
1 cup blueberries	
1 eating apple, peeled, cored, and diced (such as Fuji, Gala, Granny Smith, or Honey Crisp)	***3*** In a separate small bowl, mix the sugar or stevia and the cinnamon.
2 tablespoons honey	
1 teaspoon lemon juice	***4*** Place the tortillas on a baking sheet, baste them with butter, sprinkle them with the desired amount of sugar and cinnamon, and then turn them and do the same on the opposite side.
3 tablespoons no-sugar-added fruit preserves, any flavor	
½ cup sugar (or 3½ tablespoons of stevia for a sugar-free option)	***5*** Stack the tortillas on top of each other and cut them into 8 wedges. Then spread the chips out in one even layer and bake until crispy, approximately 8 to 10 minutes. Repeat with any remaining tortilla wedges.
2 teaspoons ground cinnamon	
One 8-count package whole-wheat tortillas	***6*** Allow the tortilla chips to cool approximately 15 minutes before serving with the chilled fruit salsa.
½ stick butter, melted (or butter-flavored cooking spray)	

Per serving: Calories 211 (From Fat 48); Fat 5g (Saturated 3g); Cholesterol 12mg; Sodium 140mg; Carbohydrate 45g (Dietary Fiber 5g); Protein 3g.

Tip: Don't have the time or energy to make the tortilla chips? The salsa is also good with cinnamon-sugar pita chips and cinnamon graham crackers.

Frosty Yogurt Bowls

Prep time: 2 min • **Yield:** 2 servings

Ingredients	*Directions*
2 cups plain low-fat Greek yogurt	*1* Blend all ingredients in a blender. To incorporate all ingredients, you may have to add additional juice, but add very slowly. If you add too much, you'll end up with a smoothie and you'll have to add more frozen fruit or yogurt to get a thicker consistency.
2 tablespoons honey	
1 cup frozen fruit or berries	
¼ cup orange juice	
	2 Pour into two bowls and add any desired optional toppings to your liking.

Per serving: Calories 287 (From Fat 43); Fat 5g (Saturated 3g); Cholesterol 17mg; Sodium 77mg; Carbohydrate 40g (Dietary Fiber 2g); Protein 23g.

Tip: Before adding more juice, see if frozen fruit has gotten stuck on the blade. Shut the blender off, open the lid, and use a spatula to move the fruit and other contents around. Try to reblend. If blending is still an issue, add a drop more juice and try again.

Vary 1t! Here are some ideas for toppings: chopped nuts, sliced fresh fruit, berries, granola, wheat germ, honey, dark chocolate chips, or crushed graham crackers.

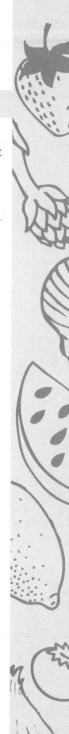

Chapter 15

Sinless Sweets

In This Chapter

▶ Eating sweets in moderation

▶ Whipping up cold desserts in a snap

▶ Baking delicious desserts

You don't need to avoid desserts at any time in your life, least of all while you're being treated for cancer. In fact, desserts can serve as the highlight of your meal, make a welcome snack, or provide a bit of comfort when you're on a rocky road. Now, we're not telling you to devour a whole gallon of ice cream or three slices of cheesecake. Ultimately, that wouldn't be good for your body, and you'd likely get a stomachache. Plus, you'd probably feel guilty for having ate them, and you shouldn't have to feel bad about what you eat.

In this chapter, we provide recipes for sweets that you can feel great about eating! In addition to being delicious, these recipes are packed with vitamins, minerals, fiber, and phytonutrients, providing your body with an additional source of nutrition. These desserts not only satisfy the taste buds, but also do your body good. What more could you ask for in a dessert?

Conquering Your Sweet Tooth

When you think of dessert, you probably think of sugar- and fat-laden treats, like piled-high ice cream sundaes and molten chocolate lava cakes. These desserts are artery clogging and send your blood glucose levels through the roof. But a dessert doesn't *have* to be a sugar or fat bomb to satisfy your sweet tooth. In fact, a range of flavors can be enjoyable for dessert, including tart and even bitter (as with dark chocolate).

The desserts in this chapter feature a range of flavors, which come from their wholesome ingredients. We've minimized their sugar content while maximizing flavor and texture, so they all still feel, look, and taste like desserts, but you get a range of flavors beyond sugar.

 If you find that a recipe isn't quite sweet enough for your tastes, feel free to add a little more sweetener, such as honey, pure maple syrup, agave nectar, or stevia, to suit your palate. Everyone's preferences differ to begin with and cancer treatment may also affect your sense of taste, so you may need to make modifications. The recipes in this chapter are all very versatile — feel free to tweak them as you like.

If you find that you're constantly having to up the sugar levels and you're used to craving super-sweet foods all the time, instead of always giving in, try cutting back. Cutting back on sugar may be difficult at first, but some people find that, eventually, they have fewer sugar cravings and are satisfied with foods that are less sweet.

Enjoying Cold Desserts

Cold desserts are awesome, particularly for novice chefs, because they're incredibly easy to make. No baking is required — but this doesn't mean you'll be avoiding the stove altogether. Some of the recipes in this section do require cooking; others require some blending or food-processing action.

 You can have a lot of fun experimenting with these recipes. In fact, experimenting and tasting as you go along can be part of the fun! When you strike a balance of ingredients that get your taste buds singing, be sure to write down what you did.

Homemade Fruit Gelatin

Prep time: 5 min • **Cook time:** 10 min • **Yield:** 8 servings

Ingredients	Directions
4 cups 100 percent grape or cranberry juice	*1* In a medium saucepan over high heat, mix the juice, agar flakes, and sea salt. Bring to a boil.
4 tablespoons agar flakes	
1 pinch sea salt	*2* Reduce the heat and simmer for 3 to 4 minutes, stirring to dissolve the agar. Add the fruit slices, if desired.
½ cup sliced fresh fruit or canned in juice (optional)	
	3 Pour the mixture into a gel mold or container and refrigerate for 60 to 90 minutes or until set.

Per serving: Calories 79 (From Fat 1); Fat 0g (Saturated 0g); Cholesterol 0mg; Sodium 22mg; Carbohydrate 19g (Dietary Fiber 0g); Protein 1g.

Frozen Pumpkin Treats

Prep time: 15 min • **Yield:** 9 servings

Ingredients	Directions
18 graham cracker squares	*1* Line a 9-x-9-inch baking pan with 9 of the graham cracker squares and set aside.
One 15-ounce can pumpkin	
One 15-ounce carton vanilla frozen yogurt (softened in the refrigerator)	*2* In a large mixing bowl, mix the pumpkin with the softened frozen yogurt, cinnamon, and ginger.
1 teaspoon cinnamon	*3* Spread the pumpkin mixture on top of the graham cracker squares.
⅛ teaspoon ground ginger	
	4 Top the mixture with the remaining graham cracker squares.
	5 Freeze until frozen.

Per serving: Calories 127 (From Fat 21); Fat 2g (Saturated 1g); Cholesterol 3mg; Sodium 116mg; Carbohydrate 24g (Dietary Fiber 3g); Protein 4g.

Triple Antioxidant Yogurt Popsicles

Prep time: 10 min • **Freeze time:** 3 hr • **Yield:** 12 servings

Ingredients	Directions
1 cup strawberries	**1** In a blender or food processor, combine all the ingredients and process until smooth, scraping down the sides as needed.
1 cup blueberries	
1 cup blackberries	
2 cups vanilla yogurt	**2** Pour the mixture into 12 popsicle forms (that hold at least 4 ounces each), following the product's instructions, and freeze for at least 3 hours before serving.
¼ cup orange juice	
1 tablespoon honey	

Per serving: Calories 59 (From Fat 6); Fat 1g (Saturated 0g); Cholesterol 2mg; Sodium 28mg; Carbohydrate 12g (Dietary Fiber 1g); Protein 2g.

Vary It! This recipe is exceptionally versatile. Switch the fruits, yogurt flavor, and/or juice and you'll have a whole new tasty concoction! You can even opt to change the texture by not pureeing the mixture until completely smooth or by adding some chopped fruit into the mix. A bit of bananas, for example, are excellent frozen and provide a touch of creaminess.

Popsicle forms: Store-bought or do-it-yourself

You can find popsicle forms at supermarkets, craft stores, and department stores, as well as online retailers. All kinds of popsicle forms are available, from plastic varieties in virtually any shape to stainless-steel versions.

If you're not sure you want to invest in a popsicle form just yet, you probably already have the equipment you need to make mini popsicles at home:

✔ An ice cube tray

✔ Aluminum foil

✔ Toothpicks

Simply fill each cube halfway, cover the tray with the aluminum foil, and then poke a hole through the foil to insert a toothpick into the middle of each cube. This makes about 24 cubes, depending on the size of your tray. You can even make a few without the toothpicks and use the cubes to make super-quick smoothies in the morning. All you'll need to do is add these cubes and some juice to a blender.

Cranberry Snow

Prep time: 5 min • **Cook time:** 10–12 min • **Yield:** 4 servings

Ingredients	Directions
3 cups 100 percent cranberry juice	**1** In a large saucepan, bring the cranberry juice to a boil over moderate heat and stir in the agave nectar.
⅓ cup agave nectar	
½ cup uncooked farina	**2** When the juice has come to a boil, slowly add the farina, stirring briskly with a wire whisk. Reduce the heat and simmer for 6 to 8 minutes, stirring occasionally, until the mixture becomes a thick puree.
	3 Using a rubber spatula, transfer the puree to a large mixing bowl. Whip the pudding for 10 to 15 minutes using an electric mixer set to a high speed. The pudding will triple in volume and become fluffy and a light pink color.
	4 Pour the pudding into a large bowl or individual dessert bowls. Serve immediately or cool in the refrigerator until ready to serve.

Per serving: Calories 217 (From Fat 1); Fat 0g (Saturated 0g); Cholesterol 0mg; Sodium 4mg; Carbohydrate 53g (Dietary Fiber 3g); Protein 3g.

Tip: This Finnish dessert is often served with milk on the side — a good way to add protein and extra calories.

Vary It! You can make this recipe with virtually any juice, but apple juice works particularly well. If you decide to use apple juice, add a tablespoon of lemon juice or omit the agave nectar. Made with apple juice, this recipe is easy on the stomach and can even be eaten as a meal when you're experiencing stomach upset or queasiness.

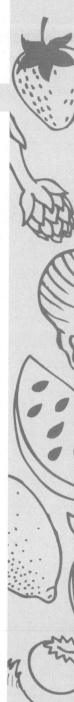

Apricot Orange Fool

Prep time: 20 min • **Yield:** 4 servings

Ingredients	Directions
½ **cup dried apricots (about 16 medium)**	*1* In a medium saucepan, combine the apricots, orange juice, and honey. Bring to a boil, and then reduce the heat and simmer for 20 minutes.
1 cup orange juice	
¼ **cup honey**	*2* Cool the mixture in the refrigerator. Once it's cool, puree the mixture in a food processor or blender until smooth. If desired, remove 1 tablespoon of the apricot puree for garnish.
1 cup plain Greek yogurt	
1 cup cottage cheese	*3* Add the remaining ingredients to the food processor. Blend until well incorporated, scraping down the sides as needed. The cottage cheese curds should disappear.
1 tablespoon flaxseed oil (optional)	
	4 Spoon the mixture into serving dishes and garnish with the remaining apricot puree, if desired. Drizzle additional honey on top, if you like. This recipe is also delicious made ahead and served chilled.

Per serving: Calories 214 (From Fat 23); Fat 3g (Saturated 2g); Cholesterol 11mg; Sodium 214mg; Carbohydrate 38g (Dietary Fiber 1g); Protein 13g.

Note: A fool, which was once spelled foole, is an English dessert that basically involves folding pureed, lightly sugared fruit into whipped cream. In this recipe, the cottage cheese and yogurt mixture replace the whipped cream to make a healthy treat.

Vary It! Try using some fresh fruit in this recipe instead of the apricots and orange juice. Strawberries and raspberries work particularly well. You want about 1 cup of pureed fruit.

Gingered Fruit Salad

Prep time: 25 min • **Yield:** 8 servings

Ingredients	*Directions*
¼ **cup honey**	*1* In a microwave-safe cup, combine the honey, ginger-root, lime peel, and lime juice. Mix well, and then microwave on high for 30 to 45 seconds or until thoroughly heated. Set aside approximately 15 minutes or until the dressing has completely cooled.
2 teaspoons grated gingerroot	
½ **teaspoon grated lime peel**	
3 tablespoons fresh lime juice	
2 cups seedless watermelon, cubed	*2* In a large serving bowl, combine the watermelon, pineapple, grapes, strawberries, and raspberries. Pour the dressing over the fruit, and toss gently to coat.
2 cups fresh pineapple, cubed	
2 cups seedless red or green grapes	
2 cups strawberries, quartered	
1 pint fresh raspberries	

Per serving: Calories 114 (From Fat 2); Fat 0g (Saturated 0g); Cholesterol 0mg; Sodium 3mg; Carbohydrate 32g (Dietary Fiber 2g); Protein 1g.

Vary It! Add additional interest and nutrients to your fruit salad by adding some unsweetened chopped dried fruits, like apricots, cranberries, and cherries; unsweetened toasted coconut; and minced fresh herbs, like mint or basil. You can also sprinkle on some toasted nuts before serving.

Vary It! Switch up the fruits to suit your palette. Kiwis, honeydew melon, blueberries, apples, pears, peaches, and cut-up citrus fruits all work well in this recipe.

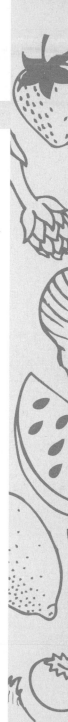

Chilled Minty Strawberry Soup

Prep time: 10 min • **Yield:** 4 servings

Ingredients	Directions
1 cup unsweetened apple or orange juice 2 cups strawberries 3 tablespoons honey ¼ cup fresh chopped mint ½ cup plain yogurt 4 ginger snaps, crumbled (optional)	*1* Place all the ingredients except for the ginger snaps in a food processor or blender and blend until well combined. *2* If desired, strain the soup through a mesh strainer to remove any seeds. *3* Chill well. When ready to serve, pour into individual bowls and top with crumbled ginger snaps, if you like.

Per serving: Calories 124 (From Fat 5); Fat 1g (Saturated 0g); Cholesterol 2mg; Sodium 29mg; Carbohydrate 29g (Dietary Fiber 2g); Protein 3g.

Tip: For a pretty presentation, consider some additional garnishes, such as a dollop of vanilla yogurt for a contrasting color, a drizzle of honey, a few mint leaves, and/or a sliced strawberry. If you have an egg slicer, you can use it to easily make a pretty strawberry garnish. Simply place the strawberry stem-side down into the slicer, and bring the slicer down onto the strawberry just shy of the leaves. When you remove the strawberry from the slicer, you can fan out the cut segments to make a pretty presentation.

Baking Wholesome Treats

Sometimes you just want something warm and sweet to sink your teeth into. Almost nothing feels more homey than having a yummy dessert baking in the oven. The smell just permeates your home, filling your nostrils with soothing scents that also start to whet your appetite. Then there's the anticipation of discovering how your treat turned out. This wonderful process culminates with getting to enjoy the efforts of your labor (and your patience).

But even if the only desserts to have graced your oven include frozen pies and prepackaged cookies and cakes, don't hesitate to try out the recipes in this section. Expert baking skills are not required, and you may just discover the hidden baker in you!

As you get started making these baked treats, keep in mind the following:

✔ To keep things simple, the recipes that follow include either all-purpose flour or whole wheat flour, with many including a combination of both. As you get more comfortable baking, feel free to experiment with the flour. There are many types of specialty flours on the market that you can try, such as buckwheat, rice, soy, oat, and coconut, all of which have different nutrient profiles. When substituting flours, just be sure to read the package instructions for recommendations on making the substitution. For instance, coconut flour can replace 10 percent to 20 percent of the flour used in most standard recipes, whereas buckwheat flour can be used as a full replacement in many recipes.

✔ When using spices, make sure they have a good smell. If their smell is faint, they may have lost their potency and won't lend much flavor. Ground spices and extracts, which are generally used in baked goods, tend to last two to three years (four years for extracts). If a recipe calls for a spice you don't like, omit it.

✔ The fruits are all very versatile. Feel free to use what you have on hand — fresh or frozen are fine. If using frozen, be sure to thaw them first. When using frozen fruit for dessert recipes, buy them in a bag rather than a box. Boxed fruits aren't individually quick-frozen, so the fruit ends up becoming encased in an ice block, which makes the fruit have an excess concentration of water.

Blueberry Crumb Bars

Prep time: 25 min • **Cook time:** 30–40 min • **Yield:** 12 servings

Ingredients	Directions
3 cups blueberries	**1** Preheat oven to 350 degrees.
1 tablespoon sugar	
2 tablespoons water	**2** In a medium saucepan, combine the blueberries, sugar, water, lemon juice, and cinnamon. Bring to a boil.
1 tablespoon lemon juice	
½ teaspoon cinnamon	**3** Reduce the heat and simmer uncovered, about 8 minutes or until slightly thickened, stirring frequently. Remove from the heat and set aside.
1 cup all-purpose flour	
1 cup quick oats	
⅔ cup packed brown sugar	**4** In a large mixing bowl, stir together the flour, oats, brown sugar, cinnamon, and baking soda.
½ teaspoon ground cinnamon	
⅛ teaspoon baking soda	**5** Stir in the melted butter until thoroughly combined.
¼ cup butter or soft margarine, melted	**6** Set aside 1 cup of the oat mixture for topping. Press the remaining oat mixture into an ungreased 9-x-9-x-2-inch baking pan. Bake for 12 minutes.
	7 Carefully spread the filling on top of the baked crust. Then sprinkle with the reserved oat mixture, lightly pressing the oat mixture into the filling. Bake for another 20 to 25 minutes or until the topping is set.
	8 Cool in the pan on a wire rack.

Per serving: Calories 170 (From Fat 51); Fat 5g (Saturated 3g); Cholesterol 10mg; Sodium 18mg; Carbohydrate 31g (Dietary Fiber 2g); Protein 2g.

Vary It! For a fall treat, consider substituting apples for the blueberries.

Tip: If you're short on time or energy, you can use one 10-ounce jar of an all-fruit spread as the filling.

Super Antioxidant Peach Raspberry Crisp

Prep time: 20 min • **Cook time:** 30–35 min • **Yield:** 14 servings

Ingredients	Directions
5 cups sliced peaches	*1* Preheat oven to 375 degrees.
2 cups raspberries	
½ cup canola oil	*2* In a medium mixing bowl, combine the peaches and raspberries. Then place in a 9-x-9-inch glass baking dish.
1 cup uncooked rolled oats	
½ cup whole wheat flour	*3* In a separate medium mixing bowl, combine all the other ingredients and mix until it resembles coarse crumbs.
½ cup wheat germ	
¼ cup honey	
¼ cup chopped almonds	*4* Spread the crumb mixture on top of the fruit.
½ teaspoon cinnamon	
⅛ teaspoon nutmeg and/or cloves (optional)	*5* Bake for 30 to 35 minutes.

Per serving: *Calories 184 (From Fat 88); Fat 10g (Saturated 1g); Cholesterol 0mg; Sodium 1mg; Carbohydrate 23g (Dietary Fiber 4g); Protein 4g.*

Vary It! Try substituting apples for the peaches and other berries for the raspberries.

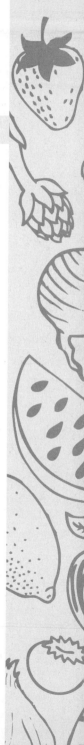

Baked Pumpkin Pie Pudding

Prep time: 15 min • **Cook time:** 45 min • **Yield:** 8 servings

Ingredients	*Directions*
One 15-ounce can pumpkin puree	**1** Preheat the oven to 425 degrees.
¾ cup granulated sugar	**2** In a large mixing bowl, cream together the pumpkin and sugar.
½ teaspoon salt	
1 teaspoon ground cinnamon	**3** Add the salt, cinnamon, ginger, cloves, and blended tofu, mixing until thoroughly blended together.
½ teaspoon ground ginger	
¼ teaspoon ground cloves	**4** Pour the mixture into a greased 8-x-8-inch baking pan.
10 ounces soft silken tofu, blended in a blender until smooth	**5** Bake for 15 minutes. Then lower the heat to 350 degrees and bake for an additional 30 minutes.

Per serving: Calories 113 (From Fat 11); Fat 1g (Saturated 0g); Cholesterol 0mg; Sodium 150mg; Carbohydrate 25g (Dietary Fiber 3g); Protein 3g.

Making your own pumpkin puree

If you don't like the idea of using canned pumpkin, you can make your own puree. All you need is one or two small pumpkins. Try to find sugar pumpkins or pie pumpkins, but if you can find only regular pumpkins, those will work, too. If you can't find pumpkins, you can substitute another squash, like butternut or even acorn. To make the puree, follow these steps:

1. Preheat the oven to 350 degrees.

2. Chop off the top of the pumpkin, so that the stem is removed and the top is flat.

3. Cut each pumpkin in half and scoop out the seeds and as much of the stringy matter as possible. An ice cream scoop works well for this purpose.

4. Cut each pumpkin in quarters and place on a baking sheet, skin side down.

5. Place in the oven and roast for 35 to 45 minutes, or until the pumpkin is fork tender.

6. Let cool slightly and then remove and discard the skins. They should come right off.

7. Place a few de-skinned chunks at a time in a food processor or blender and puree until smooth, scraping down the sides as needed. Repeat until all the pumpkin has been used.

8. If you think the consistency is too watery, place the puree into a cheesecloth-lined strainer over a bowl to remove some excess moisture.

Banana Date Walnut Drops

Prep time: 5 min • **Cook time:** 20 min • **Yield:** 12 cookies

Ingredients	Directions
2 cups uncooked rolled oats, divided	*1* Preheat the oven to 350 degrees.
2 ripe bananas, peeled	*2* Place 1 cup of the oats into a food processor or blender and process until they become fine, like flour.
¼ cup canola oil	
1 teaspoon vanilla extract	*3* Add the bananas, canola oil, and vanilla extract to the food processor or blender and process until well combined.
½ cup walnuts, chopped	
½ cup dried dates, chopped	
	4 Transfer the mixture to a medium mixing bowl and stir in the remaining oats, walnuts, and dates until well combined.
	5 Roll the dough into 12 balls, place on a nonstick or parchment-lined cookie sheet, and press to flatten slightly.
	6 Bake for 20 minutes.

Per serving: Calories 164 (From Fat 80); Fat 9g (Saturated 1g); Cholesterol 0mg; Sodium 1mg; Carbohydrate 20g (Dietary Fiber 3g); Protein 3g.

Vary It! Instead of the walnuts and dates, use any other dried fruits, such as raisins, cranberries, or cherries, or add dark or semisweet chocolate chips.

Tip: The key to this recipe is really ripe bananas, because they give the drops their sweetness. If your bananas aren't quite ripe enough, you can still make this recipe, but you may want to add a bit of honey, agave nectar, or stevia to compensate.

Note: If you're dealing with taste changes, these cookies may be appealing to you because they aren't overly sweet.

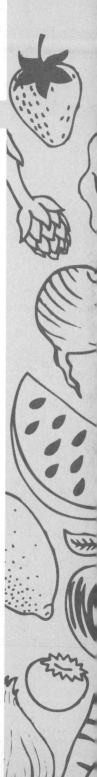

Nutty Strawberry Cream Cheese Sponge Cake

Prep time: 15 min • **Cook time:** 15–20 min • **Yield:** 6 servings

Ingredients	*Directions*
1 teaspoon cinnamon	*1* Preheat the oven to 375 degrees and grease and line two 8-inch round cake pans with parchment.
1 cup whole wheat flour	
½ cup ground almonds	
4 eggs	*2* In a medium mixing bowl, sift together the cinnamon and flour. Then stir in the ground almonds. In a separate medium mixing bowl, beat the eggs and 3 tablespoons of the honey or agave nectar together until thick, using an electric mixer. Carefully fold the dry mixture into the wet mixture until well combined.
10 tablespoons honey or agave nectar	
1 tablespoon almonds, chopped or sliced	
One 8-ounce package low-fat cream cheese	*3* Divide the batter evenly between the two cake pans and top one of the pans with the chopped or sliced almonds. The cake with the sliced almonds is the top layer of the cake.
½ teaspoon vanilla	
3 tablespoons lemon juice	*4* Bake for 15 to 20 minutes, or until the cakes spring back when lightly pressed. Remove the cakes from the pan and let cool on a rack.
2 cups strawberries, sliced	
	5 In a medium mixing bowl, use an electric mixer to beat together the cream cheese, vanilla, lemon juice, the remaining 4 tablespoons of honey or agave nectar, and 1 cup of the sliced strawberries.
	6 Once the cakes have cooled, spread the cake without the nuts on top with half the cream cheese mixture, and arrange the remaining 1 cup of strawberry slices on top of it. Then spread the remaining cream cheese on the bottom part of the top cake layer (the side with the nuts faces up). Sandwich the haves together to form the cake. Serve soon after you assemble it.

Per serving: Calories 389 (From Fat 153); Fat 17g (Saturated 6g); Cholesterol 177mg; Sodium 186mg; Carbohydrate 52g (Dietary Fiber 5g); Protein 13g.

Cocoa Walnut Brownies

Prep time: 15 min • **Cook time:** 30 min • **Yield:** 18 servings

Ingredients	*Directions*
½ cup all-purpose flour	**1** Preheat the oven to 350 degrees. Lightly grease a 9-x-13-inch brownie pan and set aside.
½ cup whole-wheat flour	
¾ cup unsweetened cocoa powder (natural or Dutch process)	**2** In a large mixing bowl, sift together the flours, cocoa powder, sugar, and baking powder.
1⅔ cups sugar	
½ teaspoon baking powder	**3** Then add the egg whites, applesauce, buttermilk, and vanilla extract, and beat with an electric mixer until well combined. Fold in the walnuts, if desired.
1⅓ cups liquid egg whites (or egg whites from 7 eggs)	
⅔ cup unsweetened applesauce	**4** Transfer the batter to the brownie pan and bake for approximately 30 minutes; the brownies are done when they start pulling away from the pan.
¼ cup buttermilk	
2 teaspoons vanilla extract	
⅔ cup walnuts (optional)	

Per serving: Calories 117 (From Fat 6); Fat 1g (Saturated 0g); Cholesterol 0mg; Sodium 37mg; Carbohydrate 27g (Dietary Fiber 2g); Protein 3g.

Note: Dutch-process cocoa is reddish brown, has a mild flavor, and is easy to dissolve in liquids. This form of cocoa has been treated with an alkali to neutralize its natural acidity. As a result, it doesn't react with baking soda and should generally only be used in recipes calling for baking powder. In contrast, unsweetened natural cocoa has a more complex chocolate flavor, and when it's used in recipes that contain baking soda (an alkali), it causes the batter to rise as it's baking.

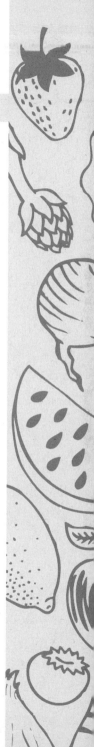

Whole-Wheat Citrus-Infused Apple Cobbler

Prep time: 25 min • **Cook time:** 40–45 min • **Yield:** 8 servings

Ingredients	*Directions*
⅓ **cup sugar**	*1* Preheat oven to 350 degrees.
1 tablespoon cornstarch	
½ **teaspoon ground cinnamon**	*2* In a large mixing bowl, combine the ⅓ cup sugar, cornstarch, cinnamon, nutmeg, and orange juice. Add the apples and toss to coat. Transfer the mixture to an 11-x-7-inch greased baking dish.
¼ **teaspoon ground nutmeg**	
⅓ **cup orange juice**	
4 cups sliced peeled tart apples (about 4 large)	*3* In a separate large mixing bowl, combine the flours, ¼ cup sugar, baking powder, baking soda, and salt.
½ **cup all-purpose flour**	
½ **cup whole-wheat flour**	*4* Cut the butter into the flour mixture until a coarse meal is formed. Add the buttermilk and orange rind, stirring just until moist.
¼ **cup sugar**	
1 teaspoon baking powder	
¼ **teaspoon baking soda**	*5* Drop the dough onto the apple mixture to form mounds, and then sprinkle mounds with the remaining 2 teaspoons of sugar.
¼ **teaspoon salt**	
6 tablespoons chilled butter, cut into small pieces	*6* Bake for 40 to 45 minutes, until the apples are bubbly and the topping is lightly browned. Let cool for 10 minutes before serving.
⅔ **cup buttermilk**	
½ **teaspoon grated orange rind**	
2 teaspoons coarse finishing sugar (optional)	

Per serving: Calories 241 (From Fat 81); Fat 9g (Saturated 6g); Cholesterol 24mg; Sodium 184mg; Carbohydrate 39g (Dietary Fiber 2g); Protein 3g.

Part IV
Staying Strong for the Long Haul

Top Five Ways to Keep Your Strength Up

- **Ask for what you want at restaurants.** When dining out, never be afraid to ask for clean substitutions or to make special requests, even for something not specifically on the menu. Most establishments are accommodating, and the worst they can say is "no."

- **Eat carryout foods right away.** If you pick up a quick meal at the supermarket or from a restaurant, make sure to eat it within an hour or two to prevent foodborne illness (but avoid picking up items from salad bars or buffets if your white blood cell count is low). If you can't eat it that soon, place it in a refrigerator or in an insulated lunch box or bag with an ice pack to prevent spoilage.

- **Get moving!** Try to get 30 minutes of physical activity daily, with a goal to get 150 minutes of moderate-intensity or 75 minutes of vigorous-intensity activity every week.

- **Be smart about the sun.** Get 15 to 30 minutes of unprotected sun exposure two to four times a week to boost your vitamin D levels (unless your oncologist tells you to avoid the sun), but use protective clothing and/or SPF 30 sunblock as needed the remaining time to protect against skin cancer.

- **Keep stress in check.** Reduce your stress levels as much as possible by finding activities that relax you and provide a sense of well-being. Some possibilities include meditation, yoga, or even a hobby like knitting or woodworking. The key is to find something that relaxes *you.*

 Find out how to avoid the gym and still get the exercise your body needs by exergaming, in a free article at www.dummies.com/extras/cancernutritionrecipes.

In this part . . .

- ✔ Eat healthfully and safely when dining out, no matter where you're grabbing a meal.

- ✔ Discover why physical activity is essential for health.

- ✔ Identify some exercises that have shown benefits for cancer.

- ✔ Find out how you can protect yourself from environmental hazards and toxins and reduce your exposure.

- ✔ Discover how you can help a loved one on his or her cancer journey.

Chapter 16

Dining Out or on the Road

. . . .

In This Chapter

▶ Getting a handle on restaurant fare and knowing what to order

▶ Finding wholesome quick eats at the supermarket

▶ Handling eating over the holidays and during social events

▶ Making your own transportable healthy lunches and snacks

. . . .

According to the National Restaurant Association, every year Americans obtain almost a quarter of their meals at full-service or fast-food restaurants. When you factor in lunches away from home and eating at parties, estimates are that two-thirds of meals may be eaten outside the home. Not only is this way of eating expensive, but it makes it more difficult to stick to a clean eating lifestyle and get all the disease-fighting nutrients you need. Plus, you can easily exceed a day's worth of calories, fat, and sodium in just one sitting.

But this doesn't have to happen to you when you eat away from home. There's a famous saying that "failing to plan is planning to fail," which couldn't be more true when it comes to nourishing yourself on the road. This chapter provides you with the information you need to plan your meals so that you can regain some of the control you lose when you leave your kitchen and venture out to eat food prepared by others.

First, we examine how to assess menus and make healthy choices in restaurants, fast-food establishments, supermarkets, and parties. No matter where you go, there are wholesome or, at the very least, better-for-you options and solutions to help you meet your goals. Then we review how to pack clean lunches and snacks. *Remember:* Snacks are particularly important when you're undergoing treatment, so you shouldn't skip them even when you're not home.

Understanding Restaurant Fare

Who doesn't like eating in a restaurant? Someone else does the shopping and cooking, and cleans up after the meal. Restaurant fare is often fancier than what you would prepare at home. It offers the opportunity to try foods that require extensive preparation that you don't have the time or energy to make yourself.

But restaurants also often prepare food in unhealthy ways and serve super-sized portions, which can easily derail a clean eating plan. In addition, restaurants strive to get you to order as much food as possible, which may lead to overindulging. Bread is brought to your table and you're encouraged to order an appetizer, entrée, dessert, and alcohol.

So, one of the most important things you can do to eat clean and optimize your nutrient intake when dining in a restaurant is to do your homework and formulate a plan. Here are some simple strategies to get you started:

- ✔ **Review your options ahead of time.** Most restaurants have their menus and nutritional information online, so you can review your options, plan what you'll order, and decide on any special requests or substitutions before arriving. Also, some chain restaurants have started adding calorie counts to their menus or using icons to designate healthier options, so keep your eyes peeled for this information.

- ✔ **For more complex food requests, call the restaurant in advance to gauge its flexibility.** Most restaurants are willing to take special orders or to make substitutions, albeit sometimes charging you slightly more for this service. But if your food request is more complex (for example, you want them to make something that isn't on the menu), it may be helpful to see how accommodating the restaurant is willing to be prior to your arrival. If the restaurant isn't willing to work with you, consider taking your business elsewhere.

Having a plan ahead of time will make it easier and less stressful to make wholesome choices when dining out. Restaurants want repeat business, so don't be afraid to ask for what you want.

In the following sections, we help you decipher food preparation techniques and how to control your portions. Armed with this information, you'll be able to make more wholesome choices when dining out.

Familiarizing yourself with menu lingo

Restaurant menus are filled with all kinds of words to get you salivating. So that you can decipher this lingo and order the most nourishing fare, we start by looking at the terms that are most likely to designate items that fit into a clean eating plan. Thereafter, we cover terms that usually describe cooking methods that are more likely to add extra fat and sodium to your meals.

The stuff to look for

The following menu descriptions are generally consistent with healthier eats:

- ✔ **Baked:** Baked protein foods generally don't have a lot of fat added to them. Your best choice would be a baked fish with lemon, which many restaurants have on their menus. Order salmon for a healthy dose of omega-3 fatty acids. Also, if you order baked poultry, remove the skin prior to consumption to reduce your intake of saturated fat.

- ✔ **Braised:** Braised foods are cooked slowly in a small amount of water, broth, or other liquid. Herbs are commonly used for seasoning. The cooking liquid may also be reserved and used to make a sauce, meaning you'll get all the nutrients that leach out into the cooking liquid. Just be sure the restaurant uses a low-fat, low-sodium braising liquid and that it doesn't first brown the meat in an unhealthy oil.

- ✔ **Broiled:** When food is broiled, it's cooked by exposure to direct radiant heat, such as under an oven's broiler. This is considered a healthy preparation method when the food isn't charred and is seasoned with fresh herbs and spices, rather than unhealthy fats and an excessive amount of salt.

- ✔ **Grilled:** Grilled foods can be an occasional healthy choice, because grilling is usually a low-fat cooking method. Just avoid eating any charred parts on grilled foods, particularly meats, to reduce exposure to potential cancer-causing compounds. Your best options are grilled veggie or fruit kebobs with a little tofu, if available. Grilled lean meats, poultry, and fish can also be healthy.

- ✔ **Oven-fried:** Foods that are traditionally deep-fried in a lot of oil can be cooked in an oven with less oil, making them a better choice. Look for oven-fried fish, chicken, potatoes, or sweet potatoes.

- ✔ **Primavera:** These dishes typically contain lots of fresh vegetables, often in combination with pasta. When served with pasta, ask if you can have a whole-grain pasta, provided you aren't having to watch your fiber intake (like if you have diarrhea), and pay attention to any seasonings and sauces.

- ✔ **Poached:** Foods that are poached are cooked in liquid with a temperature ranging from 140 to 180 degrees. This cooking method is typically reserved for cooking delicate foods like eggs and fish. When ordering poached eggs, avoid fatty sauces like Hollandaise.

- **Steamed:** Steaming is a method of cooking food in a basket removed from the cooking water or liquid. It's one of the best methods for cooking vegetables to retain their nutrients. Order steamed veggies as a side dish, but ask that they be prepared without butter or oil.

- **Stir-fried:** Stir-frying is a way of cooking foods very quickly with a small amount of oil. You may want to request that the chef use as little oil as possible. Look for veggies stir-fried with tofu, chicken, or seafood. Many restaurants also have brown rice or another whole grain available upon request for your stir-fry to be served over.

The stuff to avoid

The following menu descriptions typically indicate foods that have been prepared in an unhealthy way and that are unlikely to contain many, if any, cancer-fighting nutrients. In addition, most of these foods are high in fat, which can aggravate many gastrointestinal symptoms or conditions, including heartburn and irritable bowel syndrome. They also tend to contain lots of sodium, which can cause fluid retention and high blood pressure.

That said, if you're dealing with cancer-related weight loss or have little appetite and any of the following appeal to you, then by all means go ahead and order whatever you want. This is the time when your primary goal needs to be quantity. For more about the quantity goal versus quality goal, turn to Chapter 4.

- **A la king, Alfredo, butter sauce, carbonara, cheese sauce:** All these terms designate different types of heavy, fatty sauces. Dishes that include these sauces may provide more than a day's worth of fat, calories, and sodium.

- **Au gratin:** These foods are topped with buttered, seasoned breadcrumbs and cheese and are then baked or broiled to achieve a crisp crust.

- **Battered, breaded, crispy, fried, tempura:** Battered (like tempura) or breaded foods are usually fried, and their coatings add empty calories. These foods may also be described as "crispy." Fried foods, whether pan fried or deep fried, contain a lot of fat and may be high in the worst fat of all: trans fats.

- **Creamed:** Foods that are creamed are usually served in a fatty sauce made of butter, flour, milk, and spices.

- **Parmigiana:** These foods are often coated in breadcrumbs and cheese, fried, layered with tomato sauce and additional cheese, and then baked. As a result, they may have more than a day's worth of fat and sodium.

- **Prepared with prosciutto:** Prosciutto is a salt-cured ham. It's a common ingredient on today's menus because it adds a lot of flavor, but with all that flavor come added fat and sodium.

✔ **Smoked:** Although smoked foods have a nice flavor, the smoking process produces compounds that have been associated with cancer, at least in animals. To err on the side of caution, avoid these foods.

✔ **Smothered:** Foods that are smothered are usually covered in a rich gravy or sauce that is high in sodium and fat.

✔ **Stuffed:** Stuffed foods are usually filled with cheese, breadcrumbs, and other unhealthy, high-calorie ingredients.

If you're ever unsure of a menu description, don't hesitate to ask clarifying questions. A good restaurant will make sure its service staff knows how the food is prepared or even bring the chef to your table to answer questions.

Watching portions

Restaurant portions are often up to three to four times the size of recommended healthy portions. This may seem appealing because bigger portions feel like a better value, but you need to ask yourself, "Is it worth it to eat more calories, fat, and sodium than recommended and compromise my long-term health?" If the answer is "No," here are some ways to manage portions:

✔ **Order a wholesome appetizer, side salad, and/or cup of soup.** Any combination of a small appetizer, side salad, and soup can make a satisfying meal while helping you control portions.

✔ **Look for "small plate" items.** Many restaurants now have "small plate" items on their menu, which designate more reasonable portions. You can also look for lunch-size portions instead of dinner-size portions.

✔ **Split an entrée with someone.** This strategy saves money, leads to a more communal eating experiences, and prevents you from wasting food if you don't want to take home leftovers.

✔ **Bag up at least half the entrée.** Ask for a doggie bag as soon as your meal arrives and bag up at least half of that entrée, or ask your server to bring only half to the table and to bag the rest. This makes the decision of what to have for lunch the next day quite simple.

Considering alcohol

Restaurants often encourage patrons to order a cocktail before dinner, wine with dinner, and even an after-dinner drink. That's a lot of alcohol! Most cancer institutes and societies recommend that women have no more than one drink per day and men have no more than two drinks per day. A drink is defined as 12 ounces of beer, 5 ounce of wine, or 1.5 ounces of hard alcohol. And these are not like Weight Watchers points — you can't save up these allotments to drink larger amounts on fewer days of the week.

If you drink at all, red wine may be the best choice, because it provides the powerful antioxidant resveratrol.

If you're undergoing cancer treatment, talk with your oncologist before having a drink, because alcohol may increase the risk of side effects or interact with medications. Convincing evidence also suggests that alcohol use may increase the risk of cancer or a recurrence. It also adds empty calories, which may make achieving and maintaining a healthy body weight more difficult, further increasing cancer risk.

In addition to alcohol providing empty calories, many mixers (like soda, juice, and tonic water) added to these drinks add calories. Stick with the lowest-calorie options for mixers; for example, opt for mixed drinks that add club soda rather than soda. Another option is to have a nonalcoholic drink, like a club soda with lemon or lime, a nonalcoholic beer, or a virgin Bloody Mary, so that you still feel like you're enjoying the "cocktail hour."

Making special requests

If you want to eat more healthfully, don't be afraid to ask your server what can be prepared that isn't on the menu, or whether you can order off the children's menu if your appetite is small. Most restaurants are used to dealing with food allergies and intolerances. It's a rare restaurant that can't make you a simple piece of baked chicken or fish with some steamed veggies or won't let you order off the children's menu. Restaurants want you to enjoy your food and feel good about what you're eating so that you'll be a repeat customer and maybe even send other customers to dine there.

If you're uncomfortable talking about your clean eating plan, you can always explain your special request by saying you have a food allergy or an intolerance. It's often easier to explain, and no chef or restaurant wants you to have a reaction or become ill in their establishment.

Considering substitutions and omissions

Substitutions and omissions to existing items can often turn an unhealthy eat into a healthy bite. The following is a list of substitutions and omissions that can clean up menu items if you're looking to enhance the quality of the foods you eat:

✔ **Order sauces and salad dressings on the side.** Sauces usually contain fat, salt, and even sugar. By ordering these items on the side, you can minimize the amount used. As for salad dressings, ask for oil-and-vinegar-based dressings and use them sparingly. Even a little balsamic or some fresh lemon may be sufficiently pleasing to the palate.

✔ **Ask for fruit, veggies, or a side salad instead of fries.** Although this is often included as an option on menus, these more wholesome options may be provided sparingly. So, don't hesitate to ask for a double portion. You may pay a little more, but it's worth the nutrient boost.

✔ **Ask for brown rice, whole-grain pasta, or another whole grain instead of the refined alternative.** Even if they aren't listed on the menu, the chef may have them in the kitchen, so be sure to ask about them, provided you can tolerate them.

✔ **Omit cheese.** Cheese adds extra calories and fat and often covers up the taste of the food it's covering. The only time cheese should stay on an item is if it's the only source of protein in the dish. Even then, asking for half the portion is probably a good idea.

✔ **Keep the bread basket off the table.** Most restaurants still serve refined bread, so you're not getting a lot of nutrients other than calories. Save your calories for something more wholesome.

Making the most of fast food

Many of the suggestions in the previous sections, such as having condiments on the side, may also help at fast-food establishments. In addition, here are some of the best choices you can make if you find yourself needing to eat fast food:

✔ **Pizzerias:** Choose vegetarian pizza and load up on veggies. Try to find pizza places that use part-skim mozzarella cheese or that can substitute it for whole-milk mozzarella. Also, ask if your pizza can be prepared with whole-wheat crust and half the cheese. Although you want some cheese for the protein, each ounce adds at least 5 g of fat.

✔ **Mexican:** Try fajitas; bean burritos (as long as the beans are prepared without lard); soft chicken or fish tacos without cheese; and burrito bowls with brown rice, vegetables, a lean protein, and without cheese or fatty dressings (guacamole is okay).

✔ **Asian:** Choose seafood or chicken stir-frys. Ask if brown rice is available. Steamed vegetable dumplings are also an okay choice.

✔ **Fast-food chains:** Plain grilled chicken sandwiches or a small hamburger are acceptable options. Also, don't be afraid to ask for the kid's meal with the fruit option instead of fries. Some chains also offer salads with light dressings, yogurt parfaits, and even fruit smoothies, which can make for a good accompaniment.

✔ **Sandwich shop:** Order a turkey breast, lean meat, or cheese sandwich on whole-grain bread with mustard and all the vegetables available. Add a side of vegetable soup, if available.

If your white blood cell counts are down, it's best to avoid delis. Because the foods are not cooked, there is a higher risk of a foodborne illness.

One chain's burger or fish taco may have significantly different nutritional stats than that of another chain. Most fast-food establishments make their nutrition information available online or in the store, so be sure to make full use of this information.

Checking out the Supermarket

In addition to shopping for groceries for the week, today's supermarket has become a destination for grab-and-go lunches and dinners. The same rule applies in the grab-and-go situation as when shopping for groceries (see Chapter 7) — shop the perimeter of the store, where the freshest, cleanest foods are usually housed.

Grab-and-go items to consider

When grabbing quick bites at the supermarket, here are some more wholesome options to look for:

✔ **Amy's or Kashi frozen meals:** Many supermarkets carry these brands of frozen meals or single-serving burritos. Although these processed foods are not as wholesome as preparing your own foods, they're a reasonable option for a quick, hot meal.

✔ **Salad bars:** Many supermarkets now have salad bars. Load up your salad with dark greens, other fresh veggies, and fruits. Add some beans for protein or diced tuna or chicken. If these aren't available, pick up a small can of garbanzo beans or tuna so that you have some protein on your salad. Finally, use oil and vinegar or a light dressing. If you're undergoing treatment and have low immunity, you may instead want to look for similar ready-packed salads to reduce your exposure to salad-bar germs.

✔ **Prepared hummus with raw veggies:** Most deli sections have several options for prepared hummus. Pick the one with the least fat, and grab whatever cut-up raw veggies you can find. Carrots, celery, broccoli, cauliflower, pea pods, and cherry tomatoes are almost always available.

✔ **Smoothies:** Supermarkets may sell different types of bottled smoothies, some with protein. These may be found refrigerated by the produce or in the areas where dairy or refrigerated juices are stored.

✔ **Vegetable steamers:** Numerous frozen vegetable brands offer vegetable combinations that can be steamed in the microwave directly in the bag they come in. Some even include whole grains like brown and wild rice. Add protein by mixing in some tuna; canned salmon; cut-up, low-fat, prepared chicken breasts (like Perdue Short Cuts); or beans, like black, kidney, or garbanzo.

✔ **Yogurt or cottage cheese with fresh fruit:** Grab a single-serving yogurt or cottage cheese and some cut-up fresh fruit.

Ensuring food safety

Always make sure you check dates on grab-and-go items. Don't buy or eat anything that is beyond its use-by date. Also, if you aren't going to eat your store-bought item within an hour or two of purchasing, make sure to store it in a refrigerator or in an insulated lunch box or bag.

If purchasing foods that need to be heated, make sure to closely follow the cooking instructions and heat them to the recommended safe temperature. If you bring already-heated grab-and-go foods home or to the office, make sure to eat them within one to two hours or reheat them to at least 165 degrees.

If your white blood cell counts are low, avoid eating from buffets, salad bars, salsa bars, and delis, because there is a greater risk of contracting a foodborne illness. You basically want to avoid any places where other consumers handle food, because there is less control over food safety.

Dealing with Social Occasions

Social occasions, including holidays, parties, and other gatherings, almost always mean lots of food. Many foods served and eaten during these times provide comfort, because they're part of our customs and may be associated with happy memories. So much about food is more than how it affects our health. Numerous environmental, social, and emotional cues also affect eating and how we feel about the foods we eat.

But you can't live in a bubble. Socializing with family and friends is healthy and enriches life, so you don't want to avoid these situations because you're afraid they'll derail your ability to nourish yourself. Instead, planning ahead to manage the cues that these events are likely to trigger can help you eat right and enjoy gatherings, whether for holidays or other special occasions.

Food at parties may not always be clean and healthy, and there are often many decadent options to tempt you. In addition, alcohol usually factors largely into the festivities. Decide in advance what allowances you're willing to make and strategies you may employ to keep yourself on track. Here are a few strategies to consider:

- **Offer to bring a dish.** This strategy ensures that you'll have something clean to eat and takes some of the burden off the host. Snack options that require little effort include vegetable platters, hummus with whole-grain crackers, and salsa and/or guacamole with whole-grain baked tortilla chips. In addition to snacks, numerous main dishes, sides, and desserts in Part III of this book may fill the bill. Bringing your own dish is also a good choice if you have little appetite or are dealing with any other cancer-related side effects that affect your ability to eat, because you can at least bring the foods you tolerate the best.

- **Offer to be the designated driver.** This way you won't be tempted to drink more than the safe amount of alcohol, or you can use this as the reason you're avoiding alcohol altogether.

- **Take advantage of the opportunity to socialize.** It's rude to talk with food in your mouth, so the more you talk and socialize, the less you're likely to eat.

- **Don't go hungry.** Don't skip meals before the party. Consider a small meal or snack before arriving, preferably one that helps you meet your fruit and vegetable quota. Trying to "save your calories" for the party almost always leads to overindulgence.

- **Use a small plate.** Try to put bite-size portions of things you want to taste on your small plate, and when it's full, walk away from the buffet table. Avoid going back for seconds, unless you're loading up on veggies and other wholesome eats.

- **Follow the 80-20 rule.** Diets often fail due to their restrictive nature. That's why you want to approach clean eating not as a diet, but as a life-style. As such, you can afford flexibility, so if you eat clean foods 80 percent of the time, you can afford to indulge in less healthy options when you eat away from home.

Preparing Wholesome, Transportable Lunches and Snacks

Preparing wholesome, transportable lunches and snacks requires careful planning and access to certain tools. First and foremost, you need clean, healthy food in the house. You also need some transportable food containers, a good insulated lunch box (particularly if you won't have access to a refrigerator), and some lunch box ice packs. Finally, you need the discipline to get up a few minutes earlier in the morning to pack your lunch and snacks or muster the energy to do it in the evening before bed.

In this section, we look at the basics of packing clean, healthy lunches and snacks so that you can nourish yourself through the workweek, as you're receiving or waiting for treatment at your cancer center, or when you're on another outing.

Making clean lunches

The following are a few ideas for making clean lunches:

- ✔ **Whole-wheat pita sandwich:** Avoid filling with lunch meats. Instead, stuff with homemade chicken, tuna, or egg salad; and load with lettuce, tomatoes, and other veggies.

- ✔ **Homemade salad:** These days, you can easily pack your own salads, especially because you can buy already chopped and washed lettuce and other veggies. Combine dark leafy greens, veggies of your liking, and a lean-protein source in a transportable container, and place the wholesome dressing of your choice in a separate container to prevent your salad from becoming soggy.

- ✔ **Nut butter and fruit spread sandwich on whole-grain bread:** If you don't have a way to keep your lunch cold, this may be your safest option.

- ✔ **Leftover soup, stew, or chili:** Pack hot in a thermos or in a container suitable for reheating in the microwave, and add some whole-grain crackers or bread. Other leftovers work well, too.

In addition, always add the following to your lunch box:

- ✔ **Cut-up fresh veggies and fruits:** If you don't have cut-up fruit, grab a banana, a piece of fresh fruit, or even a small baggie with dried fruit.

✔ **Yogurt or kefir:** An individual container or carton will add protein and calcium to your lunch.

✔ **Healthy beverage:** Pack a bottle of water, a container of unsweetened iced tea, or even a single serving of soy milk so you're less tempted to get a soda out of a vending machine.

Making clean snacks

Snacks can help provide energy to keep you going in between meals. The best snacks provide complex carbohydrate and protein. Chapter 14 provides lots of wholesome, transportable snack suggestions. Here are a few others:

✔ **String cheese and whole-grain crackers:** Grab on a daily basis or take enough for a week and keep the cheese in a refrigerator at work.

✔ **Trail mix:** Make your own by adding ¼ cup dried fruits and 1 to 2 tablespoons of nuts and/or seeds to a resealable plastic bag, or make a batch of our Fruit and Nut Trail Mix recipe (see Chapter 14) to eat throughout the week.

✔ **Celery, apple, or anything else you like with nut butter:** If you keep the nut butter in your desk, all you have to do is bring fresh veggies and/or fruit.

✔ **Whole-grain cold cereal:** Keep a healthy box of cold cereal in your desk. Snack on it dry or with some low-fat milk. If you have a refrigerator at work, bring a quart of milk to work on Monday to use throughout the week.

Chapter 17

Making Conscious Lifestyle Changes

. . . .

In This Chapter

▶ Understanding how exercise can help you through your cancer journey

▶ Taking clean living beyond the food you eat

▶ Considering environmental factors that can negatively impact health

. . . .

*L*ifestyle has a tremendous impact on health. Poor diet, being overweight or obese, lack of exercise, stress, and lack of sleep can all take a tremendous toll on your body, making it susceptible to cancer and other diseases. By eating clean, you've addressed one major lifestyle factor for the better. But there are other lifestyle factors left to tackle if you're going to truly optimize your health and well-being.

This chapter provides insights on how you can make other conscious lifestyle changes to enhance your clean-eating plan (see Chapter 6) and improve your life. First, we examine why exercise is essential and how you can be more active. Then we review some other ways to take clean living beyond the foods you eat and how to minimize environmental risks that can impact health.

Exercising through Cancer

We live in a sedentary society. We spend more time sitting at our desks and in front of the TV or computer than we spend engaged in any type of physical activity. Lack of physical activity raises the risk of cancer and other chronic illnesses like heart disease, stroke, and diabetes. It also raises the risk of being overweight or obese, further increasing the risk of developing one or more chronic illnesses. Regular exercise can protect against cancer and alleviate many of the side effects of cancer and its treatments, including fatigue, loss of muscle mass and strength, pain, depression, anxiety, and sleep disturbances. One preliminary study even suggests that engaging in exercise for several weeks after you finish chemotherapy may remodel your immune system, enabling it to become more effective in reducing the risk of cancer recurrence.

When you're going through cancer treatment, you may think that exercise is too taxing, that it may be best just to relax so that your body can recover. Although relaxation is certainly important for recovery, so is exercise. And the sooner you start engaging in regular physical activity, the better you'll feel and the fewer medications you're likely to need — plus, you may lower your risk for certain complications. The American Institute for Cancer Research (AICR) recommends that cancer survivors be physically active for at least 30 minutes every day. In this section, we look at how you can be more active and fill you in on some forms of exercise you may want to incorporate into your regimen.

Defining exercise and physical activity

When people think of physical activity, some form of exercise usually comes to mind. But exercise is only one type of physical activity. *Exercise* is any activity that requires physical effort and is performed to specifically improve health and fitness, whereas *physical activity* is any bodily movement that results in energy expenditure. Both are important for maintaining a healthy life. If you get 30 minutes of exercise daily but you're sedentary the rest of the day, the benefits reaped from the exercise are negated by the inactivity.

Exercise and physical activity can be performed at various intensity levels: light, moderate, and vigorous. Light activities require minimal energy expenditure and may include activities like housework, shopping, or gardening, whereas moderate activities require as much effort as taking a brisk walk. Vigorous activities use large muscle groups and result in a faster heart rate, deeper and faster breathing, and sweating. According to the American Cancer Society (ACS), adults should get at least 150 minutes of moderate-intensity or 75 minutes of vigorous-intensity activity each week (or a combination of these), preferably spread throughout the week.

What follows are some exercises that have shown promise in the cancer arena and that can be used to meet the physical activity goals of the AICR and the ACS.

Before starting these or any another regimens, consult with your healthcare team.

Cardiovascular exercise

Cardiovascular exercise (also known as *aerobic exercise*) includes any exercise that increases your heart rate for 10 to 30 minutes. Cardio is important to preserve heart and lung function and can also help burn body fat, lower blood pressure, improve cholesterol levels, boost the immune system, decrease stress, and prevent depression and anxiety. It can also help to protect against complications from cancer treatment, such as fatigue, and the cardiovascular effects of certain chemotherapeutic agents, which impair the heart's pumping function and reduce the ability of red blood cells to carry oxygen throughout the body.

Popular cardiovascular exercises include walking, running, swimming, rowing, and bicycling. Because cardio has numerous benefits, it's often included in cancer rehabilitation programs.

Strength training

Strength training uses resistance to induce muscular contractions to build strength, increase *anaerobic endurance* (a form of endurance that doesn't hinge on oxygen consumption and increases performance of short-duration activities), and grow muscles. It also increases bone, tendon, and ligament strength, reducing the potential for injury; boosts metabolism, making it easier to maintain an ideal body weight; and improves cardiac function.

Although many cancer rehabilitation programs focus on endurance training, several studies have shown that strength training can address the two most common lingering effects of treatment: muscle loss and fatigue. But strength training is most effective when combined with cardiovascular exercises. One study showed that participants who did 18 weeks of rehab with cardio and strength training starting six weeks after their last chemotherapy session were less tired, stronger, and fitter. A cardio and strength-training regimen is also ideal to maintain for life, because it can help keep your body weight under control, which is important to prevent a recurrence or a secondary cancer.

Stretching

Stretching increases the range of motion for joints, reducing the risk of injuries. The goal of stretching exercises is to increase flexibility.

Stretching can be static or dynamic:

- ✔ **Static stretching** lengthens a muscle to an elongated position and holds that position for a period of time. An example is reaching down to touch your toes.

- ✔ **Dynamic stretching** propels muscles toward their maximum range of motion while the body is in motion. An example is doing repetitive karate kicks.

 If you have a job that requires you to sit at a desk all day, be sure to periodically stretch. This also helps with blood circulation. The Mayo Clinic provides a great slideshow of static stretches you can perform right at your desk at www.mayoclinic.com/health/stretching/WL00030.

Aquatic exercises

Aquatic exercises are performed in water, making them a low-impact activity that takes the pressure off your bones, joints, and muscles. When you exercise in water that comes up to your neck, your joints are only supporting about 10 percent of your body weight, so age, body weight, and physical condition usually aren't issues in the water. Aquatic exercises can include swimming, walking, and strengthening maneuvers.

A recent study showed that an aquatic exercise program conducted in deep water reduced cancer-related fatigue and increased strength in breast cancer survivors. To find an aquatic exercise class, contact your local YMCA, sports club, or community college.

If you're receiving radiation therapy or if you have a low white blood cell count related to your chemotherapy, you should avoid swimming pools because they can expose you to waterborne bacteria that may cause infections and the chlorine may aggravate irradiated skin.

Yoga

There are many types of yoga, but a fundamental goal of each is to unify the mind, body, and spirit through a series of poses (referred to by yogis as *asanas*), meditation, and breathing. Yoga has been shown to help relieve some of the more distressing symptoms of cancer, including pain, depression, anxiety, and sleep disturbances. It may also decrease blood pressure and heart rate, increase energy levels, and improve mood. Some postures may be difficult to achieve because they require extreme stretches or tremendous balance (like one-legged stands), but you should never stretch beyond your limits and should always adjust poses to reflect your capabilities.

If you're interested in finding a yoga class, look for a Hatha yoga program (it's considered a gentler form of yoga) or Hatha yoga classes at your local YMCA. To learn more about yoga and its many types, visit `www.american yogaassociation.org`.

Ta'i chi

Ta'i chi, considered a martial art, uses a sequence of precise body movements, meditation, and synchronized breathing to improve health and well-being. There are five major styles: Yang, Wu, Chen, Sun, and Wu/Hao. The differences among styles range from varying speeds to the manner in which movements are executed. Although ta'i chi is a moderate physical activity, its movements are gentle, so it can be performed by anyone. Ta'i chi movements can improve stamina, muscle tone, agility, and flexibility, while its breathing component may reduce stress. Studies have shown that ta'i chi also reduces pain and improves physical functioning, sleep, and balance.

To learn more about ta'i chi or to find a class, visit `www.americantaichi.org`.

Increasing physical activity

Sometimes being more physically active isn't as difficult as it may seem. Even a seemingly small change can make a big difference. Here are just a few simple ways you can increase your daily physical activity levels:

✔ **Limit sedentary behavior.** Many of us spend a lot of time sitting down, between our desk jobs, TV watching, and computer time. Instead of sitting down to watch your favorite TV show, do some gentle exercises. If you're at your desk, take time to stretch to keep the blood circulating.

✔ **Park a little farther away.** Whether it's the parking lot at your work, the mall, or the doctor's office, make a habit of parking farther away, provided there are no safety hazards. The benefits of all those extra steps will accrue over time.

✔ **Avoid labor-saving devices.** If you can, take the stairs rather than an elevator or escalator. Mow the lawn with a push mower instead of a riding mower. Rake leaves by hand instead of using a leaf blower.

✔ **Take a short walk during lunch.** Instead of remaining chained to your desk during lunch, get out and take a short walk to get the blood circulating.

✔ **Tackle the home tasks you've been putting off.** Maybe you've been meaning to clean out the garage or prepare the new plant bed in front of your house. Dedicate a little time each day to such tasks until they're accomplished. Your home will thank you for it.

✔ **Find an exercise you enjoy.** Find an exercise that you enjoy and add it to your routine. Exercise is more than doing sit-ups and push-ups. There are countless options to consider, from belly dancing to bicycling. Be adventurous and learn something new!

Look for every opportunity to boost your ability to be active. Engaging in any physical activity beyond your usual activities, no matter what your general activity level is, can have many health benefits.

Considering cancer

Before starting any exercise program, talk to your healthcare team. They'll be able to direct you to the types of exercise and physical activities that are most appropriate for you depending on where you're at on your cancer journey. For example, if you're receiving radiation treatment, they'll likely tell you to avoid aquatic activities, and if your white blood cell count is low, you may be instructed to avoid exercising in a gym. There are many factors to consider, and only your healthcare team knows your specific situation, so it's important to discuss your plans with them.

When you start any exercise program, start slowly and progress incrementally. Depending on your fitness and comfort level, you may need to start with a 10-minute walk around the block, slowly adding time until you reach the 30 minutes of daily physical activity recommended by the AICR. On the other hand, if you were a gym rat before your cancer diagnosis, you may have to lower the intensity of your workouts for a while.

If you feel too fatigued to engage in a full 30 minutes of exercise, try breaking up your routine into smaller sessions, like three 10-minute walks. And don't beat yourself up if you miss a day or more of exercise. As with clean eating, when you're ready and capable, just pick it up again. Above all, listen to your body. If you're feeling sick, running a fever, or simply feel like a walking zombie, get some rest.

Try to find exercise programs designed specifically for cancer patients, particularly when you first start and especially if exercising is new to you. Your healthcare team may be able to point you in the right direction. These classes are better equipped to address your challenges and needs. Plus, you'll meet others in the same boat, which can expand your support network.

Taking Clean Living beyond the Foods You Eat

Chemicals are all around us and in us. Not all are bad or harmful, but many can be, particularly at high doses or if accumulated over time. If you want to reduce your exposure to chemicals, there are many ways to achieve this. What follows are some key areas where you can take steps to minimize your risks. Avoiding exposure to every possible toxin is impossible, but you can limit or take steps to greatly reduce your and your family's exposure, which will help the environment to boot. There's no cleaner living than that!

Beauty and personal-care products

Beauty and personal-care products are the least regulated products under the Federal Food, Drug, and Cosmetic Act (FFDCA). The FFDCA doesn't require safety testing, review, or approval for these products before they hit the market, and hundreds of chemicals used in cosmetics and personal-care products have been reported to be toxic substances. To avoid exposure to such toxins, some of which are known carcinogens, choose products that contain the fewest ingredients and that indicate they're natural. To determine the safety risks of your cosmetics and personal-care products and to find the safest ones, search the Environmental Working Group's Skin Deep database at www.ewg.org/skindeep.

In addition to buying safer products, you can further reduce risk by cutting down on makeup use and the length of time cosmetics remain on the skin. Because skin is highly permeable, the chemicals in cosmetics are easily absorbed. One study showed that users absorbed 13 percent of the cosmetic preservative butylated hydroxytoluene and 49 percent of the carcinogenic pesticide dichlorodiphenyltrichloroethane (DDT), which is found in some cosmetics containing lanolin.

If you want to get away from mass-market products altogether, there are natural solutions for any personal-care product you can imagine. For example, you can make a nice lotion with coconut oil simply by whipping it up and adding a few drops of an essential oil if you want to enhance the scent. You can also use coconut oil or olive oil as a deep conditioner; a combination of mayo, honey, and lemon to create a face mask; and vitamin E capsules to soothe dry lips. Go online and explore the options. The Campaign for Safe Cosmetics (`www.safecosmetics.org/article.php?id=233`) is a great place to start.

Always check with your healthcare team before using any cosmetics, even homemade products made from natural ingredients. This is especially important if your skin is compromised in any way. For example, if your skin is irradiated or you're receiving certain biologic agents, products containing alcohol or that are heavily perfumed can be irritating.

Cleaning products

Natural has become a buzzword in the cleaning-products arena. But as with cosmetics, there is no regulation when it comes to these labeling claims, and many products that say they're "natural" have been found to contain toxins. If you want to browse the safety of your cleaning products, you can do so at Household Products Database of the U.S. Department of Health and Human Services at `http://householdproducts.nlm.nih.gov`.

If you want to avoid exposing yourself and your family to the potentially carcinogenic chemicals contained in cleaning products altogether, you can easily make your own nontoxic solutions. Most likely, you'll find all the ingredients you need — vinegar, baking soda, lemon juice, and detergent — right in your kitchen. The only specialty items you need are spray bottles for the all-purpose and window cleaners, but if you don't have them, you can just use a bowl and dab and wipe in the meantime.

> ✔ **All-purpose cleaner:** Mix equal parts of white distilled vinegar with hot water in a spray bottle. Shake to mix. Spray on the desired surface and wipe away with a sponge, rag, or paper towel. If you don't like the smell of vinegar, you can add citrus peels to vinegar for a few weeks, strain the peels, and then make the solution by adding the hot water.

> ✔ **Creamy scrubber:** Mix ½ cup or so of baking soda with enough water to form a paste that has the consistency of frosting. Apply the paste to the desired surface using a damp sponge. When you're done scrubbing the area, clean off the sponge and then use it to wipe away the remaining baking soda. Alternatively, if you're cleaning a flat surface, such as your kitchen counters, you can just sprinkle on the baking soda and then apply the damp sponge. The creamy scrubber works great on counters, tiles, bathtubs, and sinks.

✔ **Furniture polish:** Mix 3 tablespoons of olive oil with 1 tablespoon of white distilled vinegar or fresh lemon juice (strained) in a glass jar. Dab a small amount of the solution on a soft cloth and wipe the wood surface. If you want to add fragrance, you can add a drop or two of essential oil (such as lemon, lavender, or pine) to your solution. If your furniture is varnished, keep in mind that use of a damp cloth is all that's needed. Furniture polish is best used on wooden pieces that require conditioning.

✔ **Window cleaner:** Place ½ teaspoon of liquid soap or detergent, ¼ cup of distilled white vinegar, and 2 cups of water in a spray bottle, and shake it up to mix. Now you can use this solution as you would any commercial window cleaner: Simply spray and wipe.

Dry cleaning

The concern with dry cleaning is that many dry cleaners use perchloroethylene (*perc* for short), a chemical solvent, to clean garments and other textiles. In animal studies, perc has been shown to be carcinogenic, and several studies have shown a higher rate of certain cancers among people working in the dry-cleaning industry. As with all health effects, the potential for an increased risk of cancer depends on several factors, including how much perc exposure there is, how often the exposure occurs, and how long it lasts. So, if you don't use dry-cleaning services too often, there really is very little concern that your health will be affected.

But if you're still concerned, you can look for businesses that offer wet-cleaning services. Wet cleaning uses specially designed machines that use water as the solvent. Most garments that are typically dry cleaned — including those made of silk, wool, linen, suede, or leather — can usually be wet cleaned, sometimes with better results.

Pesticides, herbicides, and fertilizers

If you own your own home, you may find yourself applying pesticides, herbicides, and fertilizers various times throughout the year. For these agents to cause any adverse health effects, you have to come in direct contact with them, whether through the skin or eyes, by inhalation, or by ingestion. To avoid these routes of transmission, do the following:

✔ Always wear personal protective equipment, such as gloves, masks, and eye protection when applying these products or, if you can, hire someone else to apply them for you.

✔ Make sure to wash your hands after handling these agents, even if you wore gloves.

✔ If you eat any produce on which you've sprayed a pesticide, be sure to thoroughly wash that produce prior to consumption. To learn more about how to protect yourself from pesticides in produce, check out the Environmental Working Group's website at www.ewg.org/foodnews.

✔ Look for more natural products. Those marked "organic" may be a better choice. Alternatively, you can make your own pesticides, herbicides, and fertilizers. Many nontoxic homemade remedies can be found online on gardening websites.

Building materials and home goods

Most building materials and home goods these days have green, environmentally friendly options. You can now find VOC-free paints, chemical-free carpets, formaldehyde-free insulation, and everything else you could imagine. Although exposure to carcinogens from building materials is very low, particularly if you're not working with these materials on a daily basis (for example, you're not a house painter), selecting these products can make you feel like you're doing something good for the environment.

Volatile organic compounds (VOCs) are chemicals emitted as gases. They've been associated with ill health effects.

Many *big-box stores* (the big chains like Lowe's, Home Depot, and Walmart) carry green building materials, but they may be more difficult to find because nongreen items abound. To get around this, visit Green Depot at www.greendepot.com. This retailer carries only environmentally friendly building products. Although there are currently only a few Green Depot stores in the United States, you can order online or at least find products you can then look for locally.

Limiting Radiation Exposure

Radiation exposure is a known risk factor for cancer. One potential source of radiation that has been receiving quite a bit of press are cellphones. But studies thus far have not shown a consistent link between cellphone use and cancers of the brain, nerves, or other tissues of the head or neck. Still, if you want to take every measure to protect yourself, the Environmental Working Group (www.ewg.org) makes the following recommendations:

- ✔ Use wired or wireless headsets. They emit less radiation than phones.

- ✔ Hold the phone away from your body.

- ✔ Text rather than talk.

- ✔ Call when the signal is strongest. Avoid calling people when you have only one or two bars.

- ✔ Skip *radiation shields* (adhesive stickers applied to certain areas of the phone that are marketed to reduce radiation exposure; learn more at `www.consumer.ftc.gov/articles/0109-cell-phone-radiation-scams`). They reduce connection quality and subsequently expose you to more radiation.

A lesser-known source of radiation exposure, but one that poses a tremendous risk, is *radon,* a colorless, odorless, toxic radioactive gas that results from the natural breakdown of uranium in rock and soil. Radon causes thousands of deaths each year, but the only time you may hear of it is when you're buying or selling a home. If your home hasn't been tested for radon recently, you should test it, because radon mitigation can be undertaken to eliminate this risk if your levels are found to be high. Even if you live in an apartment, unless you live above the third floor, radon testing is warranted. Radon test kits are inexpensive, costing between $15 and $25. You can order a test kit online at `http://sosradon.org/test-kits`.

 Some areas of the country have higher concentrations of radon than others. To see a map of radon zones throughout the United States or to find state-specific information, visit the Environmental Protection Agency's website at `www.epa.gov/radon/zonemap.html`.

Staying Safe in the Sun

Many people love to spend time out in the sun, but getting too many rays can increase the risk of melanoma and other skin cancers. In addition to getting regular dermatological screenings (at least once a year for a full body exam) to catch such problems early, the ACS suggests that if you're going to be in the sun, you follow the catch phrase "slip, slop, slap, and wrap," which outlines key steps you can take to protect yourself from ultraviolet rays. These key steps are

- ✔ Slip on a shirt.

- ✔ Slop on sunscreen. (The American Academy of Dermatology recommends a broad-spectrum product with an SPF of at least 30.)

- ✔ Slap on a hat.

- ✔ Wrap on sunglasses to protect the eyes and sensitive skin around them.

Now, this doesn't mean you should *always* slather on the sunscreen before venturing outside. Many experts now recommend that you get between 15 and 30 minutes of unprotected sun exposure two to four times a week. This is because the sun is the best source of vitamin D, a nutrient many of us are deficient in. The safest time to get this exposure is in the morning, before the sun is at its peak.

Getting Your Zzz's

Given that we live in a constantly turned-on world, many of us are sleeping less than six hours a night. And when you're battling cancer, the anxiety and worries may make it difficult for you to get even that. Although short-lived bouts of insomnia are unlikely to affect your health, chronic sleep loss can cause a number of health problems, including weight gain, high blood pressure, and decreased immune and mental function.

Although most people need about eight hours of sleep per night, we all have unique sleep requirements. Some people require more than that to avoid sluggishness, whereas others can thrive on less. And when you're undergoing cancer treatment, you may need more sleep than usual. Be sure to get the extra sleep you need during this time. If sleep problems are preventing this, there are some things you can do to help get those zzz's going:

- Avoid consuming caffeinated foods and beverages six to eight hours before bedtime, and don't drink anything alcoholic. But do drink something warm and caffeine-free right before bedtime, like warm milk with honey.
- Do something relaxing to help you unwind right before bed, like reading a book or taking a warm bath.
- Make sure your bedroom is quiet and dark, and that your sheets are clean and neat.
- Take any prescription sleeping medicine or pain relievers at the same time each night. If you have pain that's keeping you from sleeping, talk with your oncologist.

Managing Stress

Stress is a reaction to a stimulus that disturbs a person's physical or mental equilibrium. The term is often used to describe how we feel when these disturbances have become too much to bear. Although some stress is good, too much of it can lead to a variety of health issues and affect behavior and mood. It can also lead to poorer treatment outcomes, making stress management essential. One of the best ways to conquer stress is through exercise, but whatever activities relax you can help. Some options to consider include the following:

- **Meditation:** This mental discipline attempts to move you beyond your conditioned way of thinking to achieve a deeper state of self-awareness, beating stress through relaxation.

- **Deep breathing:** By sending more air into your body, you're not only promoting relaxation, but also aiding your heart, brain, digestive system, and immune system.

- **Progressive muscle relaxation:** This technique involves systematically tensing specific muscle groups and then relaxing them to create awareness of tension and relaxation. You can find out more about this technique at www.amsa.org/healingthehealer/musclerelaxation.cfm.

- **Laughing:** Studies have shown that laughter can lower your stress response and induce relaxation. It can also improve your immune system, alleviate pain, and increase your sense of well-being. No wonder they say laughter is the best medicine!

Chapter 18

Helping the One You Love

In This Chapter

▶ Helping your loved one cope

▶ Knowing what to say at the bedside

▶ Being the support your loved one needs

Finding out that someone you love has cancer is devastating. If it's a parent, spouse, child, or someone you're really close with, your entire world may feel crushed or shaken up, causing feelings of helplessness, anger, fear, concern, or a combination of these and other emotions. If it's a more distant friend, relative, or colleague, you may not feel as direct an impact, but you still want to be there for him.

Regardless of the nature of your relationship, when you're on the sidelines, there's an overwhelming desire to do anything you can to help, even as you work through your own emotions. That's why you're reading this chapter, right? But you may not know what to say or do, particularly because cancer is such a sensitive topic. You may also worry about saying or doing the wrong things and upsetting your loved one.

There are truly no right or wrong answers, but this chapter strives to provide you with some insights that may better help you tune into your loved one's needs and situation throughout the cancer journey.

Tuning In: What You Can Say or Do

When you first heard your loved one had cancer, you may have completely tuned everything out after the word *cancer*. But to fully be there for your loved one, you'll need to really tune into everything he or she is saying and follow the cues. Are encouraging words needed? Does he just need someone to listen? Or does she want distraction? Let your loved one lead, and provide opportunities for connectedness, such as by making eye contact, holding her hand, or patting him on the back (provided this is something you're both comfortable with and accustomed to). You don't want to treat your loved one differently from before. Cancer has a way of making people feel disconnected from the world, so you want to ensure as much normalcy and connectedness in your relationship as possible.

In this section, we look at ways you can help your loved one, whether at the hospital, at home, or on a bad day.

At the hospital

Being a patient in a hospital is not a pleasant experience. No matter how friendly or understanding the staff is, there is no privacy, there are constant interruptions for hospital-related activities, the surroundings are unfamiliar, the bed may be uncomfortable, the food may taste or look bad, and the ability to engage in activities is limited. To make this situation more tolerable, your loved one may benefit from a visit, provided she's interested in and capable of having visitors.

Just keep in mind that the person you encounter in the hospital bed may not resemble or act like the person you know so well outside the hospital, particularly if he just underwent major surgery to remove a tumor. So, before visiting or entering the room, ask the floor nurse how your loved one is doing so that you're better prepared for what you'll encounter. Also, ask in advance whether you may bring anything along for your loved one, like a favorite snack, flowers, or a book or magazines to pass the time.

During your visit, let your loved one dictate the length of your stay. If he appears interested to simply listen, is actively engaged in the discussion, or otherwise appears to be enjoying your presence, you may want to continue your visit even if it appears you're doing all the talking. Your presence in the hospital can be very therapeutic, even if you're discussing items of no particular relevance to the moment, such as a planned future trip or the results of a recent ballgame.

In addition to nourishing his soul, you may consider how and if you can help nourish his body. Because hospital food is notorious for being unappetizing, ask the staff if you can bring your loved one any food from the outside, such as a favorite snack. If she has a longer stay ahead of her, this may be an especially welcomed treat. And if you notice your loved one is experiencing side effects that are impacting his nutrition, you may want to talk to your loved one about it and make sure the staff is aware of it.

If you're unable to visit your loved one in the hospital, there are things you can do to show you care, including calling, sending a thoughtful card, arranging for a gift delivery from the hospital gift shop, or even sending her regular text messages or photos, provided she has access to a cellphone (access is restricted in some hospital settings).

At home

A major advantage of being home, rather than in the hospital, is being in a familiar environment and around normal activities. But a disadvantage is the lack of access to multiple staff that'll tend to your loved one's every need. If your loved one is recovering from a hospitalization or is incapacitated from a treatment-related side effect, it may take some time before he feels well enough to resume all the normal activities of daily living, including shopping for groceries, planning for and preparing regular meals, or taking care of other household chores. If your loved one lives alone or with someone who is overwhelmed by caregiver burden or has limited ability to offer assistance, this may lead to an exceedingly stressful situation. This is the perfect opportunity for you to step in and show your support by making visits and offering to help with chores, preparing wholesome meals, or simply lending an ear.

Even if your loved one is able to take care of herself or has this assistance covered, knowing you care can make all the difference in the world. Calling, visiting, or even sending a thoughtful card can bring a bit of cheer into the day. You don't have to talk about or focus on the cancer either. If you visit your loved one, do an activity together, like a craft project or making a meal or snack together. Even if your loved one's cancer is advanced and unlikely to be cured, focusing on noncancer issues can be therapeutic.

If you live with or live close to your loved one, think of fun activities you can do together. For example, if the medical team recommends that your loved one engage in increased activity to help with recovery, think about appropriate activities you can do together. Taking walks around the neighborhood or mall, swimming leisurely laps in the community pool, or taking a yoga class together may do wonders to speed the recovery process along — and you'll be creating many new wonderful memories to boot!

While your loved one recovers or undergoes treatment, you may also consider taking over more of the mealtime chores, unless this is something your loved one enjoys doing. In that case, perhaps you can still lend a helping hand to make the activity more fun and rewarding.

Help getting meals on the table

When you're dealing with treatment and life's demands, the meals may go on the back burner, but this is also the time when it's most critical for you and your loved one to be well nourished. By nourishing your body, you're better equipped to face what's in front of you. What follows are a few resources you can look into that can help you plan, procure, prepare, and serve meals:

✔ **Meals to Heal** (www.meals-to-heal.com): This service provides weekly deliveries of wholesome, chef-prepared, cancer-fighting meals and access to experienced cancer nutrition professionals. You can also find helpful nutrition information on the website.

✔ **Take Them A Meal** (www.takethemameal.com): This website helps you set up a page that friends and families can use to bring you and your loved one meals, facilitating meal coordination.

✔ **Meals On Wheels Association of America** (www.mowaa.org): If your loved one is a senior at risk of malnutrition from hunger, this organization can help you locate a meal delivery service in your loved one's area. Although the meal may not be tailored to consider cancer, they provide nourishment, which is essential to preventing malnutrition.

✔ **Netgrocer** (www.netgrocer.com): This is an online grocery store that delivers nationwide, as well as to APO/FPO addresses (but not to post office boxes). You can shop for refrigerated, frozen, and nonperishable groceries and other supplies on the website.

If you have a favorite local grocery store, chances are, they deliver, too. Next time you stop in, ask a customer service employee if they offer such services. Or just peruse the store's website or give them a call.

On bad days

When cancer is in the equation, difficult days are to be expected. Your loved one may be fatigued, may be experiencing adverse effects from the cancer or its treatments, may have received unexpected bad news, or may simply be in an emotional rut contemplating the cancer's impact on his future. The best thing you can do during such times is to be supportive.

You can provide support in many ways, but often simply listening to concerns and being empathetic is the best therapy. Be sure to truly listen to your loved one and to acknowledge her feelings and concerns. And above all, remember that expressed concerns, even if not factually correct, are still valid, because they're affecting your loved one's inner world and sense of well-being. So, you never want to flat out say something like "You're being overly dramatic" or "You shouldn't feel that way." Instead, you want to use more sensitive and supportive language like "I can understand why you feel that way" and "I'm here for you." If you think your loved one's situation is not temporary or the sense of unhappiness is excessive, you might suggest that he also discuss these feelings with his healthcare team.

You can also help remedy bad days by providing or offering assistance if your loved one is struggling to physically get through the day because of the cancer or a treatment-related side effect. If you live together or close by, try to alleviate the burden of the daily grind. Offer to make the meals and take care of the essential chores. And if you can, engage your loved one in a fun activity, even if it's just watching a movie together on the couch.

Alleviating Caregiver Burden

Caregivers can have bad days, too! As you're caring for your loved one, you may experience a whole range of emotions — from sadness to helplessness to feelings of guilt that your loved one has cancer and you don't! If you're the primary source of support for your loved one, you may also become overwhelmed by the demands, and you may need to accept help from others or ask for assistance. There's no shame in this. No single person can manage everything! It doesn't matter how competent or capable you are. And most likely, your family and close friends would like nothing more than to be able to help you in any way possible. After all, they love *you*, too!

To ensure you get the help you need, depending on your circumstances and existing support system, you may want to consider making weekly or monthly assistance charts and assigning various responsibilities to certain people. Maybe you need someone to pick up your children from school while your loved one is receiving treatment, or maybe you need someone to sit with your loved one once a week while you run errands, or maybe you need someone to get your loved one to certain doctor's appointments. Whatever your needs are, don't hesitate to openly discuss them with your close family and friends to see what assistance they can provide. Even if they aren't able to personally provide much help, they may know of some solutions.

If you feel uncomfortable asking for help or have a limited support system, consider making use of outside services to alleviate as much caregiver burden as possible.

Fortunately, these days, lots of services are available that can help you out (see the nearby sidebar, "Help getting meals on the table"). You can order groceries, medications, and other goods online and have them delivered directly to your door. You can also drop off your laundry to be washed and folded, arrange for housekeeping services, make use of after-school programs for children, and use transportation services to get your loved one to and from appointments. Whatever your needs are, there's a solution. Go online, use your local Yellow Pages, talk to your loved one's healthcare team, or call the American Cancer Society and other cancer organizations to find local services that can address your specific needs. (Check out www.dummies.com/extras/cancernutritionrecipes for more resources.)

Brushing Up On Your Bedside Manner

When your loved one is going through treatment, a variety of unknown, unscheduled, and unexpected demands may arise. These situations will be taxing on both you and your loved one, and depending on the circumstances you find yourselves in, you may have to take on whole new roles.

Being an advocate

If your loved one receives bad news from the doctor, he may tune everything out. During such times, you can be an advocate for him by closely listening to everything the doctor is saying, asking questions to ensure you're completely clear on the situation, and writing everything down for future reference. This will help prevent any miscommunications or misunderstandings.

You may also become an advocate for your loved one when she's unable to function normally, such as may occur during a hospitalization or if she's distraught. At such times, if you notice that your loved one needs something but can't ask for it or hasn't gotten it, don't hesitate to make the request and follow up on her behalf — for example, if the pain medication hasn't been delivered despite being ordered an hour ago or lunch never arrived and she's hungry.

Although being an advocate can be straightforward, if your loved one's condition worsens and he becomes unable to make healthcare decisions, you may have to make them on his behalf, particularly if you're the spouse. During such times, you may be unclear about what your loved one would want, particularly if you haven't had such discussions. To avoid this situation, you and your loved one should establish *advance directives.* This includes two key documents: a *living will,* which outlines the desired level of medical care when the condition is terminal (such as use of CPR or ventilators), and a *power of attorney for healthcare,* which appoints the person who'll act as the surrogate decision maker.

For more information on advance directives, visit the National Institute of Aging website at www.nia.nih.gov/health/publication/advance-care-planning. In many cases, your loved one's cancer center, physician, social worker, or counselor can help with obtaining and completing these forms.

Being a nurse

There may be times when you'll need to assist your loved one in a manner more consistent with the role of a nurse. This may occur when your loved one returns home from the hospital, such as after undergoing surgery, or at a later point in the cancer journey if he develops advanced disease and is no longer able to care for himself.

During such times, you may feel ill-equipped to perform such functions, particularly if you have limited medical knowledge or you're physically unable to bear the weight of your loved one, such as you might need to do to assist with bathroom trips or simply to adjust her position in bed. Regardless of the circumstances, if you don't feel you can handle this level of care, don't hesitate to discuss your concerns with your loved one's healthcare team. It may be possible to have additional help (for example, a nurse's aide) in the home to assist in providing some level of care, particularly if you're facing a hospice situation. During such times, you also shouldn't hesitate to lean on close family and friends for support.

Being a sounding board

One of the most important functions you can serve is to be a sounding board for your loved one. It's always fine to respond, particularly if your loved one is seeking your thoughts, but it's the nonjudgmental and genuinely supportive listening that's so critical to his well-being. Having an ear to hear concerns, hopes, and fears can be therapeutic.

In fact, several studies have shown that talk therapy can help prevent depression, which is common in people with cancer. And even if your loved one develops depression, you're more likely to identify it if you're actively listening to her. Because depression can have serious consequences, preventing it from developing and intervening early when it does can maintain your loved one's quality of life and ensure better outcomes.

Part V
The Part of Tens

the
part of
tens

For a list of ten sources for even more information on cancer and nutrition, head to www.dummies.com/extras/cancernutritionrecipes.

In this part . . .

- ✔ Get your appetite back, even in the middle of cancer treatment.

- ✔ Find ways to enjoy food on your cancer journey.

- ✔ Protect yourself from *pathogens* (disease-causing agents) in the environment.

- ✔ Keep your immune system strong for the long haul.

Chapter 19

Ten Ways to Revive Your Appetite and Enjoy Food Again

. . . .

In This Chapter

▶ Ensuring you get the benefits of proper nutrition

▶ Discovering strategies for stimulating your appetite

. . . .

In Chapter 4, we explain that cancer and its treatments can contribute to loss of appetite. Because the calories you get from food are energy, if a poor appetite results in not enough food intake, you may experience fatigue. Poor food intake may also result in weight or muscle loss, which can impair your immune function and make it more difficult to recover in between treatments.

Eating can be difficult when you don't have much of an appetite, but try to think of food as part of your treatment. You wouldn't skip a treatment, would you? Food is just as important as the medicines you're taking or the treatments you're receiving. So, while you may not have the desire to eat, you have to try to use your powerful mind to get something in your body so that you can maintain your strength.

Fortunately, there are several strategies you can use to prevent a poor appetite from causing you to lose weight and become malnourished. In this chapter, we offer ten tried-and-true tips to help you meet your nutritional needs when you lose your appetite. Keep in mind that many of these tips can be combined to help you maximize your intake of nutrients.

If you have any questions about diet or nutrition, ask your physician for a referral to a registered dietitian (RD), either at your cancer center or elsewhere. The Academy of Nutrition and Dietetics website (www.eatright.org) has a "Find a Registered Dietitian" tool. Click "Search by Expertise" and select "Cancer/Oncology Nutrition" before searching for RDs in your zip code.

Stay Active

Sometimes a little activity can help stimulate your appetite. Light-intensity physical activity may increase the production of a hormone known as *ghrelin,* which is responsible for appetite and may increase food intake. Even 30 minutes of light activity has been shown to increase ghrelin production and food intake. If 30 minutes seems overwhelming, try several shorter activity sessions throughout the day.

So, what qualifies as a light activity? Basically anything that gets you moving but isn't overly taxing. Some examples include taking a casual walk around the neighborhood, yoga, light gardening (like raking or weeding), low-intensity housework, resistance training, treading water in a pool, or leisurely swimming.

Be sure to tell your physician that you're interested in getting some physical activity. Try to work with a fitness expert to help develop an individualized plan that considers your cancer, treatment, and current health status. Some hospitals offer oncology rehabilitation programs. If yours doesn't, look for an American College of Sports Medicine Certified Exercise Trainer. Some areas, particularly in the eastern United States, have LIVESTRONG at the YMCA programs; you can learn more at `www.livestrong.org/What-We-Do/Our-Actions/Programs-Partnerships/LIVESTRONG-at-the-YMCA`.

Try a Meal Replacement Drink

Sometimes when you don't feel like eating, it's easier to drink your calories, protein, and other nutrients. Try drinking high-calorie, high-protein liquids throughout the day. A number of liquid nutritional supplements are available with macronutrient and micronutrient profiles similar to what you would get from eating a meal. (That's why they're often referred to as "meal replacements.") Because these supplements are usually 70 percent to 85 percent water, they can also help you meet your hydration needs.

When looking for a meal replacement, find the one that has the most calories and protein, but don't buy it in bulk just yet. Buy just a few bottles, in different flavors, to see if you like any of them. The last thing you want to do is spend a fortune on meal replacements only to be stuck with something that makes you want to toss your cookies.

Some surveys have shown that chocolate-flavored meal replacements are preferred over other flavors, because they tend to taste less artificial.

If you don't like the commercial liquid supplements that are available, try making a homemade protein shake or smoothie. In a blender, mix a whey powder, soy powder, or other protein powder with some fruit, milk, or juice, and add some yogurt or frozen yogurt. Experiment by adding different options like tofu, nut butters, and wheat germ. Even green smoothies can be tasty — try variations that include avocado, spinach, and green tea. Chapter 10 offers some tasty smoothie recipes.

Get a Healthy Dose of Omega-3s

There are a variety of omega-3 fatty acids, but the most important omega-3 to help support normal metabolism and weight maintenance when you have a poor appetite is eicosapentaenoic acid (EPA). Some studies show that 1,500 mg of EPA per day is the optimal dose, but be sure to talk with your doctor about what's right for you.

Some physicians don't allow patients to take dietary supplements during cancer treatment. And there can be some concern about omega-3 supplements for people taking blood-thinning medication. So, don't ignore that advice about talking to your doctor before you start supplementing with omega-3s (or anything else).

Food sources of omega-3s in general and EPA in particular include salmon, halibut, sardines, tuna, cod, herring, mahi-mahi, red snapper, flounder, venison, buffalo, walnuts, flaxseeds, canola oil, and wheat germ. Although it's good to try to increase these foods in your diet, when you have a poor appetite, fish, which is the best source, may not be very appealing. In addition, it's very diffi-cult to get 1,500 mg of EPA from food sources alone. Even if you have a hanker-ing for fish, you'd have to eat something like 5 to 14 ounces of fish every day to get 1,500 mg of EPA (and at this level, you risk consuming too much mercury).

If your oncologist recommends supplementing with omega-3s, check ConsumerLab.com (`www.consumerlab.com`) to find a brand that has been tested for quality.

Flip Your Meals to Take Advantage of Your Best Time of Day

There may be a time of day or meal when you most feel like eating. If you can, try getting in two meals or a meal and a snack during these times. (For some quick and tasty snack recipes, turn to Chapter 14.)

For many people, breakfast is often the best meal of the day. If this is the case for you, try making breakfast your heaviest meal instead of lunch or dinner. If vegetables aren't appealing later in the day, try eating a vegetable omelet for breakfast or drinking a glass of vegetable juice in the morning.

Eat Frequent, Small Meals throughout the Day

Although it may sound counterintuitive, eating smaller, more frequent meals throughout the day can help you get in more calories, protein, and other nutrients. The typical portions that you're used to eating when you eat three meals a day may be overwhelming and cause you to push the plate aside without eating anything. In such cases, eating smaller amounts of food every couple hours during the day can be more manageable.

Your small meal should include a source of protein and a source of carbohydrate, if possible. Most of the foods you'll pick will also contain some fat, so you don't have to look for sources of fat. In fact, fat takes longer to digest and may leave you feeling full longer, so you don't want to consume too much extra fat during these times. Some examples of a mini meal are a tuna-salad-stuffed tomato, a hardboiled egg with toast, hummus with pita wedges and vegetables, a bowl of cereal and milk, or half a sandwich. Some of your small meals can also be drinks like protein shakes and smoothies.

Have on Hand High-Calorie and High-Protein Snacks

When you're being treated for cancer, snacking should be guilt-free. It can actually be quite healthy in place of traditional meals to help you meet your nutritional needs, so you should feel good about eating a high-calorie snack during this time.

You may need many snacks throughout the day to meet your nutritional needs. Try to snack on high-protein foods, and find ways to incorporate vegetables and fruits into your snacking plan. For example, you can add some fresh or frozen berries to Greek yogurt, dip some carrot sticks into guacamole, or dip apple or celery into a nut butter. To facilitate snacking, consider keeping trail mix (dried fruits and nuts) readily accessible.

This may also be a good time to try something new. Try snacking on a little Mochi, which is made out of sweet brown rice. You can buy Mochi in the freezer section of many health-food stores. Break off a piece and pop it in the oven for about ten minutes. Spread a little almond butter or other nut butter on it, and enjoy! If you can't find Mochi, try a mini rice cake or a cracker instead.

Boost the Nutrient Density of What You Eat

If you're only able to eat a small amount of food, you can boost the nutrient density of what you're able to eat without increasing the amount of food you have to eat. Nonfat dry milk, protein powders, dried fruits, nuts, seeds, nut butters, and flaxseed oil all can add calories and other nutrients to the foods you may be eating.

Try cooking hot cereals with your milk of choice and nonfat dry milk and adding dried fruit and nuts. Blend a nut butter into a shake or smoothie or add to yogurt. Add nonfat dry milk or protein powder to mashed potatoes or soups. You can also make healthy purees by blending various veggies and legumes and adding this to some of your favorite recipes. You'll be amazed at how great mac and cheese can taste with some pureed beans or carrots added in.

Relax Before Mealtimes

Dealing with cancer and its treatments is stressful, and trying to eat when you don't feel like eating adds to that stress. Well-meaning family and friends who love you may coax you to eat, creating more stress. Try not to let this interfere with your eating. You need to do everything you can to manage stress so that you can relax before mealtimes and optimize your nutrient intake.

There are many strategies for relaxing before mealtimes. For example, going for a walk can help reduce your stress levels while improving your appetite. You can also listen to soft music before and during meals. If you have the energy, create a fine-dining experience at home by using your nice dishes and turning down the lights or lighting a candle or two, which may make eating more enticing. Sometimes simply eating with people whose company and conversation you enjoy can make mealtime more appealing.

Consume Foods at Room Temperature

Sometimes when your appetite is poor, just the smell of foods can turn your stomach. If food smells bother you, try sticking with cold foods or foods at room temperature. Foods served and eaten at room temperature or cool often have less aroma and taste. Obviously, you don't want to leave out at room temperature foods that should be refrigerated — that wouldn't be safe. But you might, for example, opt for a sandwich filled with protein-dense salads, such as tuna, chicken, or egg salads. Or you might stuff these salads into a tomato for a great meal. Whole-grain and bean salads may also be foods you can tolerate. Even a fruit plate with cottage cheese or yogurt can be something to look forward to.

Ask Your Oncologist about an Appetite Stimulant

If the previous strategies don't work for you, consider talking with your oncologist about a prescription appetite stimulant. Medications are available that may be worth a try. As with all medications, there are side effects to consider, so be sure to talk with your oncologist about the pros and cons.

Appetite stimulants that have been shown to help stimulate appetite in people with cancer include megestrol acetate (Megace), mirtazapine (Remeron), and dronabinol (Marinol). *Note:* Dronabinal has a similar effect on the brain as marijuana, so this is something to discuss with your oncologist if it's recommended to you.

Another medication that isn't necessarily an appetite stimulant but can indirectly help improve appetite is metoclopramide (Reglan). This drug facilitates stomach emptying and may help if you have a constant sensation of feeling full.

Another option to discuss with your dietitian or oncologist includes the use of β-hydroxy β-methylbutyrate (HMB), which may help decrease weight and muscle loss. Because studies have shown HMB to be helpful in improving muscle mass, it's now added to many liquid nutritional supplements. If you're drinking your meals, you may want to consider using a liquid nutritional supplement that contains HMB, such as Juven (www.juven.com).

Chapter 20

Ten Ways to Prevent and Fight Off Colds and Other Infections

. . . .

In This Chapter

▶ Getting protection from germs

▶ Fighting off infection

▶ Keeping your body strong and resilient

. . . .

*O*ur world is made up of all kinds of germs, from viruses to bacteria to fungi. These microscopic organisms even take up residence on and in our bodies. Research has shown that anywhere from 20 percent to 50 percent of healthy people are colonized with *Staphylococcus aureus,* the strain of bacteria responsible for the dreaded and deadly staph infections you often hear about on the news. When these bacteria and other germs (technically called *pathogens*) are kept in check by the immune system, as they often are, they aren't a problem. But when the immune system is weakened, these organisms can replicate out of control and start interfering with bodily functions (a process known as *infection*), which can cause everything from a stuffy nose to diarrhea.

Because some types of cancer and its treatments can weaken or suppress your immune system, you may be more susceptible to infections and have a harder time recovering from them when they occur. That's why taking measures to bolster your immune system and prevent exposure to potentially harmful germs is so important. After all, as Benjamin Franklin once said, "An ounce of prevention is worth a pound of cure." Sometimes no matter what preventive measures you take, infection happens. In such cases, you can take steps to help the recovery process along. In this chapter, we look at ten things you can do to protect yourself from germs and fight off infections when they occur.

Practice Good Hand Hygiene

The Centers for Disease Control and Prevention (CDC) estimates that up to 16 percent of respiratory infections and the vast majority of foodborne illnesses can be prevented by the simple act of washing hands with soap and water. Now, this doesn't mean you should wash your hands every ten minutes. Washing your hands *too* much can be counterproductive and lead to other problems, including *contact dermatitis* (an uncomfortable skin condition that can leave your skin red, raw, cracked, and inflamed, while increasing your risk of an infection because your skin is compromised).

But there are situations before and after which you should wash your hands. *Always* wash your hands *before* doing any of the following:

- Eating and preparing food
- Caring for sick people
- Touching any areas of your body through which germs can enter, such as your nose, mouth, eyes, ears, and wounds

In addition, *always* wash your hands *after* doing any of the following:

- Touching raw foods like meat and poultry
- Using the toilet
- Changing diapers
- Touching animals or their waste
- Treating injuries
- Caring for sick people
- Touching soiled surfaces or items, such as dirty laundry
- Handling garbage, chemicals, and any other potential contaminants

When washing your hands, be sure to lather well and rub your hands together for a good 20 seconds, getting in all the cracks and crevices, such as between your fingers and under your fingernails. Then rinse well and dry your hands using an air dryer or a clean towel or paper towel. If possible, use a paper towel to shut off the water faucet and to open the bathroom door, particularly if you're in a public restroom, because these surfaces have been found to be among the most contaminated with germs.

Alcohol-based hand sanitizers (like Purell) don't kill all bacteria. They're better than nothing, but washing your hands with soap and warm water is best.

Get Plenty of Sleep

If you're like most people, you probably feel terrible when you don't get enough sleep and exceptional when you do. The evolutionary reason as to why we sleep is not completely understood, but studies are increasingly showing that sleep can affect both mental and physical health, with inadequate sleep increasing the risk of chronic diseases like cancer and impairing everything from memory to immune function. Some evidence suggests that lack of sleep can make you more likely to catch a cold, flu, and other viruses. There is also evidence that once an infection is present, sleep levels can affect your body's ability to fight that infection. So, as you can see, sleep is very important.

In general, seven to eight hours of sleep are recommended, but everyone's sleep requirements vary. You may do fine with fewer hours, or you may need more. Whatever amount leaves you feeling refreshed is what you need.

When you're fighting an infection or feel like you may be coming down with one, your sleep requirements may increase. During these times, you should get extra sleep whenever you can. Even a 15-minute nap at lunch may be beneficial and can help you get through the rest of the day.

Of course, cancer symptoms, treatments, and the stress of the diagnosis can impair your ability to sleep. Studies indicate that up to 50 percent of people with cancer suffer from sleep disturbances. If you find this to be the case, be sure to talk to your oncologist. Numerous interventions can be tried, including many non-drug strategies. For example, you may want to try a cup of chamomile tea or a cup of warm milk before bed to help you sleep, or you may find that practicing yoga during the day reduces stress and improves your sleep at night.

Get a Flu Shot

Influenza is devastating even if you don't have cancer. After all, millions of people around the world are hospitalized every year due to the flu, and anywhere from 200,000 to 500,000 people die as a result of it. Because cancer and its treatments weaken the immune system, you're more susceptible to both contracting the flu and suffering serious problems as a result of it. For this reason, the American Cancer Society recommends flu shots for people with cancer unless there is some reason that the shot shouldn't be administered (such as the cancer treatment regimen prohibiting it).

Before getting a flu shot, be sure to get the green light from your oncologist or primary-care physician.

Once given the green light, get the flu vaccine as soon as it's available or as close to the beginning of the flu season as possible. In the United States, flu season generally starts in October and goes through May. It takes about two weeks after getting the vaccine for your body to develop the antibodies to protect you from the flu.

When you get the flu shot, you're only protected from the strains in the vaccine. Every year, the vaccine is reformulated to offer protection against the three influenza strains that research indicates will be the most common during the upcoming flu season. The flu shot isn't a 100 percent guarantee that you won't get the flu, but it definitely helps.

Engage in Moderate Physical Activity

Studies indicate that engaging in *moderate* physical activity can improve immune function, enabling your body to fight off bacterial and viral infections. The exact mechanism behind this is unclear, but theories abound. Some scientists think that physical activity can decrease respiratory infections by flushing germs out of the lungs. Others think that exercise may increase the release of white blood cells and antibodies that target germs, enabling them to be dealt with before they cause problems. Then there are the theories that the elevation in body temperature caused by exercise inhibits bacterial growth, and that exercise reduces stress hormones, which have been associated with increased susceptibility to illness. But although these theories are open for debate, the benefits of exercise are not.

Avoid gyms or other public workout areas while undergoing or recovering from cancer treatment. These areas are germ havens and increase your exposure to other people's bodily secretions, particularly because not everyone is good about wiping down equipment when they're done using it. Plus, there is a lot of heavy breathing going on, which can release more germs into the air.

The key, however, is to do moderate-intensity exercise, not vigorous exercise, because the latter has been shown to *increase* the risk of infections. An easy way to gauge exercise intensity is by doing the talk test. At the moderate level, you should be able to talk clearly during the activity, but not be able to sing, whereas at the vigorous level, you'll only be able to say a few words before needing to catch your breath. Examples of moderate-intensity activities include walking briskly, leisurely bicycling, golfing, pushing a lawn mower, and washing your car.

Get Enough Vitamin D

Some people have called vitamin D the "wonder drug of the 21st century." This is because studies have shown vitamin D to have a wide range of effects, from supporting the immune system to maximizing muscle function to having antioxidant and anti-inflammatory effects. In addition, vitamin D receptors have been found on most cells in the body, indicating that this vitamin is essential for proper cellular function.

Although it's widely accepted that vitamin D can bolster the immune system, a recent study indicated that taking large doses of this micronutrient provides no protection against upper-respiratory infections and doesn't reduce the length of such infections. But all participants in the study had normal vitamin D levels to begin with, and the researchers acknowledged the possibility that people who are deficient in vitamin D may very well reduce their risk of colds by raising their vitamin D to normal levels.

Because vitamin D deficiency is common for all kinds of cancer, talk to your oncologist or primary-care physician about checking your vitamin D levels (through a simple blood test) and getting them to the normal range if you're found to be deficient.

Keep Nasal Passages Moist

Cold viruses tend to thrive when humidity is low, which is why they're particularly prevalent during the fall and winter. The low humidity also dries out the mucus membranes of the nasal passages, making you more prone to infections. When the nasal passages are moist, the mucus traps and attacks invading germs, preventing them from reaching your lungs. But when the nasal passages are dry, there's nothing to trap these germs, enabling them to take root and cause illness.

To prevent your nasal passages from drying up, you can get a whole-house humidifier or keep a portable cool-mist humidifier in your bedroom or next to your chair where you sit or nap. When using a humidifier, just be sure to carefully follow the instructions for operating and cleaning that come with it to ensure you don't inadvertently unleash additional germs into the air.

If your nasal passages are already dry, such as from a cold, you can moisten them by rinsing your nostrils with a saline solution/spray or by applying some saline gel or a small amount of petroleum jelly to the inside of your nostrils. Additionally, you can try taking a hot shower or steam bath to moisten and open your nasal passages.

Ensuring adequate hydration is another important measure for keeping your nasal passages moist. For more on hydration, see Chapter 4.

Incorporate Immunity-Boosting Superfoods in Your Diet

Nutrients are essential for keeping your body functioning properly, including in the immunity department. Because superfoods are nutrient-dense, containing abundant vitamins, minerals, and phytochemicals, these are the foods that have the greatest protective benefits. Most vegetables and fruits are considered superfoods, as are foods that are high in certain nutrients, like selenium and omega-3 fatty acids. Examples of such foods include Brazil nuts, wild salmon, and wheat germ.

To reap the greatest benefit, you should consume superfoods on a regular basis, rather than after the onset of a cold or other infection. These foods pack a powerful punch, but they work best before an infection takes root. Some foods that have been reported to protect against cold and flu viruses include apples (the red kind); citrus fruits; berries; broccoli, kale, and other greens; garlic; green tea; and shiitake mushrooms. To learn more about superfoods, turn to Chapter 7.

Some studies suggest that taking zinc lozenges at the first sign of a cold may help shorten the duration of the cold and its accompanying symptoms. As we mention in Chapter 4, a little zinc is good, but you don't want to take more than 40 mg to 45 mg per day, or it'll be counterproductive.

Avoid Crowded Places

The more, the merrier . . . and the more germy, particularly if you're in an enclosed environment where air circulation may not be optimal, such as a shopping mall, airplane, or restaurant. Although your body generally does a fantastic job of dealing with all the germs you may come in contact with on a daily basis, when your immune system is weakened, it's easier for the germs assaulting your system to cause an infection. And even if you take precautions, you ultimately can't control the person who coughs or sneezes in your direction.

This doesn't mean you should remain isolated at home, but if your immune system is suppressed, try to limit your time in crowded places as much as possible. These days, many tasks that previously required venturing out into crowded areas can now be handled online. For example, you can go online to order groceries (and have them delivered), pay bills, and shop for whatever you need. If you don't have Internet access, or you need something that can't be found online, see if you can enlist the help of family and friends — they'll probably be happy to help run errands for you.

When you do venture out to crowded places, be sure to avoid touching any sensitive areas (like your eyes, nose, and mouth), and wash your hands when you get home. When your immune system is compromised, it's also a good idea to avoid eating at buffets and salad bars, because germs are easily spread on shared utensils.

Keep Your Kitchen Clean and Your Food Safe

According to the CDC, every year approximately 48 million Americans get sick from a foodborne illness, and approximately 3,000 people die from them. These illnesses occur through many means. For example, a cantaloupe may have become contaminated with bacteria where it was grown, milk may have been left out too long at the grocery store before being refrigerated again, or you may have inadvertently spread bacteria to your spice jar when seasoning your burgers. You can't control what happens to your food before it reaches you, but you can control how it's handled and prepared in your kitchen.

Keep your kitchen countertops clean by regularly wiping them down, particularly after handling foods with safety hazards, like raw meat. Turn to Chapter 17 for some homemade cleaning solutions.

Be sure to wash your hands after touching raw meat and other hazardous foods, making sure not to touch anything else until your hands are clean. Be sure to thoroughly wash produce, especially if you're eating it raw, and cook your meat until it reaches a safe temperature. Consider investing in a digital meat thermometer so that you can track this. You can find out more about digital thermometers and recommended food preparation and storage temperatures in Chapter 9. Also, be sure to have two cutting boards: one for produce and the other for raw meats, poultry, and fish. Finally, be sure to follow any instructions on the food's packaging in terms of storage and preparation.

Quit Smoking

If you're a smoker, one if the best things you can do for yourself after a cancer diagnosis is to quit smoking and encourage your family members to do the same. Smoking not only increases the risk of cancer recurrence, but also makes you more susceptible to catching colds and other viruses by further impairing your immune system, which is already compromised. Smoking is thought to have this effect because tobacco smoke has been shown to paralyze the *cilia,* the microscopic hairlike cells that line the nasal passages and airways, inhibiting their ability to sweep germs and other foreign matter away from the lungs. In addition, cigarette smoke can make cold symptoms worse by irritating the respiratory tract, causing increased mucus production and coughing, and delaying your recovery.

Quitting smoking certainly isn't easy, but there are many resources at your disposal, from nicotine replacement therapy to hypnosis or acupuncture to tobacco cessation programs. It's important to discuss the options with your oncologist or primary-care physician, who can help provide guidance on which method or intervention may be best for you.

Index

• T •

• U •

• V •

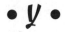

About the Authors

Maurie Markman: Dr. Markman is Senior Vice President for Clinical Affairs and National Director for Medical Oncology at Cancer Treatment Centers of America (CTCA) and Clinical Professor in the Department of Medicine at the Drexel University College of Medicine in Philadelphia.

Carolyn Lammersfeld: Carolyn is a Registered Dietitian who has spent most of her career pioneering the science of nutrition in cancer care. She is currently the Vice President of Integrative Medicine for CTCA.

Christina Torster Loguidice: Christina is a medical journalist and the Editorial Director of two peer-reviewed clinical journals in geriatrics.

Dedication

From Maurie: I dedicate this book to my loving and supportive wife, Tomes, and our wonderful children. I would also like to dedicate this book to the patients I have had the privilege to serve over the past three decades.

From Carolyn: I dedicate this book to my husband, Hugh, and my parents, Joan and Rich Lammersfeld.

From Christina: I dedicate this book to my mother-in-law, Josephine Loguidice, one of the strongest and most beautiful people I've ever known.

Authors' Acknowledgments

We'd like to thank all the folks at John Wiley & Sons, Inc., who had a hand in this project, including our acquisitions editor, Tracy Boggier, and our project editor, Elizabeth Kuball. We'd also like to thank our agent, Matt Wagner. Finally, thanks to our technical editor, Barbara Grant; our recipe tester, Emily Nolan; and our nutrition analyst, Patty Santelli.

Publisher's Acknowledgments

Senior Acquisitions Editor: Tracy Boggier

Project Editor: Elizabeth Kuball

Copy Editor: Elizabeth Kuball

Technical Editor: Barbara Grant, MS, RD, CSO

Recipe Tester: Emily Nolan

Nutrition Analyst: Patricia Santelli

Art Coordinator: Alicia B. South

Project Coordinator: Sheree Montgomery

Photographer: T. J. Hine Photography

Stylist: Lisa Bishop

Illustrator: Elizabeth Kurtzman

Cover Images: T. J. Hine Photography

Apple & Mac

iPad For Dummies,
5th Edition
978-1-118-49823-1

iPhone 5 For Dummies,
6th Edition
978-1-118-35201-4

MacBook For Dummies,
4th Edition
978-1-118-20920-2

OS X Mountain Lion
For Dummies
978-1-118-39418-2

Blogging & Social Media

Facebook For Dummies,
4th Edition
978-1-118-09562-1

Mom Blogging
For Dummies
978-1-118-03843-7

Pinterest For Dummies
978-1-118-32800-2

WordPress For Dummies,
5th Edition
978-1-118-38318-6

Business

Commodities For Dummies,
2nd Edition
978-1-118-01687-9

Investing For Dummies,
6th Edition
978-0-470-90545-6

Personal Finance
For Dummies,
7th Edition
978-1-118-11785-9

QuickBooks 2013
For Dummies
978-1-118-35641-8

Small Business Marketing Kit
For Dummies,
3rd Edition
978-1-118-31183-7

Careers

Job Interviews
For Dummies,
4th Edition
978-1-118-11290-8

Job Searching with
Social Media
For Dummies
978-0-470-93072-4

Personal Branding
For Dummies
978-1-118-11792-7

Resumes For Dummies,
6th Edition
978-0-470-87361-8

Success as a Mediator
For Dummies
978-1-118-07862-4

Diet & Nutrition

Belly Fat Diet For Dummies
978-1-118-34585-6

Eating Clean For Dummies
978-1-118-00013-7

Nutrition For Dummies,
5th Edition
978-0-470-93231-5

Digital Photography

Digital Photography
For Dummies,
7th Edition
978-1-118-09203-3

Digital SLR Cameras &
Photography For Dummies,
4th Edition
978-1-118-14489-3

Photoshop Elements 11
For Dummies
978-1-118-40821-6

Gardening

Herb Gardening
For Dummies,
2nd Edition
978-0-470-61778-6

Vegetable Gardening
For Dummies,
2nd Edition
978-0-470-49870-5

Health

Anti-Inflammation Diet
For Dummies
978-1-118-02381-5

Diabetes For Dummies,
3rd Edition
978-0-470-27086-8

Living Paleo For Dummies
978-1-118-29405-5

Hobbies

Beekeeping
For Dummies
978-0-470-43065-1

eBay For Dummies,
7th Edition
978-1-118-09806-6

Raising Chickens
For Dummies
978-0-470-46544-8

Wine For Dummies,
5th Edition
978-1-118-28872-6

Writing Young Adult Fiction
For Dummies
978-0-470-94954-2

Language &
Foreign Language

500 Spanish Verbs
For Dummies
978-1-118-02382-2

English Grammar
For Dummies,
2nd Edition
978-0-470-54664-2

French All-in One
For Dummies
978-1-118-22815-9

German Essentials
For Dummies
978-1-118-18422-6

Italian For Dummies
2nd Edition
978-1-118-00465-4

e Available in print and e-book formats.

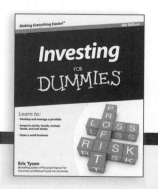
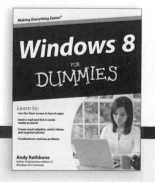
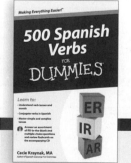
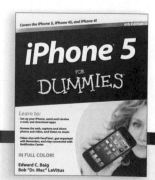

Math & Science

Algebra I For Dummies,
2nd Edition
978-0-470-55964-2

Anatomy and Physiology
For Dummies,
2nd Edition
978-0-470-92326-9

Astronomy For Dummies,
3rd Edition
978-1-118-37697-3

Biology For Dummies,
2nd Edition
978-0-470-59875-7

Chemistry For Dummies,
2nd Edition
978-1-1180-0730-3

Pre-Algebra Essentials
For Dummies
978-0-470-61838-7

Microsoft Office

Excel 2013 For Dummies
978-1-118-51012-4

Office 2013 All-in-One
For Dummies
978-1-118-51636-2

PowerPoint 2013
For Dummies
978-1-118-50253-2

Word 2013 For Dummies
978-1-118-49123-2

Music

Blues Harmonica
For Dummies
978-1-118-25269-7

Guitar For Dummies,
3rd Edition
978-1-118-11554-1

iPod & iTunes
For Dummies,
10th Edition
978-1-118-50864-0

Programming

Android Application
Development For
Dummies, 2nd Edition
978-1-118-38710-8

iOS 6 Application
Development For Dummies
978-1-118-50880-0

Java For Dummies,
5th Edition
978-0-470-37173-2

Religion & Inspiration

The Bible For Dummies
978-0-7645-5296-0

Buddhism For Dummies,
2nd Edition
978-1-118-02379-2

Catholicism For Dummies,
2nd Edition
978-1-118-07778-8

Self-Help & Relationships

Bipolar Disorder
For Dummies,
2nd Edition
978-1-118-33882-7

Meditation For Dummies,
3rd Edition
978-1-118-29144-3

Seniors

Computers For Seniors
For Dummies,
3rd Edition
978-1-118-11553-4

iPad For Seniors
For Dummies,
5th Edition
978-1-118-49708-1

Social Security
For Dummies
978-1-118-20573-0

Smartphones & Tablets

Android Phones
For Dummies
978-1-118-16952-0

Kindle Fire HD
For Dummies
978-1-118-42223-6

NOOK HD For Dummies,
Portable Edition
978-1-118-39498-4

Surface For Dummies
978-1-118-49634-3

Test Prep

ACT For Dummies,
5th Edition
978-1-118-01259-8

ASVAB For Dummies,
3rd Edition
978-0-470-63760-9

GRE For Dummies,
7th Edition
978-0-470-88921-3

Officer Candidate Tests,
For Dummies
978-0-470-59876-4

Physician's Assistant Exam
For Dummies
978-1-118-11556-5

Series 7 Exam
For Dummies
978-0-470-09932-2

Windows 8

Windows 8 For Dummies
978-1-118-13461-0

Windows 8 For Dummies,
Book + DVD Bundle
978-1-118-27167-4

Windows 8 All-in-One
For Dummies
978-1-118-11920-4

Available in print and e-book formats.

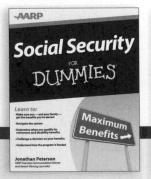

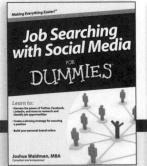

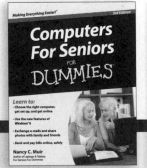

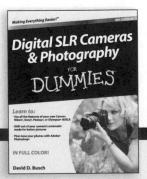